SELF-SUFFICIENT
HERBALISM

A Guide to Growing and Wild Harvesting
Your Herbal Dispensary

Lucy Jones

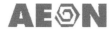

First published in 2020 by
Aeon Books Ltd
PO Box 76401
London
W5 9RG

British Library Cataloguing in Publication Data

A C.I.P. for this book is available from the British Library

ISBN: 978–1–91280–705–5

Printed in Great Britain

www.aeonbooks.co.uk

SELF-SUFFICIENT
HERBALISM

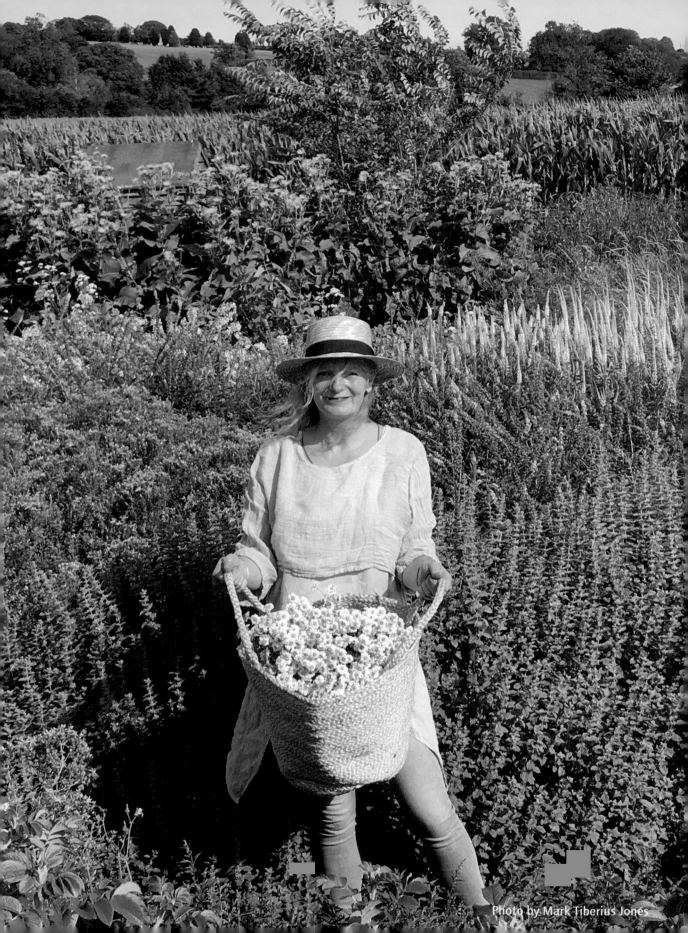

Contents

Acknowledgements

With deep gratitude to Chöjé Akong Tulku Rinpoché for his consistent encouragement and for showing me the true meaning of being a healer.

With humble thanks to my Tibetan teachers, Khenpo Troru Tsenam, Sonam Chimé, and Thubten Phuntsok, who overcame significant obstacles and travelled many miles in order to bring the very precious Tibetan medicine teachings and lineage to our little group of Western students. This teaching was truly life-changing, and its benefits continue to radiate out far beyond our own personal horizons.

I am also greatly indebted to my Western herbal medicine teachers, especially Edith Barlow, Barbara Howe, and Ifanca James, without whom I would not have been able to tread this path. Edith, in particular, has been a very great support to me throughout my time in herbal practice. I am enormously grateful to her for generously sharing her knowledge and experience.

I am very fortunate to have had so much help and support from the wonderful team at Aeon Books. Without them I could not have brought my thoughts and experience into a form that could be shared with so many others.

With much love and appreciation to my husband, Mark, and my children, Andrew and Bex, who have supported me throughout this herbal journey and have never once questioned my calling.

I am truly blessed.

SELF-SUFFICIENT
HERBALISM

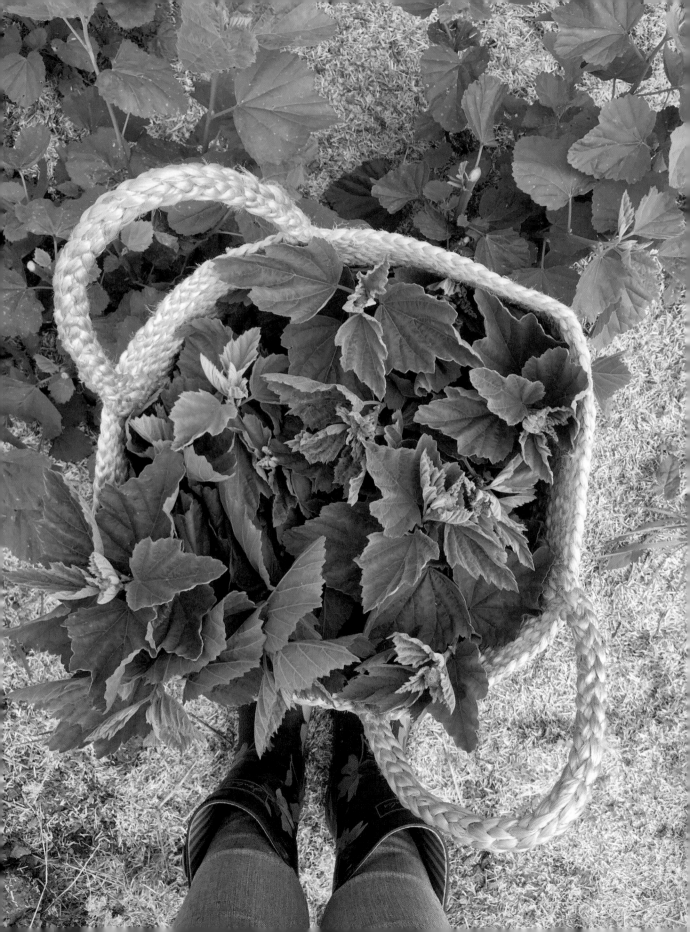

This is a guide to being more self-sufficient in your herbal practice. I have been in practice since 2006, and I have always felt that to grow and gather my own herbal dispensary is one of the most wonderful aspects of being a medical herbalist. It connects me with the plants that I work with, the ancient traditions that I come from, and the land where I am settled. It grounds and nourishes me. It provides balance to the demands and challenges that I face while carrying out patient consultations. I thoroughly recommend it.

Whether you are an established practitioner with a full patient list, newly qualified, someone who uses herbs at home to treat family members, or a small-scale herbal processor, you will find that this book offers a clear and practical guide to being more self-sufficient in terms of your herbal dispensary. Over the years I've learnt such a lot. Sometimes the learning was joyous and smooth, at other times it was the result of mistakes that seemed like frustrating obstacles at the time, but I know that the mistakes that I made have helped me to learn how to do things better. Much better, in fact. I want to share all of this hard-won knowledge with you. Within these pages I have included down-to-earth, practical guidance about growing, gathering, and preserving medicinal herbs for a working dispensary, but it does not stop there. My aim is to offer an insight into a way of practising that is much more than just sourcing herbs. I want to show you that the practice of self-sufficient herbalism can be transformative.

I have deliberately avoided writing about herbal properties or about how different herbs can be used in a clinical setting. There are many excellent books focusing on these subjects, and if that is what you are looking for, this is not the book for you. However, if you are intrigued by working traditionally and building a closer relationship with the plants that you work with, then I hope that this book will guide and inspire you.

The book is divided into three sections. The first, Part One, explains 'why' self-sufficiency in herbal practice is a good thing to move towards. The second, Part Two, goes through the main principles of 'how' to achieve self-sufficiency, divided into the different processes involved and the factors to consider. The third, The Herbal Harvesting Year, is a glossary of detailed notes on the cultivation, harvesting, and processing of 108 particular herbs. It is arranged by the seasons, so you can use it as a reference when you are starting out. Everything that I write here is based on my own experience.

Before beginning, what I should say is that very few medical herbalists will be able to be truly 100% self-sufficient in herbal medicines. Self-sufficiency is something to aim for: it is a way of working and a move away from large-scale cultivation and wildcrafting practices. It is a broad aim. It is the keeping alive of a vibrant and grounded connection with the herbs that we find ourselves working with. Even if you decide that you can only practically be self-sufficient in two or three herbs, I would encourage you to make this happen and feel proud of yourself for achieving it.

I reckon that in my busy full-time practice I achieve 75% self-sufficiency in terms of the herbs that I prescribe. I can say, however, that I do make every single litre of tincture, every capsule, and every topical treatment that I use.

So why only 75%? I grow and gather as much as possible, but I do choose to buy in, in some bulk, herbs from responsible and environmentally sustainable sources. I like to make and use some traditional Tibetan medicines, which contain herbs like Cloves, Cardamom, and Nutmeg, none of which I have a way of cultivating in this country. I can, in theory, grow Ginger and Turmeric in a heated greenhouse, but I do not have access to one. I have only a very small garden and an allotment in which to grow my herbs, so I need to prioritize which herbal crops I grow. As a result, if there are certain things that would take a lot of space to grow but I can buy in from good-quality sources, I will do so. Caraway and Garlic are two examples of these.

With such limited growing space, I wildcraft as many medicines as it makes sense to. Occasionally there will be a bad year for something, and I will find that I need to buy additional supplies to last until next gathering or harvest season. To be honest, I cannot remember when I last had to do this. It is a rare occurrence. I prefer to travel further afield and spend more time searching for suitable populations of the plants that I need. If wildcrafting sufficient for my needs is unreliable or potentially unsustainable, I will establish a population of that species at my allotment or in the garden. This usually gives me plenty of what I need the following year, especially as I can manage it like a horticultural crop and take a heavier harvest than I would do with a wild population.

Having said all of this, the last thing I want to imply is that herbal wholesalers are to be avoided or that they are in some way undesirable or untrustworthy. There are many really lovely wholesalers out there who make every effort to source high-quality, sustainably sourced herbs. I have a good relationship with the wholesalers that I buy from, and I appreciate their integrity, efforts, and customer service. I just do not want to rely on them for the majority of the medicines I use for my patients.

It is also worth mentioning that a busy herbal practice needs bottles, jars, bags, and other packaging materials. I minimize the need for these by recycling medicine bottles, but they still need to be bought in the first place. I also purchase 96% proof alcohol, printer paper, ink cartridges, and packaging materials for postage. There is no way that I can claim to be fully self-sufficient, but that is not my aim. My aim is to be as self-sufficient as possible in terms of herbs.

Let me take you on a journey to explain why I do this and how this can be achieved within your own situation.

Note

This book uses metric and Imperial units. The equivalent units in the United States are the following:

1 litre	=	2.1 US pints
1 Imp. gallon	=	1.2 US gallons
1 Imp. pint	=	1.2 US pints
1 Imp. cup	=	1.18 US cups
1 Imp. fl oz	=	0.96 US fl oz
1 Imp. tbsp	=	1.2 US tbsp
1 Imp. tsp	=	1.2 US tsp

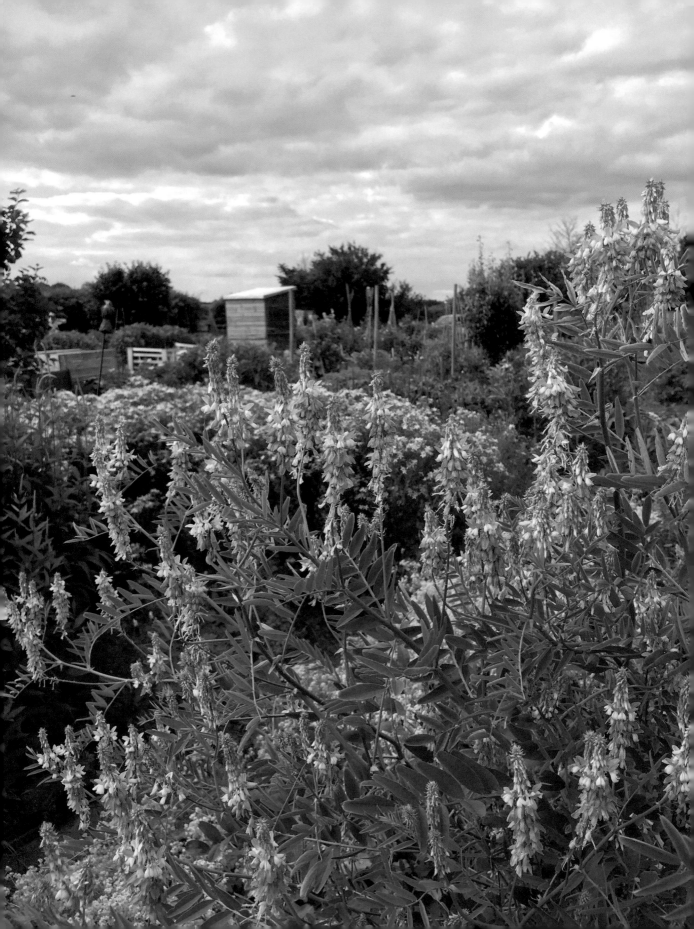

Part one

WHY SELF-SUFFICIENCY?

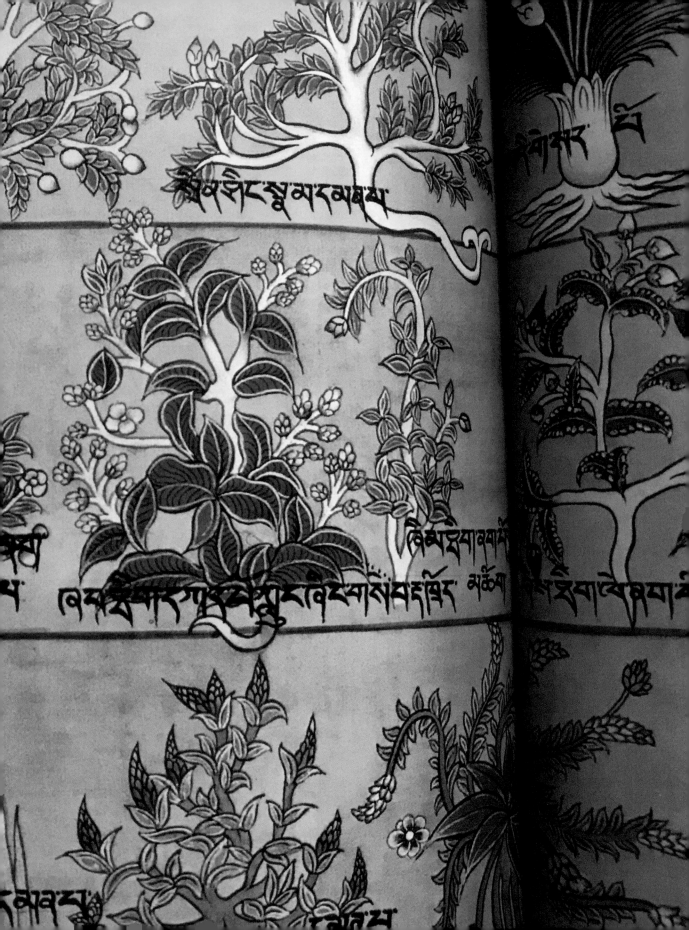

1

Environmental benefits

Herbal medicine is a health system that relies on an understanding and recognition of interconnections. As herbalists, we use whole plants rather than isolated constituents. We blend multiple herbs to create tailor-made prescriptions for each patient, and we consider whole body systems rather than isolated organs. We recognize that a person's health is greatly affected by lifestyle, habitual thought patterns, and external influences. We know that different foods and drinks suit different people, and this varies significantly according to the prevailing weather conditions and the seasons. Much as it would make things more straightforward to compartmentalize these factors and predict linear causes and effects, we cannot. Sooner or later herbal practitioners have to embrace interconnectedness.

Herbs are natural living products. Whether they come from cultivated or wild sources, they are intimately connected to the environment in which they had grown. Their medicinal qualities are affected by the climate, the prevailing soil type, and the availability of water, for example. People gathering herbs will, to a greater or lesser extent, influence the ground on which they walk or drive. Distribution, packing, shipping, and storage will each have their own environmental impacts and influences. It is, as they say, complicated. Every action that we take has an effect on the world around us. The good news is that since there are so many steps in the chain between herbs being planted and being used as medicines, there are a great many opportunities for us to lessen potential environmental harm and to create a positive contribution to the health of our planet.

Just as we can improve our health by gradually making positive lifestyle changes, so we can also gradually rethink the way we source our herbs. We need to look beyond the orders of sweet-smelling medicinal herbs that arrive on our doorsteps. Understanding how those herbs have been grown and produced gives us an opportunity to positively influence the wider environment through our purchasing decisions. We can choose suppliers who source herbs from sustainable plant populations and who reward their workers fairly. We can avoid wildcrafted herbs that are endangered; instead, we can choose cultivated herbs that have been grown in an environmentally conscious manner. We can try to find local sources, so that shipping impact is lessened. Ultimately, we can look into growing or gathering at least some of our own herbs.

It is not an all-or-nothing process. More mindful herb sourcing will result in ripples of influence – ripples that can affect not only our own health but also that of our patients and of the environment as a whole. If we can grow or gather even just one herb ourselves, it is very significant. It may be the starting point for more over time. A 100-mile journey starts with one step.

I would like to explain a little about how I came to care so much about these things. From an early age, I loved plants and was a keen gardener. I studied agriculture and forestry at university, learning about ecology and the influence of man on the landscape, both deliberate and unintentional. After four years, I left with a master's degree in forestry and a passion for saving neglected broadleaved woodlands. I started out in farm woodland consultancy and then moved on to a job in London, working for a firm of consulting engineers carrying out environmental impact assessments of large-scale developments all over the country. After the positivity of working with the management of small farm woodlands, it was quite an eye opener – and not always an entirely comfortable process – for me to work with large developments and their environmental impacts. The building of motorways, power stations, and new towns will, even with the most careful planning and assessment, have an enormous impact on the environment. I often found myself thinking that economic factors were holding much more sway than environmental ones. I concluded that the plants and their habitats needed more human allies.

Later on, I quit the corporate world and went freelance in order to have the flexibility and availability to devote myself to studying Tibetan

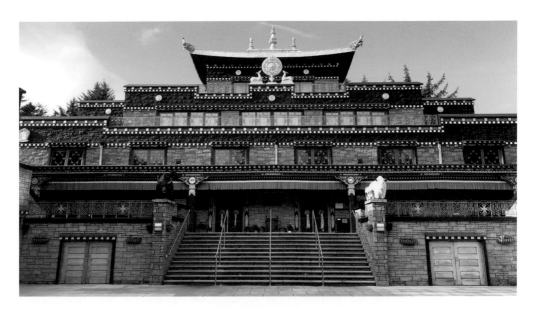

Samye Ling Temple in Eskdalemuir, Scotland.

medicine. I was incredibly fortunate to be one of a very few students able to study Tibetan medicine with the great master Khenpo Troru Tsenam at Samye Ling Tibetan Centre in Scotland for two months a year during a four-year period in the 1990s. It was an amazing time of my life. We were immersed in Tibetan language, culture, and spirituality, as well as the ancient Tibetan medical texts, including *The Four Tantras*. We were fortunate to have had the benefit of a very detailed explanation and commentary on this main text from someone widely considered to be the highest living authority on the subject. These Tibetan medical studies were hugely influential in absolutely all spheres of my life. As well as opening my eyes to a truly holistic way of healing, they changed the way that I view the sourcing of herbs and protecting the environment. In this beautiful and sophisticated system of medicine the interrelationship between patient and

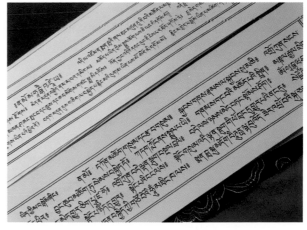

The text for Medicine Buddha practice.

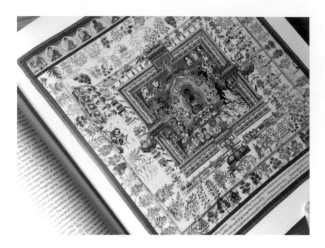

Tanaduk

external environment is considered to be the most fundamental factor in illness and recovery. Tibetan medicine teaches that the true root cause of all illness is an inability to recognize that we are intimately and irrevocably linked to the environment around us. To this end, Tibetan medicine can actually be viewed as a path to spiritual enlightenment. This excerpt from the *Root Tantra* as taught by Khenpo Troru Tsenam in 1994 illustrates the deep reverence for the environment and natural medicines taught within the Tibetan medical tradition.

In the legendary city of Tanaduk there are all the medicinal substances which can cure all illnesses. In the centre is a palace encrusted with jewels which can cure both hot and cold diseases. To the north is the 'Snow Mountain' where plants grow in a cool energy and can cure hot ailments. To the south there is a second mountain called the 'Piercing Mountain' where there is a hot energy and the plants which grow there are used to cure cold ailments. To the east is the 'Fragrant Mountain' where 'myrobalans' grow and cure many diseases. In the west is the 'Malaya Mountain' where remedies, particularly minerals, are found which cure all sorts of diseases. The whole area is very beautiful and gives off a very good feeling which is uplifting and healing in itself. In the middle of the city is a beautiful palace with a throne in the centre on which the Medicine Buddha is sitting. He is immersed in compassion and wishes to relieve all beings of suffering.[1]

I love that this excerpt exudes interconnectedness. It focuses on the relationship between the environment and the nature of the plants that it supports, the ability of these plants and minerals to cure various health imbalances depending on their nature, the link between the feeling we experience being in a particular area and how it makes us feel, as well as the fundamental role of the development of compassion within Tibetan medicine and within healing in general. You will also see that it mentions Myrobalans. These are

---

[1] Khenpo Troru Tsenam's teaching of the Root Tantra, 1994, translated by Katia Holmes, 1994.

special wild plums considered to have the ability to address all sorts of bodily imbalances. In Tibetan iconography, the Medicine Buddha is depicted as holding a sprig of Myrobalan in his right hand. It is the most spiritually significant medicine in the Tibetan pharmacopaea and the reason I chose it as the name of my clinic.

Once we are aware of it, we need to be very conscious of interconnectedness when sourcing herbal medicines. We have to accept that we have a responsibility to promote wellness and balance throughout the supply chain. By wellness and balance, I mean safeguarding wild plant and animal populations, ensuring that soil and water are cared for, and taking care of the health and well-being of the people who work in herbal growing and wildcrafting production.

So where do our bought-in herbs come from? We may know the country of origin, but that does not really tell us very much. When buying in packets of dried herbs, we are at serious risk of being disconnected from the supply chain. Our involvement in sourcing that herb may have been limited to the making of one phone call and unpacking a delivery. Yet in sourcing the herbs that we are to use as medicines, we should really be asking ourselves and our suppliers a series of questions. Were the herbs cultivated or wildcrafted? If cultivated, how did the land first come into cultivation – for example, was valuable natural habitat safeguarded or lost in the process? Has cultivation been carried out with an awareness of the need for soil conservation? We should also consider how much water is used in the cultivation of our herbs. Is this water plentiful, sourced through rainwater harvesting, or is it in short supply and come from a borehole that is relied upon for drinking water by local communities? Are pesticides and fertilizers used, and if so, which ones? If they are used, how long a time period elapses between the last application and the time of the harvest? If the herbs are wildcrafted, do we know whether the species concerned are common or scarce in their source area? Do we know whether this area is clean or polluted? Do we know whether the people gathering the herbs are harvesting sustainably, only taking a maximum of 1 in 20 plants from abundant healthy populations, or are they gathering the maximum yield possible, either unaware of the environmental damage that this causes or unable to consider it, due to their own desperate need for income? Do we know whether the plants have been identified correctly or whether batches of correctly identified material have a consistent presence of other species that were growing in close proximity to the desired one? Do we know whether the herb is insect-damaged, contains insect larvae, or is contaminated with soil?

In considering the interconnectedness of our supply chain, we cannot separate the people involved from the herbs themselves. How much do we know about the people at the beginning of the herbal supply chain? Are they part-time growers or gatherers seeking to supplement their income from other sources, or are they working as employees? Do they belong to a cooperative or growing community, or are they working alone? What are the economic circumstances in the community where the herbs are sourced? What kind of thought pattern was prevalent during the harvest? It is pretty tough to think positive healing thoughts if you and your family depend on the income from these herbs to make the difference between eating and going hungry.

There are so many questions, it would be impossible to know the answers to all of these directly for ourselves unless we grow or gather our own herbs. Perhaps what matters most is that we are aware of the issues and we recognize that as herb purchasers we are a link in the chain from soil to patient. If we are buying in herbs, we need to trust that our suppliers have asked the right questions and sourced wisely. A good interim solution is to choose herbs that have been grown or gathered according to an appropriate certification scheme.

Biodynamic agriculture and horticulture is organic in nature, but it has metaphysical and spiritual roots that organic production does not. Biodynamic certification (known as Demeter certification in the United Kingdom) does not allow the use of genetically modified organisms or the use of artificial fertilizers or pesticides. It places great importance on the making of compost, fortified by adding positive intention and carefully made preparations that are also applied directly to the land. Biodynamic production aims to create farms that are self-sustaining organisms, to farm 'regeneratively' rather than 'just' sustainably. Biodynamics is as interconnected as an officially certified production system gets. My spiritual teacher, Akong Rinpoché, liked biodynamics a great deal. He once told me that it contained elements very similar to the Tibetan understanding of respecting and caring for the environment.

Next is organic certification. Organic certification for herb growers offers a guarantee to the consumer that environmental concerns have been addressed in the growing, harvesting, processing, and packaging stages of production. The aim is for sustainability, taking care of the soil, the environment, and wider resources through the use of carefully sourced inputs and maximum use of recycling within the farm or horticultural business. Pesticides and artificial fertilizers are avoided. Natural habitats and wildlife are safeguarded. Workers are treated fairly. There are many different organic certification schemes.

In general, all certification schemes rely on checking facts and providing assurances to customers. Checking and inspections are an inevitable part of this. If you buy an organically certified product, you can be sure that it has been produced according to the organic standards of the certifying organization. Producers have to complete a significant amount of paperwork for record-keeping and in preparing for the inspector's visit to the farm. Larger businesses can afford to employ people to help with this, but smaller businesses can find it an unwelcome burden when added to the pressures of working on the land and producing a product. As a result, many small businesses opt to follow the guidelines 'unofficially' and avoid the administrative burden of compliance and inspections.

I had long felt that choosing organically produced food and herbs was a positive way in which we can make our environmentally conscious voices heard more widely. The point of certification is that it provides surety about the way each crop has been produced, so I agree that it is a very valuable attribute for growers to aspire to. Having worked for a certification body for seven years, I know the hard work that is involved and the dedication of the certification staff, but I can also see that organic produce may not always be 'better' for the environment than non-organic. Choosing to buy from local organically certified producers is, without doubt, a very sound strategy, but if there are none local to you, a little research may reveal uncertified growers producing beautiful wholesome 'untreated' crops. If these growers are local to us, we can form our own relationship with them and see their production methods for ourselves. By simply always choosing 'organically grown' in our wholesale catalogues, we may actually be ordering herbs that have been grown in quite an intensive way and may have been shipped large distances using unsustainable transport methods.

Once you start thinking about what is best, no sourcing decision is easy. The important thing, though, is to actually think about it. Just as we all do our best with our choice of the foods that we aim to eat, so we need to do our best with the information we have available about the herbs that we buy. Organic production guarantees that no pesticides have been used and workers have a 'fair and adequate' quality of life, but it does not guarantee that the herbs are, for example, free from insect larvae. To have confidence in the herbs that we intend to work with, we need to either know the circumstances of the grower or trust our supplier to build that relationship on our behalf and carry out rigorous quality control testing.

Although organic certification ensures that the workforce has a 'fair and adequate' quality of life, Fair Trade certification goes further than this. It aims to promote the sharing of benefits from trade with people all along the supply chain. The Fair Trade Foundation tends to favour small producers, although some larger producers can apply to join the standard, provided that they meet certain specified criteria.

FairWild certification has a different emphasis. It was created in 2008 in order to extend the fair ethos to wildcrafted products and to consider the people at the start of the wildcrafted herbal supply chain. By looking after those who traditionally wildcraft herbal medicines, FairWild certification aims to promote the conservation of natural habitats and herb collecting as an economically viable way of life. If precious natural resources are more economically and socially valuable, they stand a much better chance of being cared for. The FairWild standard is a really positive development in terms of sustainable and fair wild plant harvesting. It is definitely worth choosing herbs that are FairWild certified if you are buying in wildcrafted herbs. The reality, though, is that FairWild certification still applies only to a relatively small number of wildcrafted species. If you can't find FairWild certified herbs, please ask your suppliers to consider stocking them.

Table 1 shows the species listed on the FairWild Foundation website as being available in February 2017.

United Plant Savers is a not-for-profit organization established to raise awareness of, and to promote conservation of, rare and endangered plants, together with their habitats, in the United States and Canada. In recent years there has been a huge explosion of demand for herbs and herbal products, and this has placed more pressure on wild plant resources all over the world. Habitat destruction and over-harvesting is a widespread threat to wild medicinal plants. By bringing these issues to the attention of herbal consumers and

Table 1
FairWild certified herb availability, February 2017

Zimbabwe	Baobab fruit, *Adansonia digitata*
Bosnia Herzegovina	*Rubus idaeus, Rubus fruticosus, Urtica dioica, Taraxacum officinale, Sambucus nigra, Tilia platyphyllos, Tilia cordata, Tilia tomentosa*
Bulgaria	*Tilia tomentosa, Rubus fruticosus, Urtica dioica, Sambucus nigra, Malva sylvestris*
Georgia	*Glycyrrhiza glabra, Rosa canina*
Kazakhstan	*Rubus idaeus* and *Glycyrrhiza uralensis*
India	*Terminalia chebula* and *Terminalia bellirica*
Spain	*Glycyrrhiza glabra*
Serbia	*Rosa canina*
Poland	*Achillea millefolium, Juniperus communis, Tilia cordata, Tilia platyphyllos, Rubus fruticosus, Urtica dioica, Sambucus nigra, Taraxacum officinale*
Hungary	*Rosa canina, Urtica dioica, Tilia cordata / Tilia platyphyllos, Sambucus nigra*

Source: FairWild Foundation.

processors, United Plant Savers are doing valuable work in encouraging more sustainable sourcing of wild medicines.

The subject of endangered medicinal plants is very close to my heart. In the early part of the millennium I was asked to attend a meeting at Samye Ling Tibetan Centre, where a group of people had been assembled to discuss how best to conserve Tibetan medicinal plants. My spiritual teacher, Akong Rinpoché, was concerned about the wild harvesting of Tibetan medicinal plants within Tibetan areas of China. With a huge surge in the popularity of Tibetan medicine, the demand for Tibetan medicinal herbs was soaring. Since wild harvesting is the traditional way of sourcing herbs in Tibet, there was increasing pressure on traditional gathering areas. Opportunistic foragers were moving in and picking herbs in order to supplement their meagre family incomes. Lack of knowledge and respect for the plants meant that many plants were unnecessarily uprooted during gathering, because it is quicker to do it that way. Having studied medicinal plants in Amdo, I can report that it is very easy to inadvertently uproot plants at high altitude because the soil is so thin and dry in the summer months. Plants that are traditionally gathered for their roots are even more vulnerable to population depletion, and many are becoming very scarce. There is no established tradition of growing medicinal plants in Tibet; in fact, it has always been considered less desirable due to the risk of inadvertently killing small beings that inhabit the soil. It is also considered that medicines that have grown in the wild are more potent than those that have been cultivated. Unfortunately, with many medicines critically endangered or officially extinct in the wild, we need to encourage a shift in sourcing patterns, even if it is somewhat of a compromise. Akong Rinpoché had the foresight to start to change this pattern. He decided to sponsor young Tibetan doctors to come to the West and learn horticulture. Once they had been trained in the production of herbs, he encouraged them to set up small herb gardens in Tibet, in the areas where they would be practising. He also planned to establish two larger herb-growing areas, in order to improve supplies of herbs and to gain experience in cultivation and harvesting practices. At that time, he asked me and a friend, Betty Richardson, to start to grow medicinal herbs in the United Kingdom. The aim was for us to build up knowledge about how to grow the herbs at lower altitude and in the softer growing conditions in Europe. In time, the European-sourced herbs could help to supply Tibetan medicinal practitioners based in the West. He specified that this initial herb growing should take place in Somerset, although at the time I was living in Dorset and Betty was living in Gloucestershire. We thought it was odd, wondering whether he was mistaken, since the counties are adjacent. A few years later Betty had moved her growing operations to Spain, and my family and I found ourselves unexpectedly having to move away from Dorset. We ended up in Somerset.

I now grow some Tibetan medicinal plants in my garden. Each year of growing adds to my knowledge about how to care for and propagate these herbs in the West. My efforts are especially focused on plants that are scarce, and one, Himalayan Burdock (*Saussurea lappa*), is officially extinct in the wild. *Saussurea lappa*, also known as Costus ('*Ruta*' in Tibetan), is gathered for its root, which is a warming bitter, particularly valuable for people with a nervous disposition who are suffering with digestive weakness. It is a very popular medicine and is used in a great many important traditional formulae. In consequence, it is in great demand. Although officially extinct in the wild according to the Convention on International Trade in Endangered Species of Wild Fauna and Flora [CITES], there may possibly be some remote populations still existing at high altitudes, accessible only to those who know the locality. It does worry me that wild harvesting may still be continuing, as there is such a strong demand for these plants. The way forward for this plant is definitely to encourage the availability of good-quality cultivated stock, and hopefully in time wild populations may begin to recover.

It is definitely food for thought to be growing and harvesting seeds from a plant that is so precious and scarce. My trips to Tibet and this small-scale conservation work has really brought home to me the reality of how our demand for medicinal herbs affects the habitats and plant populations far from where we live. Many plants used by medical herbalists are at risk in the wild. Take Golden Seal (*Hydrastis canadensis*), Slippery Elm (*Ulmus fulva*), Blue Cohosh (*Caulophylum thalictroides*), Ginseng (*Panax ginseng* and *Panax quinquefolius*), Beth Root (*Trillium erectum*) and Black Cohosh (*Actaea racemosa* or *Cimicifuga racemosa,* as it was formerly known), for example. It is not all doom and gloom, though: great conservation work and awareness-raising is being done by United Plant Savers and other conservation bodies. Growers are stepping up to the challenge and growing these endangered and scarce species, so that there are sustainable sources for practitioners to buy stock from. It is also inspiring to see the work being done by the Sustainable Herbs Program. It would seem that plants do, in fact, have people speaking up for them.

As herbalists, we source and work with a wide range of medicinal plants other than those that are endangered. Some will be relatively common, others will be scarcer. Certification schemes can be a helpful guide to how herbs have been produced, but availability of certified stock may be limited, and we cannot know everything about how they have been produced and the social and environmental impact that has been created. Ultimately, the best way to ensure that we take care of the environment while sourcing our herbs is to form relationships with local growers or to start to grow them or gather them ourselves. When we do this, we know that our actions will not have contributed to the destruction of a habitat or to the depletion of a scarce plant population. The herbs will not have been shipped long distances using fossil fuels. Their production will not have contributed to social inequality or exploitation.

We may not be able to grow or gather all that we need, but each herb that we can source in a self-sufficient manner will result in a significant positive contribution to the environment, along with many other benefits.

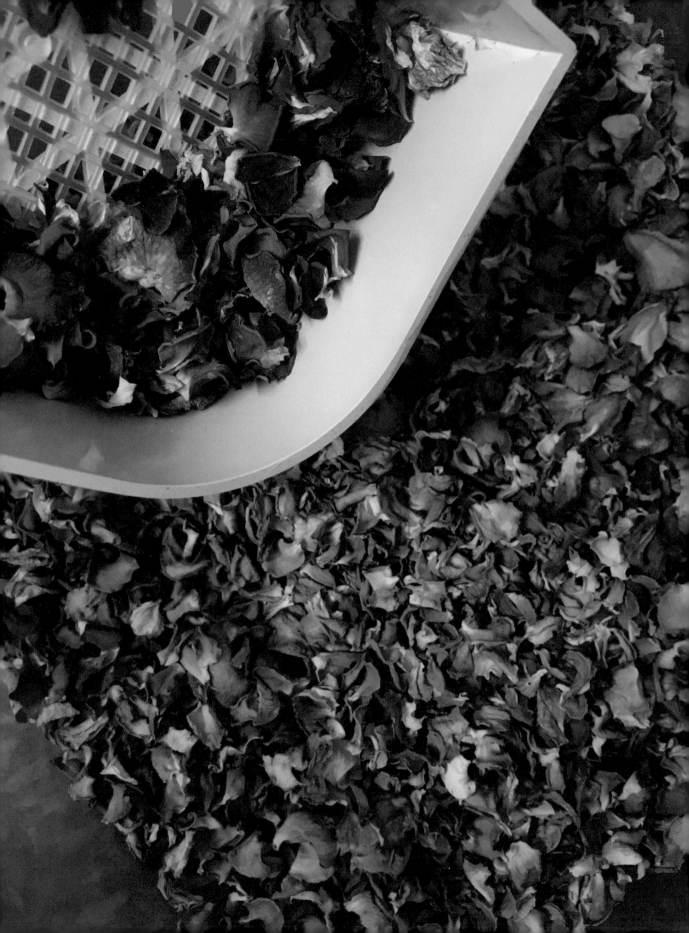

2

Quality of plant medicines

When I first started growing and gathering my own herbs, I was motivated by factors other than quality. I had come to herbal medicine through my love of herbs, and it was only natural that I should wish to spend time with them. By growing and gathering the herbs that I was using to treat patients, I could build a real connection with them and get to know them much more deeply than if I had been relying on bought-in dried herbs. At first, I gathered only relatively few herbs. Each year, as I came to know my local area better, I was able to increase the number of species that I could collect. In the early years, though, I relied more on a mixture of bought-in herbs combined with those that I had grown or gathered myself. In those days, I was not as proficient as I am now at estimating the quantity of each herb that I would need during the year ahead. I would often start the season with my own herbs and then buy in replacement stock when it was needed. As a result, I had numerous opportunities to compare my own home-grown and wild-harvested herbs with those that were provided by herbal wholesalers. I immediately realized that the quality of my own herbs seemed markedly better than those that I was buying in.

Even though large-scale herbal suppliers make every effort to source the highest possible quality herbs for sale, they would be the first to agree that batches arriving at the warehouse vary, in both medicinal and keeping qualities. In order to safeguard quality and safety, suppliers have to put into place sophisticated, costly, time-consuming procedures to assess each batch of herbs that they purchase. It is worth noting that the certification schemes that were outlined in the previous chapter do not guarantee the quality of herbs. They simply give assurances about how they have been grown and harvested. For example, we touched on the issues surrounding wild harvesting and the efforts to address social inequalities in traditional gathering populations by FairWild certification. Very impoverished gatherers, paid by the weight of herb collected, may be tempted to adulterate their harvest with rocks or soil in an effort to earn enough to feed their families. This is described officially as 'economic adulteration', in recognition of the pressures that arise when growers and gatherers do not feel that they are getting a fair price for what they are supplying. Likewise, wildcrafters gathering herbs in less abundant years may be under pressure to include plant material that is faded, past its best or infected by insect or fungal pathogens. They may even be tempted to gather similar-looking plants that are not related to the target species. We know that we should not gather herbs growing by the side of busy, dusty roads, in cemeteries or growing in waste water from settlements, but wholesale gatherers may make the decision to overlook such restrictions on the basis of economic necessity. Problems with quality are not restricted to wild-harvested herbs. Cultivated herbs can also be subject to unexpected inclusions. Although it has never happened to me, herbal colleagues have reported the presence of soil, cigarette butts, plastic ties, and even, perhaps most disturbingly, animal faeces in some batches of cultivated herbs that they had bought in. Needless to say, in all cases those batches were immediately returned to the supplier with a complaint.

In order to safeguard quality standards, many wholesale suppliers are investing huge sums of money in complying with 'Good Manufacturing Practice' (GMP). Batches of herbs are tested for adulteration with foreign objects and for adulteration with other species of plants. They may be tested for pesticide and heavy metal contamination, as well as the presence of fungi and insects. Sometimes shipments are rejected outright if they are below the required standard, and at other times remedial action can be taken. Remedial action may include sieving out physical adulterants such as soil and rocks and irradiating or freezing the herbs to kill insects and larvae. In the latter case the dead insects and larvae remain within the batch of herbs. I find it rather disconcerting to think that there is a certain level of insect larvae that is considered officially acceptable to be present in GMP-compliant herbs.

It is perhaps surprising to find that GMP does not actually require testing for the level of therapeutic compounds in herbs. As long as a herb is what is says on the bale or sack and it passes safety and adulteration checks, it is officially good to go and can be described as GMP-compliant. Knowing how variable the quality of herbs can be, many wholesalers do go to the extra effort and expense of checking the levels of active ingredients using thin-layer chromatography and other laboratory techniques.

There are a great many variables that need to be considered in sourcing herbs, and this brief review is by no means a comprehensive list of all the quality considerations that suppliers have to deal with. I honestly think that our herbal wholesalers are doing a heroic job in trying to navigate an increasingly complicated regulatory environment while maintaining a reasonable catalogue of herb species and trying to stay economically viable at the same time. I do not envy their challenges and the pressures they are under. I am very grateful for their efforts to provide good-quality herbal medicines, and I appreciate the option of being able to supplement my dispensary with bought-in stock when needed.

Wholesalers may be doing a great job, but if we grow or gather our own herbs, we can be much more actively involved in preserving quality at all stages of the process, from growing to medicine making. The medicinal potency of herbs varies according to the way that they have been grown, the soil type and aspect of the growing site, the season and the way that they have been harvested, handled, and stored. A huge number of factors can have an impact on the final quality of the batch. In growing our own, we can have a close relationship with the crop, and we can respond to changing circumstances in order to safeguard quality. Just as a home-grown carrot is always going to taste better than a carrot produced in a large-scale horticultural operation, so carefully produced home-grown herbs will seem more vibrant and will keep longer than mass-produced bought-in dried herbs.

My study of herbs has been lifelong so far and shows no sign of abating. I know that I am not unusual in this. It seems as though one lifetime is not enough to fit in all of the study and experiential learning that we are drawn to. We come across herbs with which we are not yet familiar, and it is only natural to want to understand how they can help people. As we research herbal properties, we start to discover that there are differences in therapeutic properties between similar species of the same

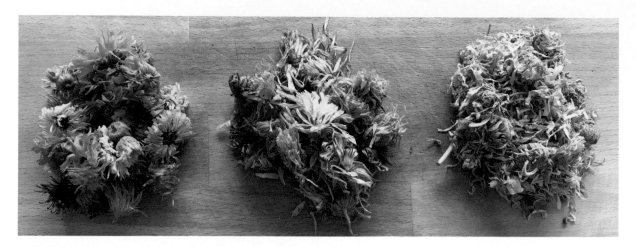

There is quite a difference visually between the different batches of dried Calendula flowers according to their age and source. On the left are this year's flowers, and you can see that year-old home-grown flowers (*middle*) still have a superior colour and appearance compared to the current year's bought-in stock (*right*).

genus – the Echinaceas, for example. We find it fascinating to learn how different plant parts within a particular species provide different degrees of therapeutic actions. We study various extraction techniques and see how they can change or enhance the therapeutic properties of the herbs that we are working with. We may build up a library of studies that provide evidence for the way that herbs work, or a spreadsheet cross-referencing various sources about herbal actions. There is nothing wrong in this – in fact, it is a great way to learn. I am an unashamed herb nerd. With all of this learning, though, whether through formal study or by experience, we can become so focused on the properties and actions of each herbal species that we may start to assume that all batches of a particular herbal species will act in exactly the same way. The stark reality is that not all batches of the same herb are equal. Herbs are naturally variable products.

I lose count of the number of times that people have told me that they had tried a certain herb for a particular symptom, but it made no difference. Whenever I hear that, I do not automatically assume that the herb was inappropriate for that person. Instead, I wonder about the quality of the herb and the form in which it was taken. When I was first a Western herbal medicine student, I tried various courses of herbal self-medication for symptoms that I experienced. Looking back on my attempts now, I can see how

I rather missed the point, since I focused totally on symptoms rather than understanding why those symptoms were arising. Nevertheless, it was a very valuable learning experience to take herbs and to feel their effects first-hand in my body. On one occasion, I had decided to take Dandelion (*Taraxacum officinale*) leaf for its diuretic effects, because I had some water retention. In those days, I was right at the beginning of my herbal course, and I had only just started to build up a home dispensary. I did not have any Dandelion leaf to hand, so I bought some pills from my favourite independent health-food shop. I know the folk who run this shop, and I am aware of how carefully they source their products. The product I bought was of excellent quality. I noticed an immediate effect and continued to take the pills until the pack finished. When they did run out, I was nowhere near my favourite shop, and so found myself buying a replacement pack from a large high-street health chain. After a few days I noticed that the Dandelion leaf seemed to have stopped working. Either there was too little Dandelion leaf in the formulation, or the Dandelion leaf that was used was of much lower quality than the one I had been taking so far. It was a real eye-opener. I had assumed that all Dandelion leaf was Dandelion leaf.

Aside from different amounts of a herb being present in a prepared formulation, why might batches of herbs vary in quality? All plants begin to deteriorate once they are harvested, no matter whether you are harvesting a tonne or just two or three plants. The speed of that deterioration can vary from almost imperceptible in the case of roots to very rapid in the case of flowers. If we are to preserve maximum quality in our herbal medicines, we need to understand how to slow that process down. The deterioration, or potential deterioration, is caused by various factors that can come into play during different stages of harvesting and processing. If we are aware of the potential for herbs to deteriorate at each stage, we can take steps to avoid this deterioration, or at least to minimize it.

It is a fact of life that large-scale growing and harvesting means that each crop has to be treated more as a whole than as a collection of individual plants. Once harvested, the plant material is transported from the field to the processing area. Whether or not the operation is mechanized, dealing with increased volumes means that it is more difficult to make fine-tuned adjustments for different parts of the harvest. There is consequently a greater risk of the herbs deteriorating in quality. It is, of course, perfectly possible for large-scale operations to incorporate management practices that preserve maximum quality in the harvested crop, and I am sure there are conscientious growers who do this skilfully. Equally, I am sure there are many growers who do not.

Take temporary storage following harvest, for example. If freshly harvested or gathered herbs are piled up in crates or in a trailer, there is a risk that the lower layers will become compressed and will start to heat up through natural biological degradation. This process takes place alarmingly quickly, especially on a hot day. You do not want to include herbs that have begun to turn into compost in your medicine. Once the herbs get back to the processing area, there are many other factors that can result in changes to their quality. These include the temperature used to dry them, their exposure (or not) to light, the amount of cyclical rehydration they experience during the drying process, their vulnerability to insects and fungi, the amount they are cut, whether they are handled once wilted, and much, much more. These factors and how to avoid them impacting on the quality of the herbs that we are growing or gathering are discussed in detail in Part Two.

When we grow or gather our own herbs, there is so much that we can do to improve the end quality of the medicine that we produce. We can make sure that at each stage of the process the herbs are treated with knowledge, care, and respect. First, we can harvest the herbs at the optimal stage of growth, on a day when the weather is suitable. We can ensure that they are not piled up too deeply or for too long after gathering, instead being transported quickly to the processing area before decomposition starts to take place. We can avoid excessive handling of the plant material so that bruising and consequent fermentation do not happen. We can choose to dry our herbs as uncut as possible, to avoid the loss of medicinal compounds. We can store them in the dark in a cool place. There are a great many stages in the process between harvesting a herb and processing it. If you contemplate the potential for loss in quality at each stage, you can see that there is an equal and opposite potential for preservation of quality at each one. All of these add up to create a significant difference in the end product.

If you have any doubt about the effects of handling fresh plants after harvest, think about the efforts that farmers go to in order to maximize the quality of their hay crops. I have first-hand experience of this from my time spent running a small sheep dairy farm in North East Scotland.

Nowadays I no longer need to make hay, but I do need to provide the best possible quality and the most effective herbal medicines for my patients. The principle is the same. The time lapse between cutting and drying makes a huge difference to quality, as do the many ways that plants are handled and treated during processing and storage.

Let me give you a couple of specific herbal examples to illustrate the difference in quality between home-grown or wild-harvested herbs and those that have been mass-produced. When I first started on the road to self-sufficient herbalism, I noticed significant differences in scent and efficacy between batches of Cramp Bark or Guelder Rose (*Viburnum opulus*) that I had wildcrafted compared to batches that had been purchased from herbal wholesalers. Cramp Bark should ideally be harvested in early spring, just before the buds burst. As its name suggests, it is the bark that is used for medicine since it contains the highest concentration of medicinal constituents such as valerenic acid. In early spring, the potency of the medicine is at its peak, and the bark is much easier to strip away from the stems. The Cramp Bark that I gather consists of pure bark. It is fragrant and musky, smelling slightly of Valerian due to the valerenic acid present. It consistently works quickly and effectively when I use it to treat patients. Once, when I purchased a batch of

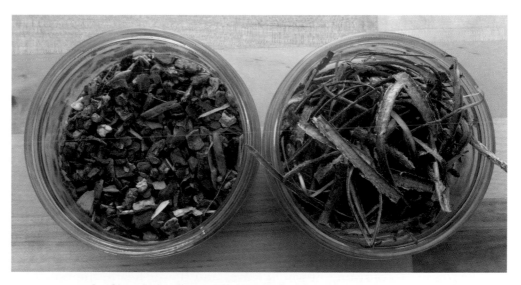

A sample of bought-in *Viburnum opulus* on the left, and one of home-grown bark on the right.

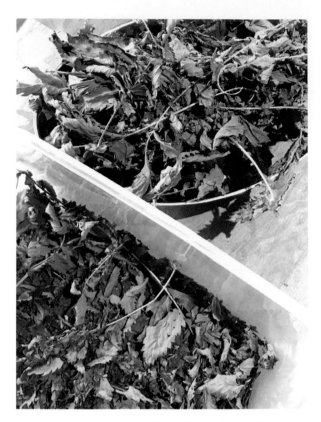

Home-grown and carefully dried Agrimony being weighed for a prescription blend.

Cramp Bark from a large-scale wholesaler, I was shocked to see that it consisted not just of bark but of small bark-covered branches that had been chipped. The bought-in batch looked totally different and was much milder in aroma than my own Cramp Bark. My batch had a very pronounced fragrance; the bought-in batch had the same fragrance, but it was considerably fainter. I cannot tell you how well it worked therapeutically, because I could not bring myself to use it. After much thought, I decided to gather additional Cramp Bark, even though it was the 'wrong' time of the year. It was harder to remove the bark, but after drying I found that the end product still seemed far superior to the bought-in batch. I resolved to harvest a greater volume of Cramp Bark the following spring.

The second example is Agrimony (*Agrimonia eupatoria*). Agrimony is a member of the Rose family with a beautiful subtle lemony fragrance. I never like to admit to having favourite herbs, but what I can say is that Agrimony is one that I know very well and use often. Its lemony scent makes it a delight to work with, and I feel that this aromatic element is an important part of its therapeutic action. Every time I open the storage box containing my own dried Agrimony, I smile because I smell its gorgeous fragrance. I use my Agrimony frequently in teas and prescriptions, and I think it is fair to say that I find it very effective. I have never bought in Agrimony from a wholesaler, but I have handled and inspected Agrimony from different wholesale sources on a number of occasions. Each time the bought-in samples belonging to fellow herbalists had a completely different appearance to my own home-grown stock. Instead of being a bright green colour consisting of whole leaves and flower heads, the bought-in Agrimony was a pale greenish-brown colour, and it had been cut quite finely, so it was not possible to see the individual plant parts. It did not smell lemony, or if it did, the scent was only extremely mild, almost as though I was imagining it because I was searching for it.

In these two examples, differences in the way batches were handled and prepared had a significant impact on their resulting fragrance and appearance. In the case of the Cramp Bark, there was less of the desired plant part in the sample, and other factors that came into play during processing may have reduced its overall potency further. In the case of the Agrimony, the fact that the lemony scent was absent or very faint would indicate that the volatile components had been lost or considerably reduced. This can happen when the drying period is prolonged or has been carried out at too high a temperature. It can also be the result of poor storage, or of exposing too great a surface area of the herb to degradation by cutting it finely before drying. It can also be due to stock being old and past its best. The fact that the colour of the samples I looked at was pale green or brownish could have indicated either poor drying practice or old stock.

I have never gone as far as carrying out laboratory testing, such as thin-layer chromatography, to prove that my home-grown or wild-harvested herbs are superior to bought-in stock. I do not see that as necessary or helpful, especially as it would entail considerable financial cost. Every batch will vary, and the quality of herbs from different suppliers in different years will vary, just as the quality of my own herbs will vary to some extent. In the two examples above my aim is to illustrate the differences that can arise from the way in which herbs are handled. It is my consistent experience that home-grown or wild-harvested herbs that have been dried carefully have a superior appearance and fragrance to those that have been bought in from bulk sources in a finely cut form. I have been using my own herbs in therapeutic practice since 2006, and I have always been delighted by how well they work. I think that it is completely justified to assume that fragrance and appearance are very good indicators of medicinal potency, but if you have doubts, then I would encourage you to try for yourself and form your own conclusions.

In addition to issues of physical quality, I firmly believe that each person who comes into contact with a herb will have an energetic impact on the quality of the medicine. Tibetan medicine teaches that the attitude during harvesting and the preparation of medicines is a very important factor in their eventual effectiveness. A gatherer who is struggling to earn enough to feed his or her family and who feels exploited and underpaid is going to find it hard to infuse the plant material with loving and healing energy when it is picked. Equally, if herbs are handled by stressed or overworked members of staff within a herbal wholesale business, I believe that this could have a negative energetic effect. We, as small-scale self-sufficient producers, can make the picking process into a beautiful, healing, positive experience if we feel so inclined. We can avoid harvesting or processing if we are feeling out of balance or unwell. We can be careful of our state of mind even when just handling our herbs. Once herbs become simply an 'economic product', disconnected from their end use, there is an increased risk that they have been handled by people who are feeling fed up, resentful, or angry.

Personally, I think that the best way to preserve maximum quality in the herbs that we work with is to source them from small batch production sys-

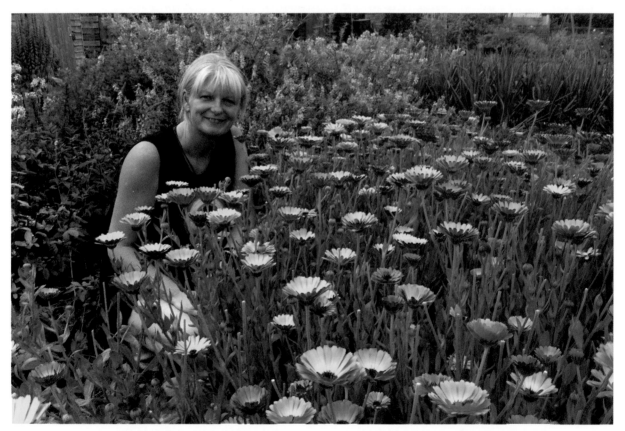

The picking process can be a beautiful, healing, and positive experience when we harvest our own herbs.

tems. This may mean growing or wild harvesting our own, or it may mean herbalists working together in small collaborations to source their own herbs. We may not be able to be self-sufficient in all of the herbs that we need, but we can at least be aware of the potential issues surrounding variability in quality and the factors that influence that. If we need to buy in herbs, we can choose herbal suppliers who take extra care over safeguarding the quality of the herbs they produce or trade.

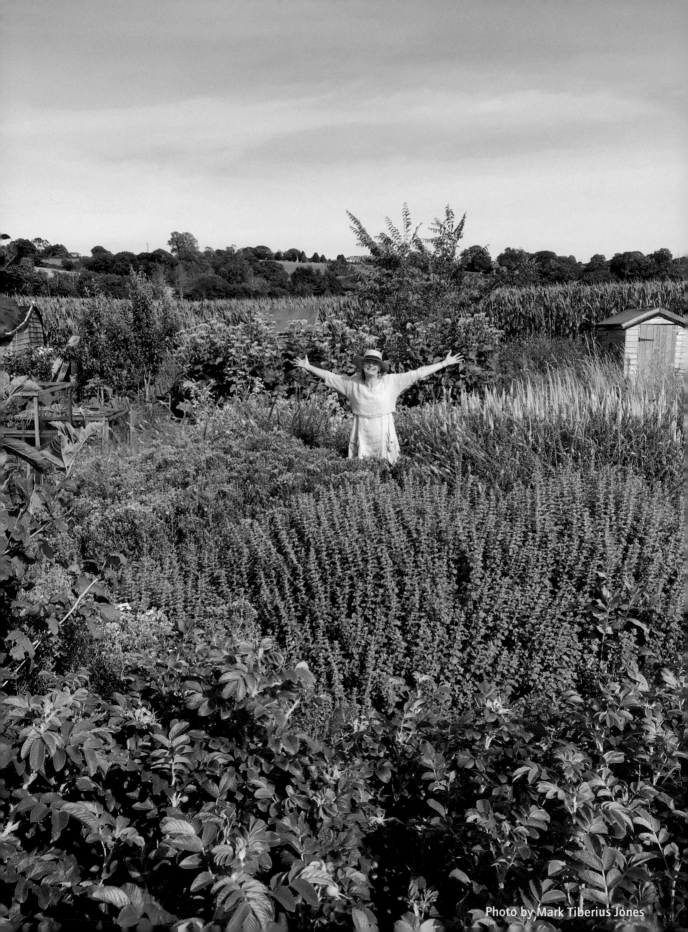

3

Connection with plants

When we grow or gather our own herbs, it is inevitable that we develop a warmth and familiarity towards them. In the case of growing our own, we have to source our plants, perhaps buying in from a nursery, taking cuttings from a friend's garden or growing from seed. We tend them, watch them grow and mature, water them during dry spells and go out anxiously after high winds or hail to see if they have escaped without damage. If we gather herbs from the wild, we have to seek out each species that we need, quartering the area months before the plants are ready to harvest. As we get to know the area in which we live and practice, we build up a mental map of where to find various plant medicines. Hours of pleasurable time exploring green lanes and wild habitats are rewarded by a deep sense of understanding the local landscape and why the plants thrive where they do. Sometimes we set out looking for a particular plant, but it is equally valuable to just wander and explore. Plants call out to us when we need them, if we give them the chance.

We learn to visit different gathering locations throughout the year to see how our plants are doing. Sometimes we can help them by a bit of judicious pruning of overhanging branches or the invasion of brambles into a precious patch of wild St John's Wort (*Hypericum perforatum*), for example. As the harvest season approaches, we will have had to visit our chosen patches several times to make sure that we do not miss the perfect time for harvest. It is only natural that we begin to feel very connected and responsible for the land around us, as well as the plants that grow there.

It can be difficult to find what we need in any given year. Wild medicines have good years and bad years, and sometimes catastrophic events such as harsh hedge trimming or development can destroy a favourite gathering area, along with the plants that grow there. I remember the first time this happened to me. Cramp Bark or Guelder Rose (*Viburnum opulus*) grows in hedgerows and is not considered particularly rare, but it was not common where I lived in West Dorset – at least, not in a form and location where harvesting of usable stems was possible. Over a period of five or six years I had built up a mental map of all the accessible Cramp Bark trees and shrubs that I could find in my local area. I had four especially favoured locations, and each year I rotated small harvests between them. I began to prune some stems from the bottom of bushes in order to encourage long straight stems to grow up, long stems being much easier to strip bark from. This worked very well, and each year I managed to gather sufficient for my needs, until one year a whole section of one of my favourite Cramp-Bark-containing hedges was brutally and severely cut back, using a hedge flail. I actually cried when I saw the devastation. The beautiful wide grass verge alongside the hedge was muddy, rutted, and churned up. Precious Cramp Bark branches were lying all over the verge and the lane, chopped into tiny pieces, irrevocably mixed with random other species, completely unusable and covered in mud. I knew that the plants would recover in time, but I cried because of the missed opportunity for those plants to offer medicine to the people that need them. I cried because it was such a waste, and, most of all, I cried because as a society we have become so very disconnected and ignorant about the value of the wild plants that surround us.

As well as the bitter disappointments over losing a favourite gathering place, we can also experience the euphoria of coming across a sizeable population of a plant that we need just when it is needed. These unexpected finds are always totally thrilling and magical. A few years ago, I stumbled upon a huge population of Wild Oats (*Avena sativa*) at the perfect stage for harvesting in an abandoned arable field scheduled for development. I had been searching my area for a couple of weeks, aware that it was coming up to Wild Oat season, but every time I walked the field edges, green lanes, and footpaths in likely locations, there were no Wild Oats to be seen. All of the usual organic arable fields had been ploughed up or put down to pasture. None of the headlands had been left unsprayed. Land had changed hands, and the new management regime discouraged Wild Oats. As my dispensary stock dwindled and my patients' needs continued to grow, I was beginning to think that I might have to actually buy some in. Salvation came as I was following up a lead from a patient who mentioned a patch of Coltsfoot (*Tussilago farfara*) next to a footpath along which she often walked. I made a note of the directions, and at the first opportunity I set out to follow them. I can still remember the thrill of rounding a corner and seeing a whole field of Wild Oats waving majestically in the breeze. As it happens, I did not find the Coltsfoot until a couple of weeks later, but I was in Wild Oat heaven for a few days while I harvested and dried enough to last my patients for at least the following two years.

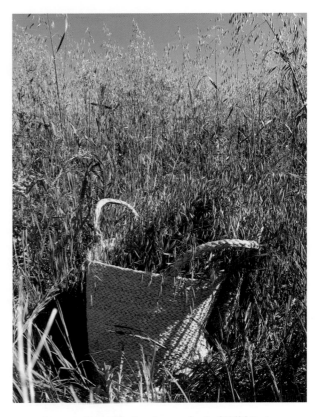

An unexpected but welcome find of Wild Oats.

When we grow or gather our own herbs, we have plenty of time, maybe a whole year or several years, to build a relationship with them. It becomes impossible to view them simply as a business input after that. At first, we may not notice that this shift has happened, but then we start to notice that when we open each herb storage container and smell the distinctive fragrance of each herb, we are instantly transported back to the day that it was harvested. We will probably remember the exact location, the weather and the sounds around us. Perhaps we remember the bird song, the sound of cows grazing or even our own singing. I feel that the memory of the harvest is a reminder of our shared bond. In that moment, it is as though the herb offered itself to be an agent of healing, and we agreed to help make that happen.

I often think that being in the presence of herbal medicines somehow seeps into our psyche and connects us with something ancient – something that is part of our history as human beings if we only open the door to it. I suppose you could call it our collective herbal consciousness. In Tibetan medicine, we

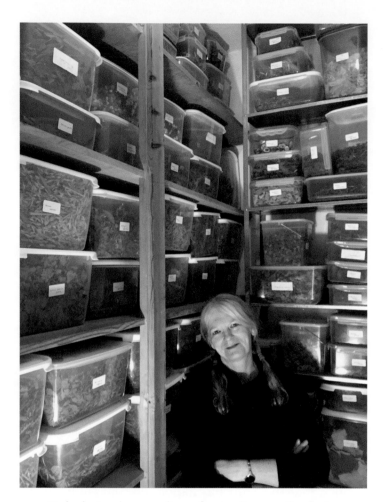

My herb store is a repository of memories as well as herbs.

are encouraged to view herbal medicines as sacred and precious. To take a substance into our bodies with the intention of making us well is a potent act of self-care. The more we value and respect that substance the more potent the act and the greater the potential for healing. If, as practitioners, we have an attitude of respect towards our medicines and if we value them, then this attitude tends to be transmitted to our patients. A medicine that is valued, appreciated, and respected will be much more effective than one that is not. Admittedly, it is totally possible and desirable to generate respect towards herbs that have been bought in or that have been gifted to us by friends. This is definitely an excellent mind set to cultivate. My point here is that, in sourcing our own herbs direct from the land, we inevitably generate this value and respect without any effort. It flows quite naturally, due to the amount of time, care, and intention that goes into the process of growing and gathering.

When I first started in practice as a medical herbalist, I had the attitude that I was 'using' herbs to help people get better. Over time, I gradually realized that I was thinking more along the lines of that I was 'working with' herbs to help people get better. Now I am convinced that I am 'working for' the herbs to help them to fulfil their healing destiny and to get them to the patients who need them. I am sure that I am not the only one who thinks in this way.

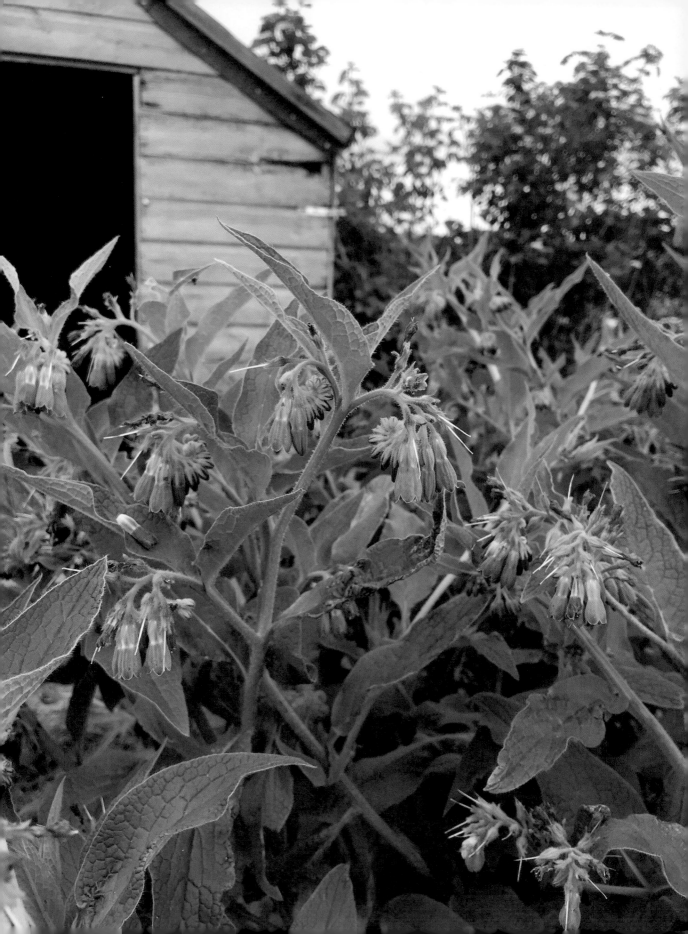

4

Continuity of supply

Three main factors affect the continuity of supply of herbs. The first is the fact that, by their very nature, they are natural, seasonal products. They are ready to be harvested at a certain time, and at this time enough needs to be harvested to last the entire year. The second, less predictable, factor is that the availability of herbs in a given season can be affected by the climate. There may be wet years, dry years, pest outbreaks, or natural disasters. Each of these will affect the abundance and availability of the herbs that we need. The third is that the supply of herbs through wholesale channels can be affected by changes to the regulatory, trading or legislative landscape or simply through supply and demand. If the demand for a particularly herb falls below a certain threshold, it may not make sense for a supplier to stock it.

As people who work with herbs, we have two main ways of dealing with continuity of supply. One way of tackling it is to treat each herb as a seasonal product that is available only at certain times of the year. This attitude is especially suitable for small artisan businesses producing high-value handmade herbal products. Seasonality can be woven into the story of the business and can become an asset. Limited availability of the products adds a sense of exclusivity, preciousness, and connection with the seasons. Customers understand the need to purchase when things are available, and they do not take year-round availability for granted. However, the 'when it's gone it's gone' model is not suitable for therapeutic herbal practices: continuity of supply represents continuity of treatment. Patients doing well on a particular prescription are likely to be disappointed if they are told that no more is available until the herb is ready for harvest the following year. In a therapeutic setting, continuity of supply is very desirable, if not essential.

In harvesting herbs, then, the aim is to store or process sufficient quantity to last the year ahead. Whether you are a family carer, a medical herbalist harvesting for your own needs or a herbal wholesaler sourcing herbs from all over the world, you have to make an informed guess as to how much of each plant you will actually need. A wholesaler will be guided by supply, demand, price, previous sales of particular species, as well as by other factors, such as profit margins, storage space, and keeping quality. Medical herbalists will be guided by the number of patients they expect to see in the course of the year, the frequency of certain presentations and their own prescribing patterns. Someone treating their family with herbs will also need to think about common health situations they are likely to encounter over the year ahead. In all situations, working out quantities that will be needed is most definitely an art, but over the years it is possible to get a pretty good feel for what will be needed. A self-sufficient herbalist has to make a judgement about whether it is feasible to grow or gather all or part of their requirements for each herb. It does not have to be an all-or-nothing scenario. Self-sufficiency is as much an attitude and a goal as it is a definitive statement of sourcing policy.

In practice, the quantity of each herb harvested is guided by the abundance in field and hedgerow. In 'good' years it makes sense to harvest extra stock, to act as a buffer for leaner years. I have concluded that being self-sufficient in herbs for a medical practice is a dance within the ebb and flow of the seasons. It is helpful to cultivate an acceptance that herbs present themselves more abundantly in certain years for a reason. I have lost count of the number of times that I have waited anxiously for a herb to be ready for harvest as stocks in my dispensary dwindled. Just when I think that I will have to buy in more stock of that particular herb, I spot the first signs that it is nearly ready to harvest. I rush out to my usual gathering spots and harvest just enough of the early flowers or leaves to keep me going until the main harvest can be taken. There is nothing quite like the satisfaction of bringing in a herb just in time for a patient who needs it.

It is not always possible to get quantities right, but there is a great deal of scope among our herbal community to help each other out. We live in different areas with different climatic factors and habitats. What is abundant in one person's area may be scarce in another's. We can swap herbs or purchase each other's surplus stock. We also have the option to research and buy in high-quality, ethically sourced herbs from wholesalers when needed.

We cannot always rely on being able to source all that we need through wholesale suppliers, however. When I was first studying Western herbal medicine, my tutors often spoke of potential threats to availability of herbs due to regulatory changes and political policies. One of my main herbal tutors and inspiration for my self-sufficient practice, Barbara Howe, would often say that if 'They' try to take away our herbs, we need to be able to defy 'Them' and grow them ourselves. I remember being surprised the first time I heard her talking in this way. It seemed at odds with the image I had of her as a gentle, wise herbal elder. Images can be misleading, though, and Barbara most definitely had a fire in her belly when it came to protecting herbal medicine and the herbs that she had worked with for years. She was quite right to pass on her concerns to her students. During my time in practice I have seen just how fragile the supply chain for herbs is, and how wider political agendas can have a swift and devastating influence their availability.

At the time that I was studying Western herbal medicine, the implications of pyrrolizidine alkaloids in Comfrey and the risk of it causing veno-occlusive liver disease were first being discussed within the herbal profession. The issue was the subject of many very heated debates among students as well as among our tutors and the different professional associations. Older, more established herbalists seemed more likely to be outraged by what they saw as ill-informed meddling in the traditional practice of herbal medicine, while many newly qualified or student herbalists felt pressure to abide by new guidelines in order to safeguard their future ability to practise. Professional herbal associations differed in their approaches, some preferring to have an ongoing relationship with the regulatory bodies in order to maintain an influence and others feeling it was much better to stay outside any regulation and to fight the process. At the time, these issues became enormously divisive in the field of herbal medicine in the United Kingdom – understandable among a group of people all of whom share a deep passion for herbal medicine and patient care. Discussions about herbs containing pyrrolizidine alkaloids were made more complicated by the enormous variability in the structure of these compounds, a lack of definitive knowledge about their action on the body and differing ideas about how they are broken down. It remains a very complicated issue to this day, and more research is being carried out to increase our understanding of these biological pathways and their implications. The spotlight is now also falling on other constituents, such as arbutin, which is present in Bearberry (*Arctostaphylos uva-ursi*) and Damiana (*Turnera diffusa*), among others. Arbutin is a glycoside of hydroquinone, and some sources claim that there is a theoretical possibility that it could hydrolyse into free hydroquinone. As hydroquinone is restricted in terms of how it can be used and prescribed, some countries have taken the step of also restricting arbutin-containing herbs.

Herbs that trigger safety concerns due to potentially toxic (or psychotropic) ingredients – whether or not we feel that these concerns are justified – will inevitably become less available through wholesale channels. In fact, in the United Kingdom, the Medicines Health Care Regulatory Agency actively counsels against wholesalers stocking herbs that are under review or subject to a voluntary ban on their use. Even if the restrictions are billed as a precautionary measure while further research is carried out, there is a real risk that we will lose knowledge of how to source and work with that herb if it is removed from circulation and herbal teaching syllabuses. A period of 10–15 years when a herb is out of regular use is probably enough to significantly change the prescribing habits and knowledge of an entire generation of herbal practitioners.

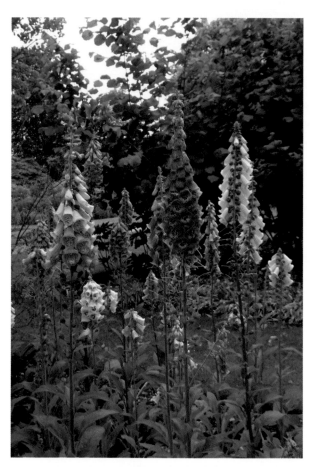

Foxglove (*Digitalis purpurea*)

Growing restricted herbs, even if we choose not to prescribe them, is a way of preserving them and staying connected to the tradition and knowledge of our ancient art. I grow several species of plants that I cannot use legally as internally prescribed medicines in my practice. These include Mandrake (*Mandragora*), May Apple (*Podophyllum*), Monkshood (*Aconitum*) and Foxglove (*Digitalis*). I have no intention of using them internally on my patients, but I continue to grow them and others out of a desire to learn about and connect with the plants themselves and to preserve traditional knowledge.

The regulatory and advisory picture varies between different countries and as new research becomes available. Please check the situation in the country where you are practising. This may influence your choice of what you will grow in your herb garden.

As well as regulatory restrictions influencing the catalogues of herbal wholesalers, general demand does too. Wholesalers need to choose herbs that are sufficiently in demand so that they can be sold before they go out of date. This means that it does not make sense for wholesalers to stock lesser-used herbs and herbs that are out of fashion. These herbs then become difficult or impossible to find commercially. Take, for example, herbs like Culver's Root (*Veronicastrum virginicum*) which is also known as Black Root. This is a herb that is bitter and is excellent for clearing viscid mucus from the gut. It enlivens a tired digestive system and helps to encourage a more regular bowel habit when this has become

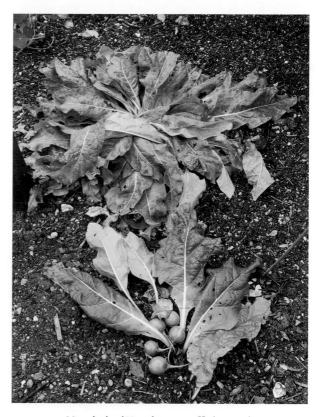

Mandrake (*Mandragora officinarum*)

sluggish. It is a herb that was much used in the era of my dear tutor and mentor, Edith Barlow. I started to grow it because she encouraged me to work with Culver's Root. I wanted to see what the plant looked like and get to know it. At the time, I did not investigate whether or not it was available through wholesalers – perhaps it was available at that time, but it certainly is not widely available now. It seems to have become a herb rarely used by herbal practitioners. I suppose it has fallen out of favour or has somehow been forgotten. Luckily, I have been growing and using Culver's Root for many years, and I am able to continue treating my patients with it.

Another herb that is difficult to source commercially, at least in the United Kingdom, is Poplar (*Populus tremuloides*) bark. In the twentieth century *Populus tremuloides* was widely used as a tonic in traditional herbal medicine. Edith Barlow taught me the value of this herb thanks to her own chain of teaching on this, which is at least 250 years old. I am someone who unashamedly loves lineage, and this appeals to me greatly. It feels an enormous privilege

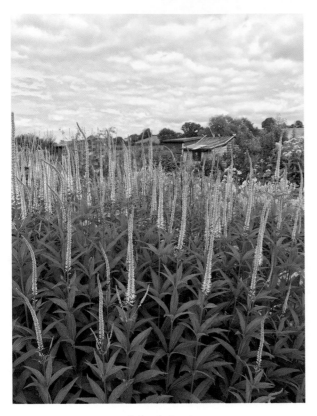

Culver's Root

to have been taught this traditional way of using Poplar bark and to be able to use it in my own practice. However, it seems that these days *Populus tremuloides* seems to be rarely stocked by herbal suppliers, and the only way that I can reliably continue to use this herbal medicine is to wildcraft it myself.

It is understandable that wholesale suppliers have to maintain a catalogue that allows them to stay economically viable, but as a practitioner I think it is sad that our prescribing practices can be moulded by market forces rather than therapeutic efficacy and tradition. By growing or gathering our own herbs, we have the option of preserving traditional ways of prescribing and maintaining access to certain less used species.

The supply of herbs can also be interrupted in unpredictable ways by market forces and climatic quirks. Even seemingly very common herbs, such as Calendula (*Calendula officinalis*) flowers, can be affected. I remember the world shortage of Calendula flowers in the summer of 2015. This was apparently due to a crop failure, but at the time I was completely unaware of the shortage, as I had been lucky enough to have a bumper crop on my allotment. With my attitude of gathering and storing extra when supplies are abundant, I had gathered and stored plenty. In 2017, inexplicably, it was Caraway (*Carum carvi*) seed that was very scarce. I never found out why. As this is a herb that I have to buy in and use regularly, I was very concerned about this. In the end, I only managed to maintain medicinal supplies for my patients by buying in Caraway in small retail packs. I suppose culinary suppliers must have had bigger stock piles.

Even when herbs are available in theory, shipments can be delayed and can be held back in suppliers' warehouses while quality control checks are carried out. If a shipment is rejected, there will be long delays while replacement supplies are ordered. If there are delays in availability of a particular herb, then as practitioners we must spend many hours contacting various suppliers to try to find supplies. If we are unsuccessful in this endeavour, continuity of patient treatment can be affected. We can, of course, use our skill and training to substitute other herbs with similar actions if necessary, but I think that it is always preferable to have access to the original herb that we felt drawn to prescribe.

I am completely in awe of the work that is put in by herbal wholesalers to maintain continuity of supply for their customers, but to rely purely on buying in herbs may leave us more vulnerable to shortages. This is especially worrying as we may only discover wider shortages once it is too late to rectify them. To grow or gather our own herbs allows us to choose which ones we want to work with and to strive to make sure that we have enough of them.

In summary then, growing and gathering our own herbs enables us to anticipate what we will require for the year ahead and grow or gather sufficient for our needs. This allows us to be shielded from sudden changes in the availability of wholesale herbs due to regulatory changes, differing crop yields or prescribing fashions. We can maintain populations of herbs that have fallen out of common use so that in the future we still have the option to bring them back into the fold if circumstances demand or allow it.

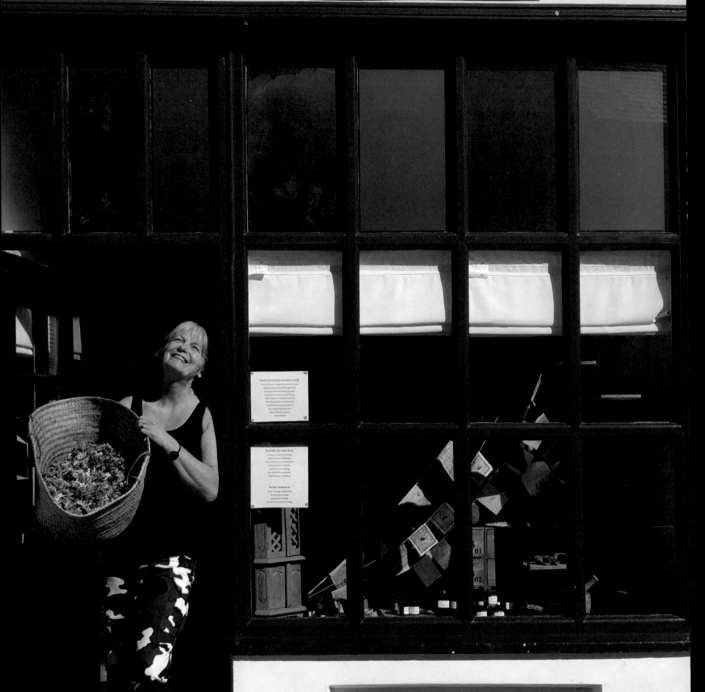

5

Favourable business model

I **have deliberately chosen** to talk about business and financial aspects last in this 'why' section of the book. I want to emphasize that I believe that the reasons for choosing a self-sufficient model of practice are much larger and much more important than purely financial ones.

I am glad to say that no one I have ever met has gone into herbal medicine with the primary motivation of making money. In my view, herbal medicine is a spiritual path on which the focus of our motivation is to help others achieve better health. If our motivation is only to generate wealth, then, I feel, this is a very unhealthy basis for therapeutic practice. I do believe, though, that economic viability is a perfectly valid secondary consideration on the basis that we have to survive and thrive in order to be in a position to help our patients effectively.

We are all in different positions as regards our need for financial suste-nance. Some people may be able to leave the question of economic viability completely out of the equation, in which case I rejoice in their ability to devote themselves to the healing arts without the constraints of financial issues. However, for most of us it is essential that our herbal practice sus-tains itself and sustains us, whether that is in a full-time or a part-time capacity. Herbal practitioners who struggle to keep a roof over their fam-ily's heads, or food on the table, are unlikely to stay herbal practitioners for long. It always saddens me when I hear about herbalists who decide that they are unable to continue in practice because they cannot support them-selves financially. I know how difficult a decision that must have been and how much they must have tried to manage on very limited income before finally giving up.

With that explanatory preamble and non-acquisitive context, let me explain that there are actually sound business reasons for choosing to establish a self-sufficient practice. To build up a dispensary based on home-grown and gathered herbs reduces the requirement for working capital, helps us to maintain stock levels, helps to ensure continuity of supply and reduces costs. Frankly, it may also give our business additional appeal in a world where more and more people wish to source locally, whether that be food or medicines. Remember, the more patients that seek our help, the more people we and our herbs can help. If we find that too many people come to us, we can refer them to fellow practitioners. Either way, we are spreading the healing wonder of herbal medicine.

First, let us look at the issue of working capital requirements. Whether we make handmade herbal products or whether we treat patients, we need to hold some stock of herbs. If we buy these in, we will have to fund that outlay until we get a return on that investment. When I first qualified, like most herbal practitioners, I realized that to build up a good dispensary with many different herbs and tinctures would involve a very significant financial cost, more than I could afford at the time. However, if I could gather and make some of my own medicines, I could substitute labour for capital and build up a wider dispensary within the budget I had available. In the early stages of being in herbal practice we have, in theory, more time available to source our own medicines. I say, 'in theory', because in my case I was actually working two other part-time jobs in order to make ends meet. It is true that there is a cost, known as opportunity cost, to the time that we spend gathering and processing herbs, because we could be using that time to do other things. However, if we love herbs, the time we spend working with them can be viewed as rest, recuperation, and inspiration for the future of our practice.

In comparison to gathering our own herbs, it is relatively costly to buy in herbs from a wholesaler. Part of the cost goes towards their profit, which is fair enough, and we also have to pay for shipping. Often, we need to pay multiple lots of shipping charges, because as companies reduce the volume of stock that they hold and reduce their product lines, it is rare these days to be able to source all that we require from one supplier. We may also be liable for pur-

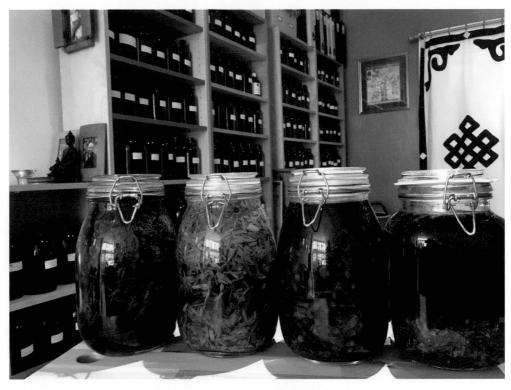

If we love herbs, the time we spend working with them can be viewed as rest, recuperation, and inspiration for the future of our practice.

chase tax, depending where we are in the world. Here in the United Kingdom, herbs are subject to Value Added Tax (VAT). If business turnover exceeds the designated threshold for registration, it becomes mandatory to charge VAT on the products and services that we supply. The threshold changes regularly, so if you are not sure of the current figure, check on the Her Majesty's Revenue and Customs (HMRC) website. If your turnover is below the designated threshold, you can still voluntarily register your herbal business for VAT, enabling you to claim back the VAT that you have paid on inputs such as herbs. This may make sense if you are a manufacturing business buying in a lot of herbs and packaging, especially if you can readily increase product prices without affecting your sales volume. If your main focus is on providing consultations, then you should be aware that if you register for VAT, you will need to start to charge VAT on your consultations, and you will have to pay

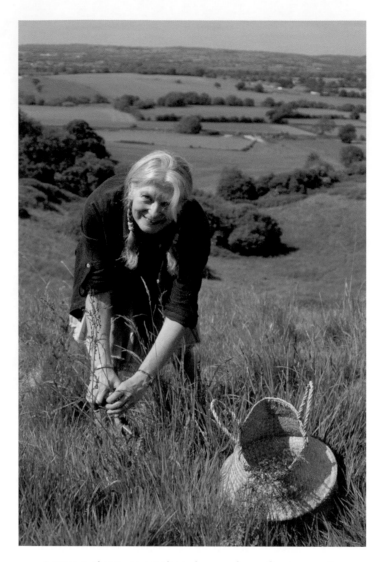

I am sure that I am not the only one who prefers to spend time harvesting and gathering herbs in preference to ordering, packing, and posting prescriptions.

this amount to HMRC. This means that it will be necessary to increase your consultation charges immediately by the amount of VAT that you will need to pay in order to maintain the level of gross income from consultations that you had prior to registering. This may not be a problem in some areas where there is a higher 'willingness to pay', but if you like to make your services as accessible as possible and you are based in an area where the average income is low, you may wish to think twice about this.

If creating a dispensary from scratch is prohibitively expensive, there is a perfectly valid school of thought that opts to hold only minimal stock and then order new supplies from wholesalers as needed, once each patient consultation has been carried out. However, a just-in-time stock control system does entail much more time spent ordering, packing, and posting, not to mention increased delivery costs (and the associated environmental impact) from the wholesaler. I am sure that I am not the only one who prefers to spend time harvesting and gathering herbs in preference to ordering, packing, and posting prescriptions.

We should also consider what our potential customers want. More and more people are excited by the idea of low food (or medicine) miles and like to feel that their herbal medicine has been grown or wildcrafted in the area local to where they are being treated. Most of my herbal medicines have been sourced within two miles of my clinic, and many of my patients mention this as something that first attracted them to my practice. By sourcing some or all of our own herbs, we may well be increasing our appeal to potential customers, and as a result of this we can bring herbal medicine to more people who need it.

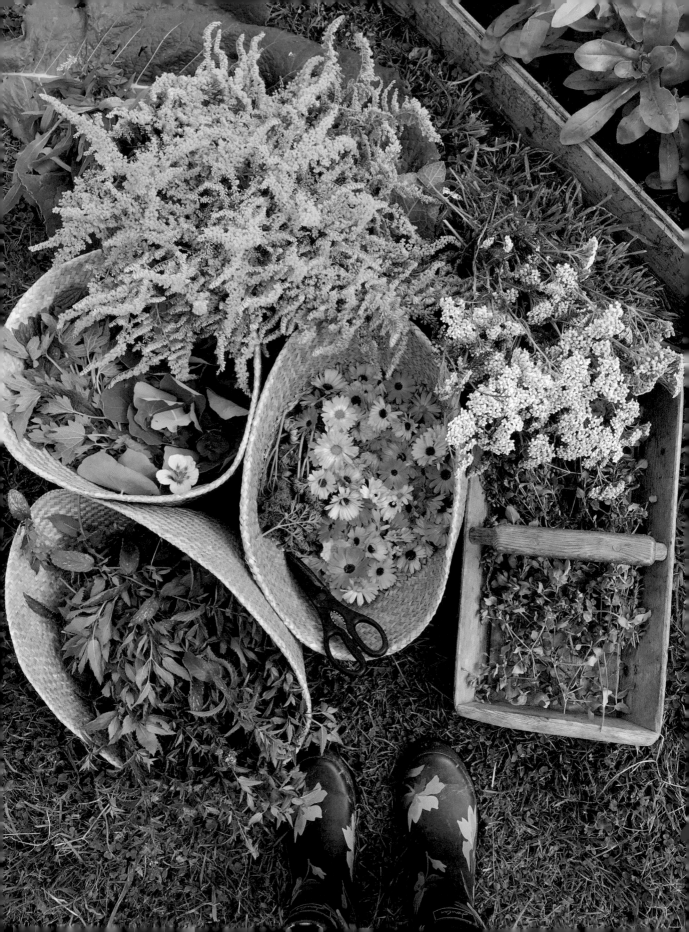

PART TWO

HOW TO BE SELF-SUFFICIENT

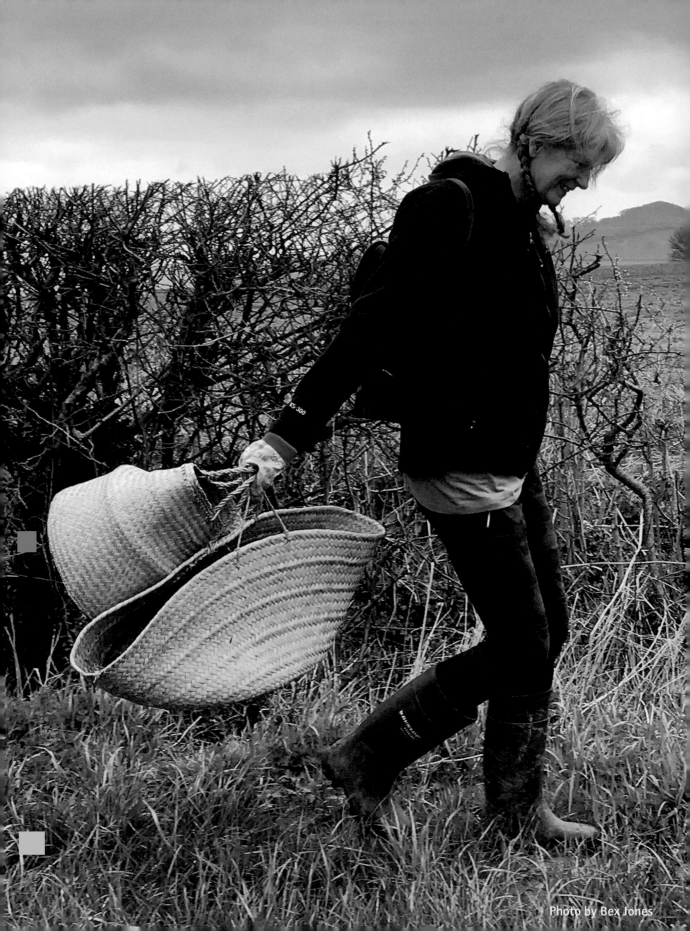

6

Wildcrafting

Gathering medicinal herbs is a wonderful, magical activity. It is glorious to wander through wild places with an open heart and an empty basket, waiting to see which herbs will announce themselves. Our ancestors gathered wild foods and medicines. Gathering is in our bones.

When I lead foraging courses, I see the strength of our pull to gather herbs. Sometimes during our shared day of exploration and learning we pause in a meadow, and I set the group the task of gathering a particular herb, such as Red Clover (*Trifolium pratense*) flowers or Plantain (*Plantago* spp.) leaves. For many people, this may be the first time that they have actually settled into gathering any quantity of a particular herb. They tell me afterwards that when they first came to the gathering location, they could see that there were a few of the plants that we were intending to gather, but there did not seem to be many of them. Once they started to gather, they looked around the area, and they realized that the plants were becoming much more visible and prominent. Suddenly what looked as though it would be 'slim pickings' became an abundant natural medicine chest. You could describe this as 'getting your eye in', or you could say that the herbs 'call to you'. It does not really matter what terms you use. The point is that as human beings we learn foraging quickly. We have an aptitude for it. It is also interesting to note that foraging course attendees often embark on the gathering task with sociable enthusiasm, enjoying the opportunity to get to know their fellow course attendees. Over time, though, they seem to drift apart, each finding their own little

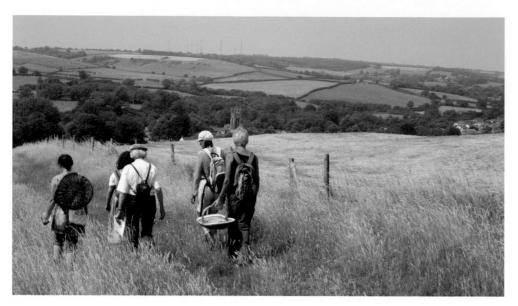

As human beings we learn foraging quickly. We have an aptitude for it.

'territory' for gathering and relaxing into a quiet, reflective rhythm. When the time comes for the group to move on, I notice that people find it hard to tear themselves away, feeling a deep urge to bend down to just pick one or two more flowers or leaves. I feel this too, whenever I am gathering. There is such a strong pull to pick just one more handful or just another couple of stems. I catch myself thinking that just one more handful would be enough for another patient's daily medicine.

Gathering is deeply ingrained within us, and it is a beautiful thing to connect with, but things have changed since we were hunter-gatherers. As modern human beings, many of us have grown up with cultural messages of entitlement over the natural world, as opposed to those of a deep respect and connection to it. We retain a strong attraction to the process of wild harvesting, but we may have lost the knowledge, confidence or opportunity to make good use of the herbs once we have gathered them. Herbs deserve to be valued and respected. If we gather them and then waste them, we are behaving disrespectfully. To avoid waste, we should at least have an outline plan for how we plan to use the herbs that we harvest. Perhaps we intend to make a tincture or an infused oil. Perhaps we wish to dry some of the leaves so that we can use them for infusions throughout the year ahead. By having a plan, we can review the quantity that we would like to harvest. We can aim to harvest just what we need and avoid the wastage caused by harvesting too much. If we do not have a plan, we may need to do a little research and come up with one. We can always return another day to harvest.

It is also really important to be aware of our wider intentions when we are foraging. By 'wider intentions' I mean our motivation. Is our motivation to share the healing properties of the herbs we are gathering for the benefit of those who need them, or is it to exploit a 'free resource' with the primary intention of making money? In the Vajrayana Tibetan Buddhist tradition, it is emphasized that having a positive and selfless intention is considered to make any act sacred and potent. Before we gather any wild herb, then, it is very positive to ask ourselves whether we have a broader aim, which makes use of the special qualities offered to us by the herbs that we are gathering. We all have our own relationship with herbs and our own reasons for gathering. It is not for me to say which intention is 'right' and which is 'wrong', but I think we should all check in with ourselves and reaffirm our intentions each time before gathering a herb. That way we will develop a habit of mindfulness about our intentions, and we will be able to say, hand on heart, that we have made peace with them.

Once we feel comfortable with our intention for gathering, we need to bring to mind a sense of gratitude and respect towards the plants we wish to wild-harvest. A good way of achieving this is to always ask their permission before starting to gather them. There are lots of different ways of doing this. You could pause, sit for a while, and inwardly explain how you intend to make use of their precious healing qualities, asking whether they would be prepared to give up some of themselves in order for you to do that. You could make a symbolic offering, such as of Tobacco or tea, to show respect and to demonstrate that you understand our interconnectedness. You could say a prayer, recite mantras, or visualize a healing archetype such as the Medicine Buddha. Each one of us will be drawn to our own way of asking permission and sensing the answer. If you are not sure about the answer, just

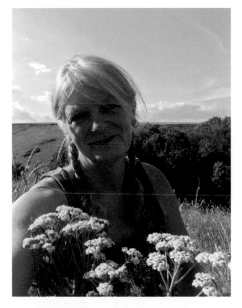

Once we feel comfortable with our intention for gathering, we need to bring to mind a sense of gratitude and respect towards the plants we wish to wild-harvest.

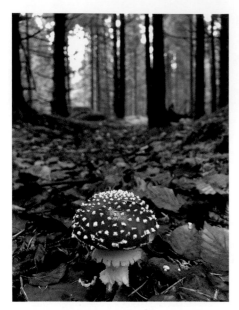

Fly agaric (*Amanita muscaria*)

relax, be still, and listen. At first you may find that you feel self-conscious and do not fully trust what you are feeling, but as your connection and confidence grows, you will learn to trust your perceptions.

Plants do not always give permission. You will know very clearly when you have been refused. It just feels plain wrong. On the other side of the coin, sometimes it can feel as though particular plants summon us, repeatedly appearing in our dreams or thoughts until we find them. This happens most often when a herb that we gather regularly is at the right stage to harvest and we know exactly where it is on our foraging patch. In cases like this we may explain away the experience by telling ourselves it is a sub-conscious tracking of the seasons, rather than a process of communication between plant and human. Sometimes it feels much more profound than that, though.

Take my recent experience with attempting to gather Fly Agaric (*Amanita muscaria*). I had not so far harvested this mushroom but had formed the intention to work with it after reading herbalist Henriette Kress's account of using it to ease the pain of sciatica. I had been keeping an eye out in the locality for a couple years but so far had not seen any growing. When autumn came around again, I started to think about my plan to harvest some. I visited some potentially suitable woodlands, finding plenty of Turkey Tail (*Trametes versicolor*) and other beautiful fungi, but not a single Fly Agaric. After a few more unsuccessful expeditions, I woke up one Sunday morning with a strong feeling that I should go to a particular woodland to search. This woodland was further afield than my normal foraging range, but I had an insistent feeling about it, and there was no way that I was going to ignore it. I was sure that this was going to be the day that I would actually find Fly Agaric. To get to the woodland, I had to drive for about an hour. When I arrived, I half expected to find some almost immediately, but I did not. There was no one else around, and I walked around for an hour or so, looking for glimpses of the iconic red caps under the trees, but there were none in sight. I was disappointed and decided that I had been completely deluded to believe that I had in some way been summoned to this place. My 'strong feeling' must have been my over-active imagination. I was just about to give up when I paused and checked in with myself. I realized that my intense desire to find the mushroom had made me forget my usual foraging attitude. I had arrived full of expectation. I needed to slow down and bring to mind my positive intentions about how I wanted to work with this medicine. I sat down by a tree and surveyed my surroundings. The dampness of the moss began to seep through my jeans, but it felt good to be there, totally alone and away from the time scales and schedules of modern human life. I began to see everything around me from a different perspective. I could see just how much all life in this woodland was deeply interconnected. Sitting there, I felt as though I was part of it rather than just an observer of it. I got up and started walking into a stand of mature conifers. There was no beaten track, and I had to twist this way and that through the trees. I had no idea where I was going, but I carried on walking. It was totally silent, the only sound being the snap of a twig when I stepped on one, something that I tried to avoid after the first time it happened. Despite my feeling of connectedness, this place felt more than a little eerie. I remember a thought popping into my head that I could be lost in these woods for days, but I immediately dismissed it. It is impossible to be lost in a wood for days in Southern England. I walked on. Suddenly I crested a small rise, and ahead of me under the trees in the soft, green stillness was a large colony of shining red-and-white-spotted Fly Agaric mushrooms. They exuded magic and mystery and intense power. It took my

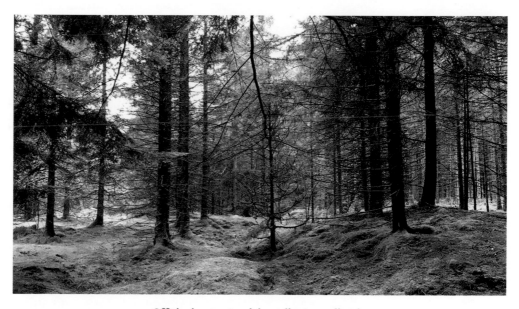

Off the beaten track in a silent woodland.

breath away to see them like that. These mushroom beings were definitely not to be trifled with or taken advantage of. Was it my imagination, or was the stillness more intense in this area? It felt as though I had wandered into another dimension. Oblivious of the damp, I sat down on the ground to take it all in. After some time, I sensed that the mushroom colony was prepared to allow me to harvest a few of their number. I carefully placed a few in my basket, thanked them profusely for the lesson and their medicine, and then set off to find my way out of the woodland.

In order to make the most of any precious plant medicines that we gather from the wild, we need to harvest them with care. You could say that harvesting herbs is a simple and natural activity and there is no need to over-complicate it; however, there are some useful techniques that are worth considering in order to make the process easier and to ensure that the quality of the plant material is preserved. The practicalities of harvesting different types of herbs are covered in chapter 9, 'Harvesting'; notes on harvesting specific herbs are given in the third section, 'The Herbal Harvesting Year'.

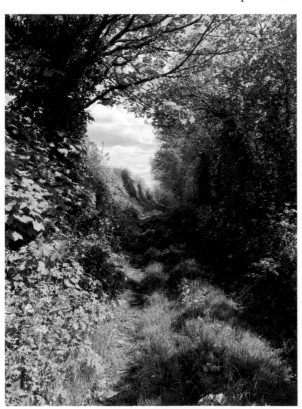

A green lane in my foraging territory.

Let us go through the guidelines for good practice in wildcrafting. These guidelines are important because they ensure that we are wildcrafting without causing harm to the environment and to the plant populations that we seek to work with. They also ensure that the plants that we gather will be of good quality, be safe to use as medicines and will not be wasted. As herbal practitioners, we also need to ensure that our actions will not cause conflict or disharmony with other people who connect with the land from which we are gathering.

Here in the United Kingdom the Wildlife and Countryside Act (1981) protects wild plants. The Act states that it is illegal to dig up or remove a plant (including algae, lichens, and fungi) from the land on which it is growing without the permission of the land owner. Small-scale responsible foraging of above-ground parts can be done along public rights of way or on land where there is free public access.

We should never collect plants that are endangered or at-risk. It is our responsibility to make sure we know which species these are if we plan to forage for medicinal plants. Wherever we live in the world, we should get hold of a good field guide and do some research on the rare or protected plants that we may come across. In the United Kingdom, Schedule 8 of the Wildlife and Countryside Act (1981) lists the species that are protected by law. It is also worth noting that the Botanical Society of Britain and Ireland (BSBI) maintains an up-to-date GB Red List showing all plants that are scarce or protected. This is really useful, because not all rare plants are protected by law, but they may be so scarce that they should not be gathered.

As well as individual species being protected, some land areas are protected under

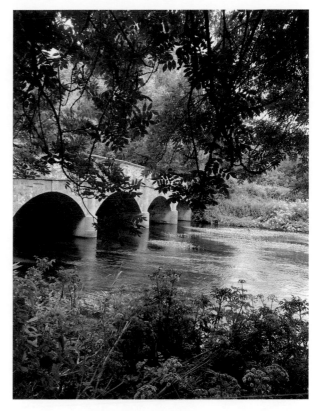

A Wiltshire river.

statutory designations. Here in the United Kingdom we have various levels of protection, including 'Sites of Special Scientific Interest', 'National Nature Reserves' and 'Local Nature Reserves', for example. On land with a conservation designation, it is not permitted to pick any plant at all.

A good guideline to remember is that if you are out walking and you come across a plant that looks unusual and is not growing in abundance, then do not pick it under any circumstances, not even to identify it later at home. It is much more responsible to carefully photograph it, including a reference scale in the shot, or to sketch it. Get into the habit of carrying a botanical hand lens with you and examine the intricate details of plants that you find. Make some notes about its features, including the arrangement of its leaves on the stems, their shape, whether they are hairy or not, the shape of the stem, any scent and the appearance of the flowers or seed heads, if they are present. These less damaging recording methods should help you to identify it later on. I should also add that if you are photographing the unusual plant, take great care not to expose it by removing surrounding vegetation in order to get a better shot. This may make it more vulnerable to grazing or wind damage.

Even when gathering species that we know are common, it is important to gather only from plant populations that are abundant, and we should never collect more than 5% of the plants that are present. We should choose plants that are in the middle of the size range for a particular population, leaving the largest and smallest members of the community. Leaving the strongest plants to reproduce ensures that we are allowing the best plants to be perpetuated and leaving the smallest ones allows the younger plants to grow and mature.

Safety and quality issues also shape foraging guidelines. It makes sense to avoid gathering plants from heavily polluted areas such as former industrial sites. If you see plants with stunted growth or affected by die-back, do a bit of research about the land-use history of the area concerned. If your foraging territory includes popular dog-walking areas, you will also need to take care. Eggs from the round-worm parasite (*Toxicara*) can survive in the soil for many months, long after the dog faeces itself has been washed away or removed.

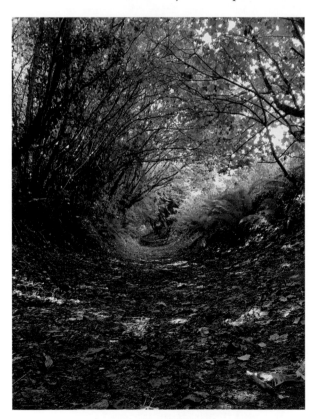

A sunken lane in Somerset.

If you are gathering from stream- or lake-sides, be aware of the water quality. If the water looks stagnant, polluted or affected by algal bloom, be suspicious about what lies upstream from where you are. For example, if you are gathering downstream from intensive livestock-rearing holdings, you could be gathering plants affected by the effluent and the chemical agricultural inputs that may have been used on the animals. Plants growing in rural hedgerows or field margins in intensively managed arable areas may have been subjected to applications of herbicides or pesticides. Orchards are especially likely to have been heavily treated with pesticides, unless they are under organic management. While cemeteries and graveyards can be really good for learning about plant identification, they are not a suitable place from which to gather medicines. The soil, and therefore the plants, in graveyards is more likely to be contaminated by toxic substances, including lead and arsenic. I also believe that these locations are unsuitable energetically.

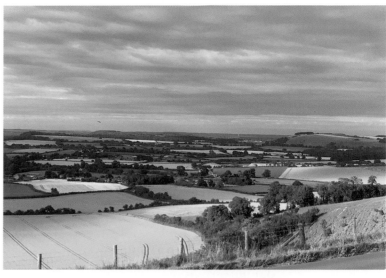

The view across the North Dorset downs.

In general, I stick to gathering from along very quiet rural lanes, bridle paths or drove roads, riversides, woodlands or from agricultural areas that I know to be under organic management. I recommend that you get really familiar with your local area. Walk the footpaths and green lanes regularly. Learn what species are present, and observe how the land is managed. Get to know your local organic land-owners, if you can. You may find that they may be very supportive of you foraging medicinal plants from their land, especially if you share the fruit of your labours with them. Aim to build up a mental map of your foraging territory. Make friends with the plants that are growing there. Watch them through their whole life cycle, and see how the population ebbs and flows in different years. If you live in an urban area, walk through and get to know your local green spaces and parks. Do not feel constrained from gathering medicines because you live in a city. The quality of plants gathered from green spaces in cities can be excellent, provided that they are not growing near a very busy road or in an area that is treated with chemicals. You can always supplement your foraging activities by making regular trips to one or two rural areas that you 'adopt' and really get to know. Your foraging territory does not have to be where you actually live.

Regardless of where you choose to forage, try not to encourage too much foraging pressure in one place. I sometimes see people suggesting that sharing exact locations of certain plant populations on apps or social media groups would be a good idea. I find this a bit worrying, because it could draw unsustainable numbers of foragers to particular places, especially if there are scarcer plants growing there. Ideally, each of us will naturally find our own preferred foraging sites, fully understanding that these sites will never be exclusive to us and that others have every right to forage there too. As we get to know our foraging locations, we each build a strong connection with the plants that grow there, and a sense of respect and responsibility naturally arises. This connection cannot be built up if we forage here and there based on map pins posted on social media.

It is crucial to always make sure that you positively identify the plant or plants that you are gathering. It is a terrible waste to gather a basket of plants only to return home to your identification guide and discover that what you gathered is not what you thought it was. Misidentification is also potentially dangerous. Some medicinal plants have leaves that are rather similar to species that are toxic. Young Foxglove (*Digitalis purpurea*) leaves, which are toxic, can easily be confused with young Comfrey (*Symphytum officinale*) leaves, for example. One distinction is that Comfrey has a smooth outline to its leaves, whereas Foxglove leaves are slightly serrated. Get to know these differences. Another potential risk is that it is possible to confuse the toxic leaves of Lily-of-the-Valley (*Convallaria majalis*) or Lords and Ladies (*Arum maculatum*) with those of Wild Garlic (*Allium ursinum*). The best way to distinguish between

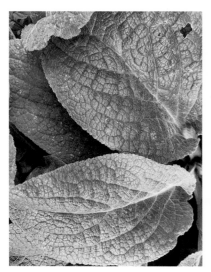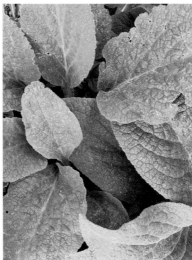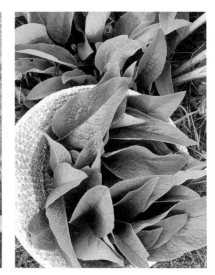

Toxic Foxglove (*Digitalis purpurea*) leaves, left and centre; Comfrey (*Symphytum officinalis*) leaves, right.

these look-alikes is through using the sense of smell. Never check the identification of a plant species by nibbling it. Wild Garlic leaves smell unmistakable. You can also look closely at the leaves and see that they are, in fact, quite different. Wild Garlic leaves arise from the base of the plant, whereas Lily-of-the-Valley bears two or three leaves on the same stem. Lords and Ladies leaves are a different shape, having downward-pointing lobes on either side of the leaf stalk. You may know these differences very well, but it is still easy to inadvertently include some of the wrong species in your basket if you are not mindful while picking.

In both of these examples the potential difficulty arises because at first glance the leaves look alike and the species grow in similar habitats. While the plants are easily distinguished when flowering, there is scope for confusion before they flower. One way around this is to get to know your foraging area throughout the year, so that you have a chance to mentally

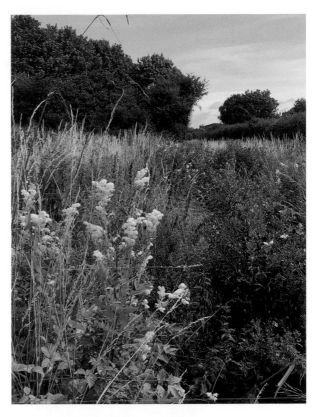

Meadowsweet growing along a small river bank.

map the location of medicinal species at a time when they are easily identified. If, for example, you come across a large flowering Comfrey plant, you can make a mental note not only of where it is but also whether there are Foxgloves growing nearby. If there are, you may need to take extra care at the time of gathering, or you may prefer to find a plant or plants that are growing in a less potentially contentious location, until you are more confident of your plant identification.

It is also important to be able to identify plants in the vicinity of the plants that you wish to gather and to take care appropriately. If you are gathering medicinal plants in areas where poisonous plants are growing, vigilance and mindfulness are absolutely essential. For example, the highly toxic Hemlock Water Dropwort (*Oenanthe crocata*) often shares a habitat with Meadowsweet (*Filipendula ulmaria*) and tends to flower at the same time of the year. The two species look completely different, but if you are gathering Meadowsweet flowers from such an area, you will need to take great care to avoid inadvertently including seed or leaf fragments from Hemlock Water Dropwort plants in with your harvest. If you are gathering mindfully, you will always be able to avoid including any unwanted species in your basket, but in the case of Meadowsweet and Hemlock Water Dropwort, there is the added risk of poisonous seeds being knocked off the plants into your gathering basket among the Meadowsweet flowers. To be absolutely safe, find areas where the Meadowsweet is not growing interspersed among Hemlock Water Dropwort plants. Definitely do not reach through seeding Hemlock Water Dropwort plants to cut Meadowsweet flowers, and do not leave your basket in a location where seeds may drop or be blown into it.

Another thing to be aware of is that the sap of Giant Hogweed (*Heracleum mantegazzianum*) can lead to photosensitive reactions, such as blistering and burning of the skin. If your gathering activities involve walking through Giant Hogweed plants, make sure your skin is well covered. It is essential to

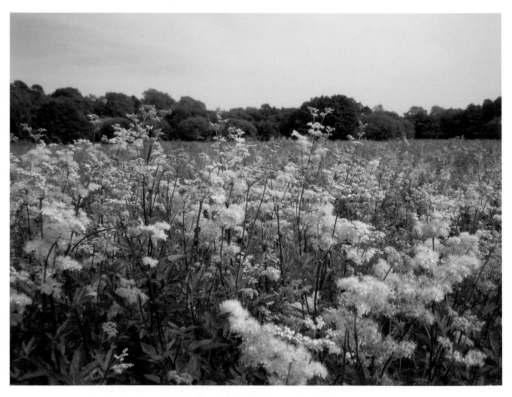

A swathe of Meadowsweet in flower.

completely avoid any contact between the plants and your bare skin.

I certainly do not want to give the impression that foraging is a highly risky activity. It really is not. My intention here is to raise awareness of potential issues. By following the simple guidelines given in this chapter, we can all have the enormous satisfaction of sourcing high-quality, beautiful and safe herbal medicines while connecting with our ancient instinct to gather plants from the wild. We can also feel confident that our wildcrafting activities are not damaging to the environment or to scarce plant populations.

Wild harvesting is a wonderfully nurturing and relaxing activity. It provides a really good counterbalance to the demands of clinical practice and restores our spirits if we are feeling a little depleted. It is most definitely in our bones, and I encourage you to learn to connect with it if, so far on your herbal journey, you have not yet done so.

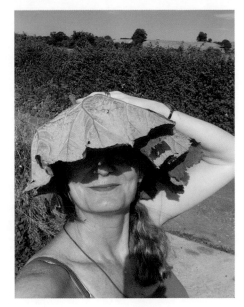

A butterbur hat!

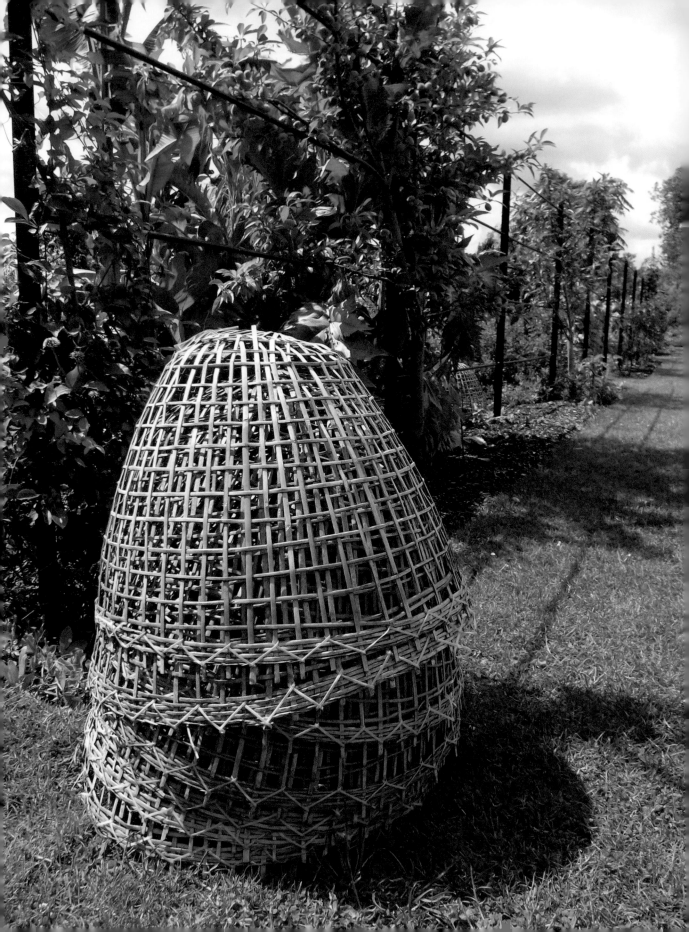

7

Planning your herb garden

At the planning stage of a herb garden it is a very good idea to assess what opportunities and constraints there are at your site. Every site has its advantages and disadvantages. It is very tempting to get stuck in and start planting straight away, but a little patience and planning will reward you with far fewer obstacles down the line as well as beautifully vibrant herbal crops.

The first priority is to understand the nature of the site that you have chosen. What is the soil like? Is the site shaded or in full sun? What climatic constraints are there: is it prone to frost or high winds, for example? If it is prone to drought, is there sufficient clean water to provide adequate irriga-

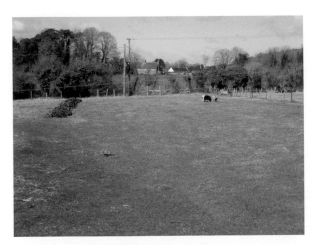 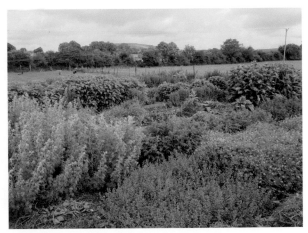

The site of my herb field in West Dorset before its creation, and nearly the same view four years later.

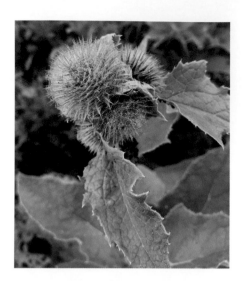

As well as common herbs, I grow Himalayan Burdock (*Saussurea lappa*), a Tibetan medicine that is officially extinct in the wild.

tion? What was the site used for before? Could it have been subject to chemical applications, or does it have a persistent weed population? What browsing animals could have access to the site, and will you need to fence it to keep them out?

Once you understand the broad physical qualities of your herb-growing site, you can move on to the second main consideration, which is to review your herb-growing objectives. Do you want to grow a wide range of medicinal herbs in order to provide a dispensary for treating your patients, or do you have specific requirements for an established herbal product range that you make? Do you intend to grow some commercial crops of herbs to supply others alongside your own needs? Is your main objective to concentrate on growing herbs that are difficult to get hold of from wholesale sources, or do you wish to focus on conservation, growing species that are endangered in the wild? Will your herb garden be ornamental or utilitarian in nature? Would you like to create a demonstration garden to teach people about herbs? Does the design of the garden need to accommodate visitor access or reflect particular themes, such as a sensory garden for the visually impaired?

Most herbs are very easy to grow and will tolerate a wide range of sites, especially if you can modify the growing conditions a little with good soil management and irrigation, as needed. This means that most of us can establish a beautiful and productive herb garden and grow the herbs of our choice. With that happy thought in mind, let us find out how to understand the physical attributes of our site.

Soil

The most fundamental thing to consider is the soil. Soil is so much more than something on which to grow our herbs. As human beings, we only survive and thrive due to our relationship with plants. Soil enables those plants to grow, and in turn we are nourished and formed by them. Yet, alongside this physical action, soil has a deeper energetic function. Soil provides us with a 'template' for groundedness and wholeness. When we take plants into our bodies as medicine, they deliver a reminder that we are part of a bigger whole. A message of wholeness and connection with the earth is a very potent agent of healing indeed.

I first learnt properly about soils while studying at Oxford University. I was taught by the legendary soil scientist, Dr Philip Beckett. Phil Beckett was a very inspiring lecturer and tutor. He was quite a character, and we all loved his lectures. He was amusing and informative, and he encouraged us to think for ourselves. He once wrote in *New Scientist* magazine:

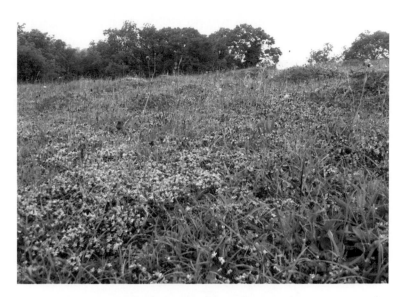

Chalk downland meadow in West Dorset.

'In research, as in life, most seminal ideas often arise before the mind and imagination have settled into a rut.'[1]

I vividly remember the magic of first seeing the relationship between the distribution of plant species and the soils beneath them. Our student cohort from the Agricultural and Forest Sciences undergraduate degree course was on a field trip to Blewbury Downs, a steeply sloping area of chalk downland near Oxford. We were divided into groups, and each group was tasked with digging a soil pit at a different point on the slope. Our location was a beautiful wildflower meadow. Around us was a hugely rich and diverse flora, including a multitude of grasses, Wild Thyme (*Thymus serpyllum*), Gentians (*Gentiana* spp.), Scabious (*Scabiosa columbaria*), Horseshoe Vetch (*Hippocrepis comosa*), Wild Carrot (*Daucus carota*), Eyebrights (*Euphrasia* spp.) and many more.

After the hard graft of digging our soil pits, we walked from the top of the hill down to the bottom, comparing the soil profiles at different locations. They varied quite a bit in different parts of the site, and we could see that the distribution of each plant species in the meadow was much influenced by soils and aspect. Not only did the plant species present vary on slopes facing to the south or to the north in the same area, but they also varied accord-

---

[1] P. H. T. Beckett & S. W. Bie, 'Diminishing Returns in Research', *New Scientist, 56* (1972), 517–519.

ing to whether they were growing at the top of the slope, part-way down it or at the bottom. It was fascinating to see that even microclimatic variations in aspect and soil type created by large anthills had resulted in different distributions of plant species compared to the overall distribution on the main slope. Suddenly, I realized that I was seeing the meadow in a new light. The arrangement of the plants had become predictable and understandable, as well as beautiful. It was as though I had been taught to read a code that had previously been illegible to me. Everywhere I looked, the connection between soil type and plant distribution was clear and visible. That moment permanently changed the way that I view the landscape around me.

The portentousness of the revelation was healthily balanced by a great deal of hilarity when we all retired to a nearby pub for lunch. Bearing in mind that we were at Blewbury Downs, some of our group had selected Fats Domino's rendition of 'Blueberry Hill' on the jukebox, and, with impeccable timing, the first iconic chords had rung out just as Phil Beckett stood up to begin a detailed explanation of our findings. To his great credit, he joined in the joke and waited until the track had played out before starting to speak.

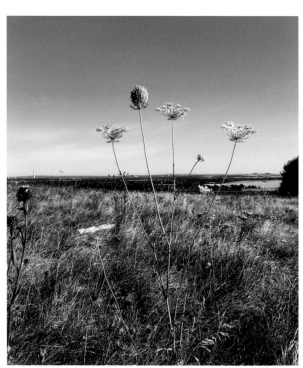

Wild Carrot growing on the downs above Blewbury.

So, while studying at university I learnt that if we understand the nature of soils, we can read the landscape around us and appreciate the intricate web of cause and effect that characterizes it. If we are aware of the link between soils, landscapes, and the plants that grow there, we automatically have a sense of place and a way of understanding different localities. Even in unfamiliar places we can find a sense of security and familiarity. We learn to associate particular plant species with certain soil types and, as wildcrafters, we learn to predict where we are most likely to find the plants that we need. As growers, when we understand our soil, we can discover which species will grow best on our land and which cultivation practices will help to ensure optimum plant growth and productivity. For a self-sufficient herbalist, soil really is fundamental.

Soils with different textures provide plants with varying levels of nutrients, aeration, and stability. They respond more or less quickly to the increasing warmth of the sun in the spring, and they vary in their ability to hold onto water or withstand being walked on or driven over without damage.

Particular soil textures are the result of the proportions of three different particle sizes: sand, silt, and clay. Pure sand feels gritty. Anyone who grew up making sand castles on the beach will know that dry sand will not stick together, but when wet it has enough cohesiveness to retain the shape that is has been moulded into. Sand is the largest of the three particle sizes. Since it cannot be packed really tightly together, water and nutrients drain easily through it. The second type of particle is silt. Silt particles are smaller than sand, and a silty soil feels smooth, soapy, and soft. If you squeeze a handful of silty soil, it sticks together better than sandy soil. The smallest particle size is that of clay. Clay particles are approximately 1,000 times smaller than those of sand. Clay is different in that it does not simply consist of weathered rock, like the first two particle types, it is actually a secondary product formed during the weathering process. Clay soils are usually described as 'heavy' because they are more difficult to cultivate than other soil types. When you squeeze a handful of a clay soil, it retains the shape of your fist and feels sticky. While pure clay soils can be challenging to cultivate, all soils benefit from the presence of some clay, as it helps to create healthy soil granules and acts as a nutrient store and a moisture retainer.

It is very rare to get soils that are made up of just one particle type. Most soils are a mixture of all three particle sizes and can be broadly divided into coarse-, medium-, and fine-textured soils. Coarse soils, which are higher in sand, allow water to drain

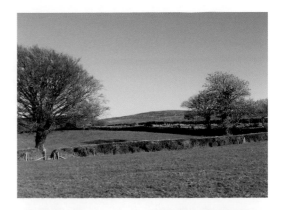

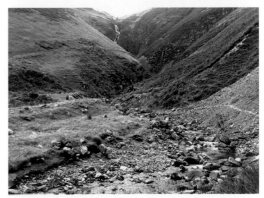

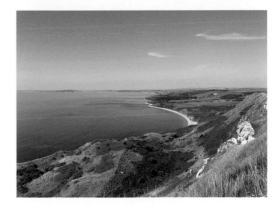

The relationship between different soil types and which plant species they naturally support is fundamental. *Top*: Dartmoor; *middle*: the Scottish borders; *bottom*: the Jurassic Coast.

through them more quickly than other soil types and have the advantage of warming up more quickly in the spring. Their texture gives them resistance to waterlogging and compaction. The downside of coarse soils is that they can be prone to drought and the loss of nutrients. If you have a very coarse soil, your management priority will be to add large amounts of organic matter in order to improve nutrient status and moisture retention. Medium soils are usually soils that are well balanced between sand, silt, and clay, so that none of these particle types dominates the characteristics of the soil. Medium-textured soils are ideal for cultivation and can be very fertile. They do not need any particular remedial management practices. Fine-textured soils are high in clay and are generally more difficult to work. Rainwater tends to collect on the surface in puddles, and the soil is slow to warm up in the spring, due to its higher moisture content. Soils with high clay content should never be cultivated or stepped on for harvesting when they are wet, as this will lead to compaction and permanent damage. When clay soils dry out, they form rock-hard segments surrounded by characteristic deep cracks, making cultivation very difficult. On the plus side, fine-textured soils retain moisture well in the summer. They can be improved by the addition of plenty of organic matter as well as by rough digging in the autumn, leaving large clods over winter to be broken down by the action of the frost.

There are many parallels between soil types and patient constitutional types in herbal medicine, whether you understand those according to Galenical humoural theory, Tibetan medicine, Ayurveda or other traditions. Each constitutional type has its tendency to moisture, dryness, inflammation, and stagnation, for example. Once we understand our own constitutional type, we can nurture ourselves effectively, staying as close as possible to an ideal healthful balance. Likewise, once we understand the soil in our herb garden, we can nourish and manage it so that we are able to grow the best possible crops of medicines.

Overlaid onto the various soil textures is the effect of its pH. Chalky soils naturally have a higher pH and will favour the growth of certain plant species such as Juniper (*Juniperus communis*), Lily-of-the-Valley (*Convallaria majalis*), Thymes (*Thymus* spp.) and Marjorams (*Oreganum* spp.), for example. Acid soils naturally have a low pH and favour other plant species such as Blueberries (*Vaccinium corymbosum*) and Camelias (*Camelia* spp.). Soils that are naturally quite alkaline, such as chalky soils, can cause essential nutrients like iron to become unavailable, even though in theory there should be plenty in the soil. Iron is an essential nutrient to plants, and when they cannot take it up, they start to form pale or blotchy leaves, often with the small leaf veins remaining green, giving the leaves a chequered appearance. This phenomenon is called 'lime-induced chlorosis'. Conversely, very acid soils can also cause problems for plants that are not adapted to those conditions. In soils with low pHs, some elements reach higher than optimal levels due to their enhanced solubility, and aluminium, manganese, and iron can be present at toxic levels. Alongside this additional toxicity, essential nutrients such as phosphorus, potassium, magnesium, and molybdenum can become deficient. When soil pH is too low, soil life becomes inhibited. This interferes both with the plants' ability to form beneficial symbiotic relationships with fungi and the overall health and balance of micro-organisms and invertebrates present in the soil. Adding more organic matter will have the effect of moving a soil closer to the neutral from either tendency. Soils with a pH that is close to neutral can support a very wide range of herbs. If you want to grow specialist herbs that prefer either low or high pHs and you do not naturally have these soils present on your site, it is quite possible to create raised beds or containers filled with appropriate soil.

Plant growth is affected by the soil not only in its surface layers, but also at deeper levels. If you are establishing a new herb-growing area, or if you do not understand your current one, it is a good idea to investigate the nature of the soil down to a depth of about 1 m / 3 ft. You can either use a soil auger, which is a hollow spike that is driven into the

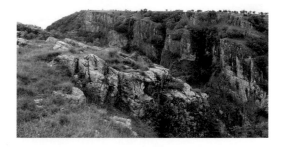

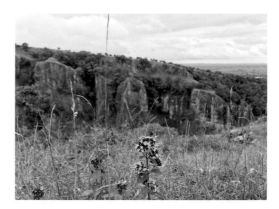

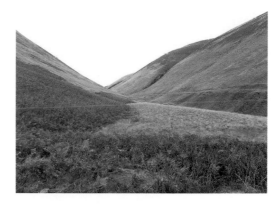

The pH of the soil will favour certain plant species. *Top*: Cheddar Gorge; *middle*: Wild Marjoram growing in alkaline soil at Cheddar Gorge; *bottom*: upland pasture on acidic soil in the Scottish borders.

ground and removes a thin core of soil, or you can dig a small soil pit. Once you start digging, you will notice that the soil consists of layers of different colours and textures. Together, these layers form what is called a 'soil profile'. The layers have been built up over centuries due to the action of vegetation, cultivation, animal or human traffic, and climatic conditions. The uppermost layer, known as the topsoil, is usually darker than the layers beneath it, due to higher levels of organic matter. You will find that the topsoil layer is absolutely teeming with life. As it is nearest the surface, it receives rainfall first, and so over time there is a tendency for nutrients to be washed down into the deeper layers. With time the higher levels of organic matter in this layer tend to increase its acidity a little and increase the solubility of mineral salts that are washed down into the lower layers. On steep slopes this top layer can be very thin, and on recently completed building sites it may be completely absent.

Below the topsoil is the subsoil. This is usually harder to dig when dry and often stickier when wet due to an inherently higher clay content. Iron oxides tend to be washed down from the top layers into the subsoil and may form hard red-coloured concretions or even a continuous hard layer, called an 'iron pan', which effectively prevents roots from being able to grow through it. If you have only a thin layer of top soil and a hard iron pan in the subsoil, it is much more difficult to grow crops, because they will have less access to water and nutrients. In wetter areas, you may notice that the soil is blueish or greenish with mottling. This is a sign that there is a lack of aeration and that the iron compounds present in the soil have been reduced to greenish ferrous oxide rather than reddish ferric oxide. Blueish-greenish anaerobic subsoils are called 'gleys' and restrict the growth of plant roots to the shallow aerated layers, unless corrected by drainage. You may find that the lower part of your soil pit is filled with water even in the summer. If this happens, you will know that your area has a relatively high water table or that the lower layers of your soil prevent free drainage. The depth of the water table has a significant influence on the plant species that will grow happily at a particular site. Land with a high water table or sub-surface compaction will reveal its true nature by the plants it naturally supports. If your new herb-growing site is covered by Rushes (*Juncus* spp.) and Creeping Buttercups (*Ranunculus repens*), you can conclude that it is naturally damp. If it also shows signs of surface damage from the hooves of grazing animals, you can suspect a high water table and compaction. On soils such as these there is much that can be done to improve them with drainage or you may decide to concentrate on growing herbs that enjoy wetter soils, such as Sweet Flag (*Acorus calamus*), Meadowsweet (*Filipendula ulmaria*), and Marshmallow (*Althaea officinalis*), for example. If you have a very wet area, then you could consider creating a pond or bog garden and grow Bog Bean (*Menyanthes trifoliata*).

Some soils are stony, or have stony layers. Provided that the water table is not too high, stones help to improve aeration and can

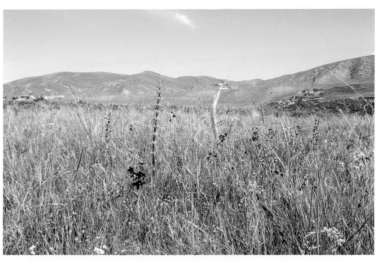

Bupleurum (the yellow umbels), growing in Amdo, China.

be a helpful source of minerals for the soil as they weather. Large stones can however make cultivation or the harvesting of root crops more difficult. If you are planning mechanized cultivation and harvesting on your land you may need to consider some stone removal. This is not usually necessary for herb growing on a small scale. If you find yourself with a particularly stony area, you can make the most of it by growing alpine plants or those that require very free-draining conditions such as Pulsatilla (*Pulsatilla vulgaris*), Bupleurum (*Bupleurum chinensis*), Arnica (*Arnica montana*), and Gentians (*Gentiana* spp.).

If you have a large site, differences in the soil profile in different parts of your growing area may help you to decide which species to grow where. While over time most cultivated sites move towards more versatile cropping, it is usually much better to let the choice of species be influenced by the soil conditions than to have a very fixed idea of what you intend to grow where. If you try to mould a site to your theoretical plans rather than working with it, you could find yourself expending a huge amount of energy and resources in trying to adapt the conditions to fit. The influence of varied soil types on your plot is a perfect opportunity to cultivate acceptance as well as to cultivate herbs. If you are lucky enough to have a medium-textured well-drained soil with a neutral pH, you will be able to grow pretty much any herb that you want, where you want.

Slope and aspect

It is easiest to manage a herb-growing area that is level or nearly level, but if you have a steeply sloping site, that need not be a negative attribute – it can be useful. Slopes lend themselves to the creation of different habitats; for example, you can create areas to grow wetland plants at the base of the slope and areas for plants that need warmer soils and more sunshine at the top. In temperate climates with high rainfall, provided the soil is free-draining and you can replicate woodland conditions, it may be possible to grow scarce woodland herbs that require free-draining, shaded conditions. Species to consider include Golden Seal (*Hydrastis canadensis*), Beth Root (*Trillium erectum*), and American Ginseng (*Eleutherococcus senticosus*).

South-facing sites will have more sunlight and will tend to get warm more quickly in the spring. If you are growing aromatic herbs for their volatile oil content, you will find that south-facing sites will be preferable. North-facing sites can be better for herbs that prefer cooler, moister conditions. Although they receive less sunlight, they are less prone to drought and the burning-off of crops.

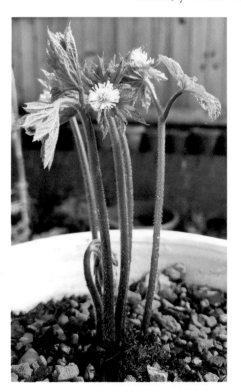

As cooler air sinks below warm air, sloping sites can influence the likelihood of frost damage in cooler climates. In winter, icy air tends to gather and stay in the lowest part of your garden. The longer this icy air stays, the more frost damage will be inflicted on your plants. Frost pockets are areas where frost collects but cannot escape: a low-lying hollow or an area at the base of a slope by a wall, for example. When planning your herb garden, it is a good idea to pay attention to where frost lingers the longest. See if there are frost pockets, and either choose these areas for hardy crops or plan a means for the cold air to flow out rather than be trapped there.

Golden Seal flowering in my garden.

Climate

Depending on where you are in the world, you will have certain parameters dictated to you by the climate. You will need to consider the frequency of frost, the volume and distribution of rainfall and the prevailing wind speed and directions. Look at what is growing naturally in your area: those plants will tell you a great deal about what species will be suited to your land. In areas with cold winters, you can extend the range of medicinal species that you are able to grow by using greenhouses, polytunnels or cloches or simply by starting off non-hardy plants indoors on the window sill. I grow Ashwagandha (*Withania somnifera*) by extending the season in this way.

If your area is prone to drought, you may need to plan for irrigation, although it makes sense to focus first on herbs that will be more drought-tolerant, such as Rosemary (*Rosmarinus officinalis*), Bay (*Laurus nobilis*) and Yarrow (*Achillea millefolium*). If you are planning to grow herbs that do require plenty of water, make sure that you have sufficient unpolluted water available. Peppermint (*Mentha piperita*), for example, requires 50 mm / 2 in of water per week, either from rainfall or irrigation, in order to thrive. Most herbs require around 25 mm / 1 in of water per week.

High winds can be damaging to young plants. In very sandy soils, high winds can even uproot surface-rooting plants from the soil and blow them away. If root

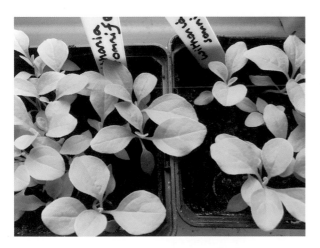 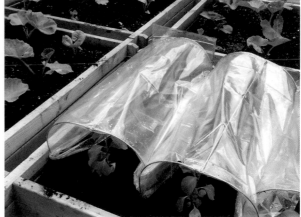

Left: Ashwagandha seedlings started off on a windowsill. *Right*: Ashwagandha planted out under a temporary cloche; the plants in the background are Himalayan Burdock.

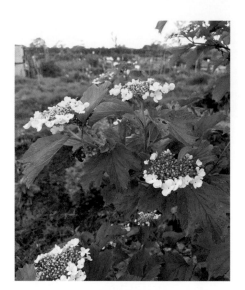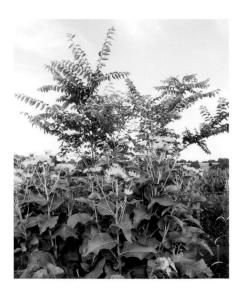

Left: Cramp Bark in flower at my allotment. *Right*: Slippery Elm growing at my allotment; the yellow-flowered plants in front are Tibetan Elecampane.

anchorage is not an issue, high winds can strip plants of their moisture, stunting their growth. Cold winds can cause dieback of plants that require warmer growing conditions, and salt-laden winds can cause burning of crops. If your herb-growing area is prone to regular high winds, you would be wise to include some shelter belts. Be aware that shelter belts, as well as buildings and walls, create their own micro-climates. The northern sides of shelter belts are shadier, the southern sides sunnier; the western sides will be exposed to more extremes of temperature, being shadier in the morning but exposed to stronger sun in the afternoon. This is not necessarily a disadvantage. A greater temperature range can encourage higher levels of essential oils in aromatic herbs. Eastern sides of buildings or shelter belts are milder than western sides, being exposed to the morning sun and the afternoon shade.

Even if you do not need shelter belts, I would still encourage you to plant some medicinal trees and shrubs. You could use them in your boundaries or establish a woodland and shrub area. Consider the following: Willow (*Salix* spp.), Birch (*Betula pendula*), Hawthorn (*Crataegus monogyna*), Elder (*Sambucus nigra*), Cramp Bark (*Viburnum opulus*), Wild Cherry (*Prunus avium*), Oak (*Quercus robur* and *Quercus petraea*), Quaking Aspen (*Populus tremuloides*), Barberry (*Berberis vulgaris*), Witch Hazel (*Hamamelis mollis*), Purging Buckthorn (*Rhamnus cathartica*), Spruce (*Picea* spp.), Pine (*Pinus* spp.), Lime flower (*Tilia* spp.), Oregon Grape (*Mahonia aquifolium*), Goji berry (*Lycium barbarum*), and Slippery Elm (*Ulmus fulva*).

Design

A well-organized herb garden will usually have a compost-making area, with a range of compost-making bays and good access for wheelbarrows. You may wish to include a shed, a greenhouse, a cold frame, or a raised propagating area. You should also consider whether or not you need to fence your garden. Is it necessary to keep deer out, or is there a large rabbit population in the area?

Each of us has our own relationship with herbs and our own way of working with them. This will influence the type of design that appeals to us. Our planting plan will also be influenced by our site and the constraints and opportunities presented by it. For example, in a small garden with heavy soils, a chequer-board design with squares of hard standing alternating with planted squares is beautiful and practical. The hard standing allows easy access to the herbs throughout the year without risk of compacting the soil. If you are going for this design, choose squares with sides 1-m long in order to allow sufficient room for the herbs. Personally, I have always wanted to create a circular astrological herb garden with an armillary sundial in the centre; I still have an old notebook somewhere with my design and planting list. Alas, so far it has never been right for my circumstances, but it was a lot of fun planning it. Another one that I would love to manifest one day is a Tibetan medicinal garden based on the tastes and properties of the herbs.

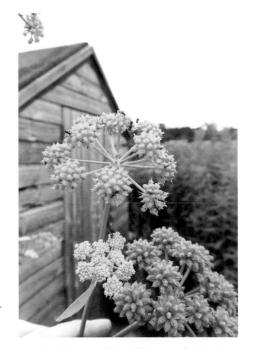

A shed is a useful addition to the herb garden. The flowers in front are those of Lovage.

If you need design inspiration, I recommend that you visit established herb gardens. In my travels, I have seen herb gardens based on therapeutic properties, affinities

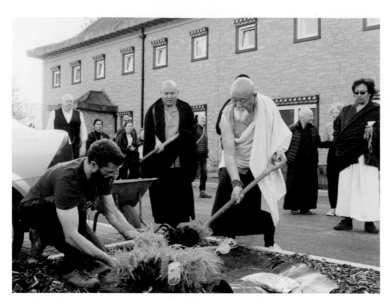

Lama Yeshe Losal Rinpoché planting Juniper at Samye Ling Tibetan Centre.

of herbs with systems of the body, and different botanical orders, as well as those arranged by colour of the flowers. All were wonderful, beautiful, and fascinating to visit. My current herb garden is rather utilitarian in design, being arranged in rows, with no paths between them. Despite this, it is still breathtakingly beautiful in the summer, when it is in full bloom. Herbs seem to have a knack of overriding our design ideas and making the place their own anyway.

Paths are a positive feature if you have room for them. They create structure in the ornamental herb garden. I have always loved the juxtaposition of hard edges with soft billowing herbs spilling over them. It reminds me vividly of my paternal grandmother's cottage garden. She had a beautiful garden, crisscrossed by neat gravelled paths. Near the house there were fragrant pinks and beds filled with roses, herbs, and other cottage garden favourites. At the bot-

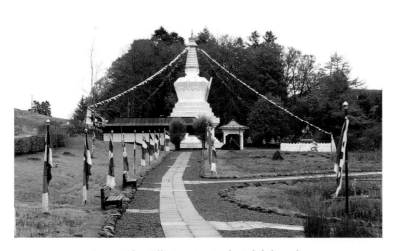

Samye Ling Tibetan Centre in Eskdalemuir.

tom of the garden, beyond a neat lawn, was a well-maintained vegetable garden, a large fruit cage filled with soft fruit, and a small orchard of apple and pear trees. I used to spend time at her house regularly while I was at boarding school, since it was too far for me to go home during exeat weekends. Although in theory there was not a lot for a young teenager to do at her house, I was always totally happy sitting in the garden among the pinks and the herbs,

or helping to pick fruit and vegetables. My grandmother's garden
was an oasis of peace amidst the
craziness and stress of boarding-
school life.

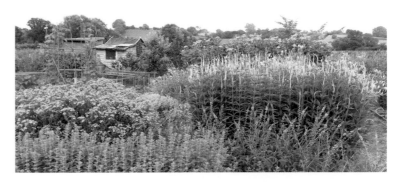

My herb garden allotment in full bloom.

Paths can be made from stepping stones, gravel, wood, bare
earth, concrete or grass. Be aware
that, unless you mow them regularly, using grass for paths within
your herb garden can result in
more weed seeds being distributed to your growing area. It may be preferable to establish gravelled paths or at least use mulched or geo-textile-covered
areas to avoid adding to your weed-control work. If you do not want to
establish permanent paths between your herb crops, using boards to stand
on when cultivating or harvesting will spread
your weight and help to minimize compaction.

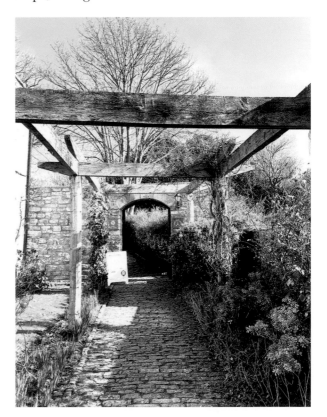

Once you have the structure of the garden,
your planting plan will be based on a number
of factors. The distribution of different soil
types may influence the siting of some of your
herb species, as we discussed earlier. Root
crops are best planted in soil that is friable, so
that they can be harvested and cleaned more
easily. Soil that is full of small stones can be
problematic when growing root crops with
small fibrous roots, such as Valerian (*Valeri-
ana officinalis*). Likewise, the prevalence of
sun and shade can influence your planting
plan. The sunniest areas of the garden are
best suited to Mediterranean herbs, such as
Thymes (*Thymus* spp.), Rosemary (*Rosmarinus
officinalis*) and Marjorams (*Oreganum marjo-
rana*), while shadier areas are better for Mints
(*Mentha* spp.), Cowslips (*Primula veris*), and
Lady's Mantle (*Alchemilla mollis*).

The Chalice Well Gardens, Glastonbury.

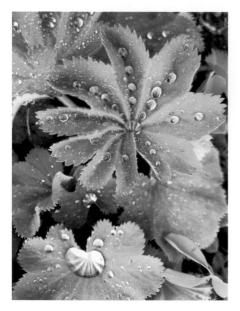

Lady's Mantle leaves.

Tall crops such as Elecampane (*Inula helenium*) and Marshmallow (*Althaea officinalis*) will cast their own shade, so this may influence your choice of where they are located. In some areas, additional shade may be desirable within the garden; in others, you will be aiming to minimize it. If you are short of space, you can plant close to each other crops that mature at different times of the year. For example, in my garden I find that Cowslips (*Primula veris*) do well next to Marshmallow. Cowslip flowers are one of the earliest crops to be harvested. Like most spring flowers, they do best if they have plenty of sunlight early in the season, but they are quite tolerant of shady conditions later on. Marshmallow starts from tiny shoots in the spring and only grows tall later in the season. The shade that it casts at that time will not adversely affect the Cowslips after they have finished flowering.

Most herbs will tolerate a wide range of planting conditions and will thrive next to all sorts of different herbal neighbours. There are a couple of exceptions, though. If you plant Fennel (*Foeniculum vulgare*) and Dill (*Anethum graveolens*) near each other, they will hybridize, as will Mints

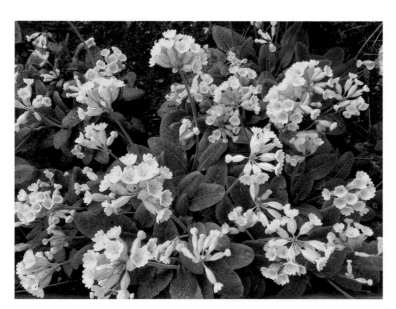

Cowslips in flower.

if they are planted together. Also, Artemisias such as Wormwood (*Artemisia absinthum*) and Southernwood (*Artemisia abrotanum*), if planted too close to Coriander (*Coriandrum sativum*), can affect the flavour (and therefore the properties) of the latter. Other than these special exceptions, you really cannot go too far wrong. In any case, if you find that one of your herbs is not thriving, you can always move it later.

Large-scale growing is easier to manage when the herbs are planted in rows, since this allows you to use mechanized cultivation or at least a hoe in order to help with weed control. Rows need not consist of just one species per row. It is possible to achieve the benefits of row planting with the benefits of a mixed cultivation system by planting parts of rows with different species.

Some growers prefer a much more informal *laissez-faire* design, allowing herbs to grow where they like. In theory, I love the idea of this, as the herbs can reseed themselves and spread around the garden, creating a beautiful informal and natural feel. In practice, though, if you do not use some judicious weeding to help your chosen cultivated herbs to thrive, you will eventually end up with a meadow of grasses and local wild herbs. It can be helpful to divide your garden into areas based on the intensity of weed control that will be required by the crops growing there. Certain areas can be designated for more intensive weeding and can be used to grow annual crops such as Calendula (*Calendula officinalis*), California

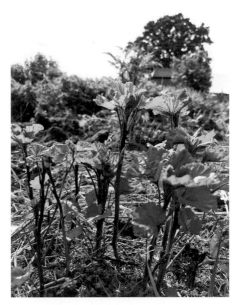

Marshmallow at an early stage of growth.

Poppy (*Eschscholzia californica*) and Nasturtium (*Tropaeolum majus*), for example. Allow sufficient spacing between the plants so that you can carry out effective weed control while the crops are establishing. Tree and shrub crops such as Cramp Bark (*Viburnum opulus*), Willow (*Salix* spp.) and Slippery Elm (*Ulmus fulva*), which are more tolerant of weeds once they are established, can be grown together in less intensively managed areas. For these, it can be a good idea to choose parts of the garden that are more prone to invasion of weeds from surrounding areas. They will form a buffer zone to protect the areas that you want to keep especially free of weeds.

Other things to consider in your layout are that perennial herbs will stay where they are for many seasons. They will form a framework within the garden around which you can rotate your annual crops. It is also worth thinking about the practicalities of harvesting your herbs. For example, if you have heavy soil, then crops that need frequent harvesting, such as Calendula (*Calendula officinalis*) and Chamomile (*Matricaria recutita*), are best planted where you can access them without having to stand on the soil.

Sometimes people ask me how much of each herb they should plant. This depends on how much you use of each species and how fertile your site is. For example, one or two well-grown Lemon Balm plants may be all that you

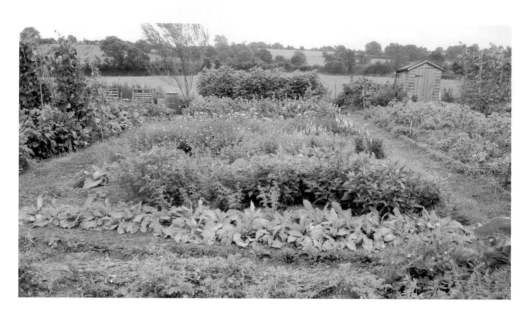

My allotment in its first year.

require to make tincture each year, but if you prescribe a lot of infusions, you may need more. I grow a lot of Lady's Mantle (*Alchemilla mollis*), because I prescribe it in sitz baths and infusions, but I only have two or three plants of Horehound (*Marrubium vulgare*) and Feverfew (*Tanacetum parthenium*) because I use less of these. I have quite a large plot (probably 50 or more

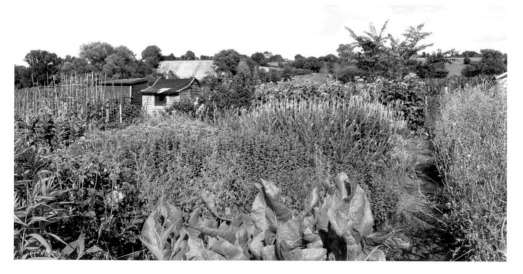

My allotment in full flower four years later.

plants) of Skullcap (*Scutellaria lateriflora*), because I need so much of it for my clinic. I also use a lot of Cramp Bark (*Viburnum opulus*) but I have found that six plants are more than enough for my needs and allow me to coppice them on a rotation. The amount of each herb we decide to plant will also be influenced by our ability to wildcraft or buy in additional supplies, should they be needed. I have a great deal of Agrimony (*Agrimonia eupatoria*) and Yarrow (*Achillea millefolium*) because I love to prescribe them and because in my location wildcrafting a sufficient quantity of these species is not easily possible. There is no hard-and-fast rule.

My advice is to establish your garden with a few plants of each herb and get to know them. Let your herb garden evolve as you learn what grows well and which herbs you most need for your family, clinic or herbal business. You can expand the number of plants as time goes on. It is easy and fun to propagate herbs. My Agrimony colony started with one plant gifted

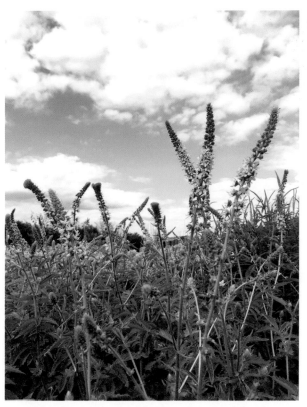

My Agrimony colony started with one plant gifted to me by my tutor.

to me by my tutor, and my Cowslip colony started with two or three plants. I do not think that I have ever bought more than two plants of any one herb.

If you want detailed guidance on designing an ornamental herb garden with suggested planting plans and the space required by each herb, I thoroughly recommend Jekka McVicar's *Jekka's Complete Herb Book*.[2] Whatever design you decide upon, I do hope that you enjoy the process. It is the first step of connecting with your piece of land. When you cultivate that sense of connection along with your herbs, your garden is bound to become a beautiful, magical place.

---

[2] J. McVicar, *Jekka's Complete Herb Book: In Association with the Royal Horticultural Society*, Kyle Cathie, 2009.

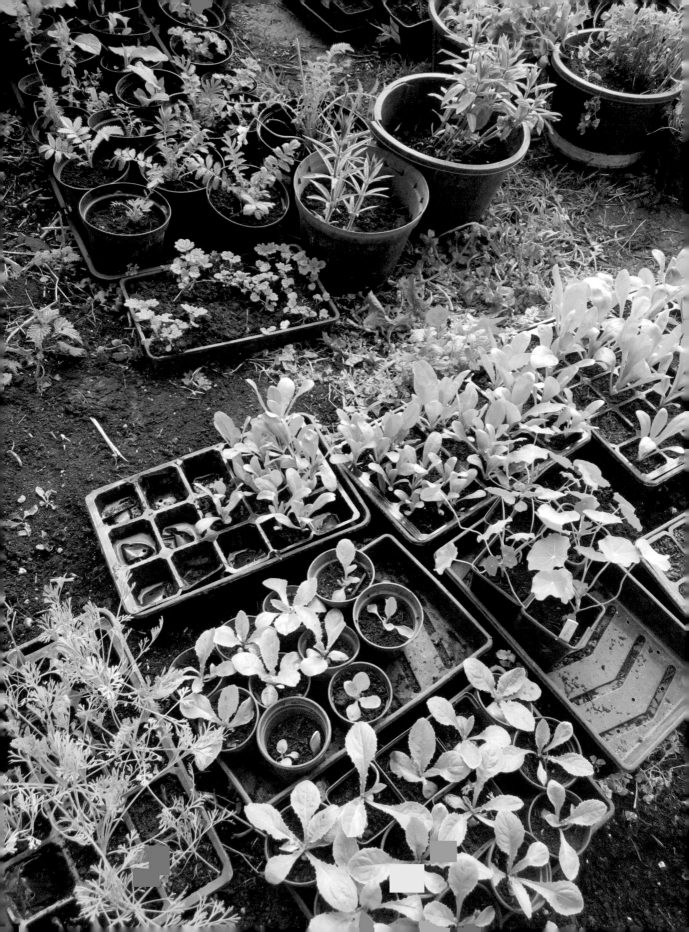

8

Cultivation and growing

To grow medicinal herbs is to experience the wonder of a true and deep connection with the earth. It is therapeutic, grounding, and magical. Whether you are an experienced grower or someone with access to a piece of land for the very first time, you will find herbs straightforward and rewarding to grow. Having said this, there are certain basic principles that it is worth bearing in mind in order to get the most out of your herb garden and the time that it takes you to look after it. You need to look after the soil, guard against compaction and ensure that the herbs growing on it have sufficient nutrients and water. You also need to maintain a balance between the different plant species that are growing in your garden through a certain amount of selective management and removal of plants that are interfering with the growth of others. This chapter is not intended to make herb growing seem complicated or to give the impression that there is a 'right' and a 'wrong' way to do it. The way that each of us chooses to grow our herbs depends totally on our own situation. We need to come to our own decisions based not only on the physical nature of our herb garden site but also our scale of operation, what we wish to grow, how much time we have available for cultivation and what the end use of our herbs will be. Over time we may find that we need to adjust how we do things in order to make our life easier or to be able to grow a wider range of species. If we understand the principles involved, we can make these adjustments in an informed manner. The aim of this chapter is to provide you with the tools to make those decisions. Growing herbs represents a shared bond between us, but it is also a wonderfully personal thing.

Starting off

When we first establish our herb garden, there are some fundamental choices that we need to consider. The first one is to choose whether we are going to use only natural inputs or whether we are going to accept the use of artificial herbicides, fertilizers, and pesticides on our plot. I will lay my cards on the table and admit that I am strongly in favour of the former option. To grow medicinal herbs brings with it a responsibility to avoid causing harm, not only to the people who will take the herbs as medicine, but also to the soil, to neighbouring wild plants, and to the environment in general. If we produce our herbs in harmony with the environment, we will be working in keeping with the holistic ethos of herbal medicine. Having said that, I do accept that in some situations some people may feel the need to have a more flexible approach, especially in the early stages of creating a garden. We all need to work with our own unique set of circumstances, both physical and environmental. What matters is mindfulness and responsibility surrounding the decision.

The second major choice is to decide whether we are going to use a traditional cultivation model or whether we are going to choose a 'no-dig' system. Traditional horticultural cultivation is based on a scaled-down agricultural production model, which requires access to cultivate the crop more or less throughout its growth period. However, when working solely with hand tools, we have the flexibility to work with a system of narrow beds that are undisturbed by cultivation or compaction through treading. This decision may be influenced by whether you are establishing your herb garden within a pre-existing garden design or whether you are starting on a previously uncultivated site.

Traditional cultivated system

First, let us consider a traditional cultivated garden system. Assuming that you are growing your herbs without the use of chemical applications, it is a good idea to give some serious thought to weed control. Weeds can be a welcome part of the herb garden, as most of them have useful medicinal properties; however, if you do not keep on top of them, you will find that harvesting becomes much slower, and within a couple of seasons weed-prone crops such as Peppermint (*Mentha piperita*) can be out-competed by Nettles (*Urtica dioica*) and grasses.

If you are starting with a piece of previously cultivated land, have a look at the plant species that are present. If you can, it is a good idea to completely remove persistent invasive weeds such as Nettle (*Urtica dioica*), Bramble (*Rubus fruticosus*), Ground Elder (*Aegopodium podagraria*), and Couch (*Agropyron repens*) before you start to plant your herbs. It is so much easier to start with a clean slate, especially as many of the herbs we wish to cultivate are perennial, and once they are established, it can be difficult to remove weeds thoroughly. Regardless of your plot's previous land use, the soil will be filled with weed seeds just waiting for their chance to break their dormancy and germinate. It may seem a good idea to plough the whole area up in one go and then plant it, but only do this if you are in a position to keep on top of the weeds. There will be a lot of them at first.

Before my family and I moved to Castle Cary in 2013, I had a herb field in Cattistock, West Dorset. The site for the field had been loaned to me by a very kind, generous local organic farming family, the Cakes. The Cakes' farm is incredibly beautiful: secluded and quiet. It is teeming with wildflowers, butterflies, birds, and mammals like foxes and deer, which have learnt that they are totally safe. As well as cultivating my field, I had free rein to wander over the farm, gathering wild medicines as needed. Mary Cake had been very close to my late maternal grandmother, Joannie, who was a healer and radionics practitioner. Mary and I would pause in our respective work to have a chat and to catch up with each other's news. Our topic of conversation was often Joannie. We would talk fondly of her, sharing our memories. Mary once told me how proud Joannie was that I had taken refuge as a Vajrayana Buddhist. I never knew that.

My herb field had been created by ploughing an area of old pasture, and this is how I know very well the effects of that establishment strategy on the weed burden in a new herb garden. As soon as the land was turned over by the plough, the weeds thrived. There were Nettles (*Urtica dioica*), Docks (*Rumex obtusifolia*), Dandelions (*Taraxacum officinale*), Couch (*Agropyron repens*), and many other grasses. Established pasture species with strong root systems simply re-grew after the ploughing. New seeds germinated. It was definitely not going to be a case of simply planting my herbs into beautiful, friable newly cultivated earth. I did not want to cause compaction by subjecting the ground to repeated cultivation with a tractor or rotavator, so

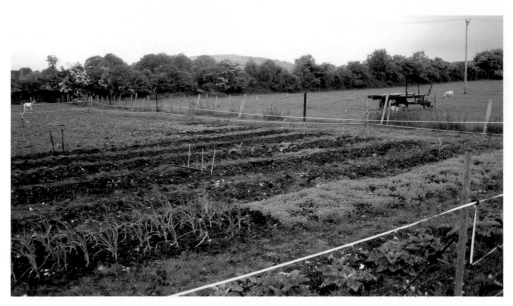

In the early days at my herb field, there were many times when I felt that I had bitten off more than I could chew.

I opted to continue with hand cultivation after the initial ploughing. There were many times when I felt that I had bitten off more than I could chew, and more than once I felt that I could no longer carry on, especially since I was working alone and managing a full-time clinical practice. On those occasions, I only continued, stubbornly, because my spiritual teacher, Akong Rinpoché, had asked me to grow Tibetan herbs in the West. I was determined not to let him down.

I learnt a huge amount from my struggles to break in that herb field, and I would definitely do it differently if I were doing it again. In the end, it took me five years of very hard graft to break the land in and to establish a system that was manageable. I started in the centre and worked outwards. The outer areas supported herbal crops that were more tolerant of weeds: Cramp Bark (*Viburnum opulus*), Phytolacca (*Phytolacca americana*), and Wormwood (*Artemisia absinthum*), for example. The inner areas supported crops such as Calendula (*Calendula officinalis*), Tibetan Elecampane (*Inula racemosa*), Echinacea (*Echinacea purpurea*), Marshmallow (*Althaea officinalis*), and Greater Celandine (*Chelidonium majus*). By trial and error, I found a way of managing the land using a combination of geotextile strips, cover crops, relentless weeding, and plenty of mulch using chopped hemp. It would have been so much

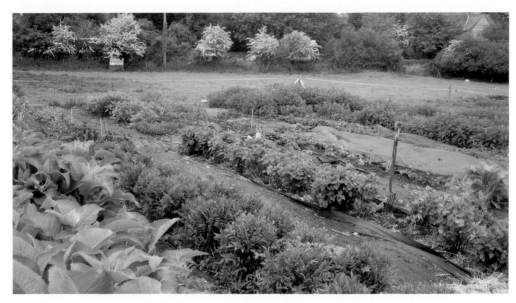

I found a way of managing the land using a combination of geotextile strips, cover crops, relentless weeding, and plenty of mulch.

easier if I had known then what I know now. Despite my formal education in agriculture and forestry, the reality of organic cultivation of a field-scale new plot by hand proved to be very tough. I poured my heart and soul and a lot of sweat into establishing that herb field.

After five years I looked around me, and I could see that I had created a beautiful and productive herb garden. I could not quite believe it: the hard work of establishment had been done, and from then on, I could continue growing my herbs on a maintenance level.

Sadly, that was not to be. Suddenly, circumstances dictated that we had to relocate. Within a few months, we were looking for somewhere new to live, and I was searching not only for a new herb garden site, but also for new schools for the children, somewhere to keep my rescue pony, and new clinic premises. There was so much to organize and absolutely no time to be emotional about it. There were no sad last goodbyes at that beautiful field. Writing this now, I have the space to feel those shelved emotions, and my heart aches when I remember how wonderful it was to sit among my crops, watching the butterflies and drinking in the scent of the earth and the fragrance of the herbs. It is sad to think of the loss of that field as a productive herb garden, but I sincerely believe that impermanence is a great gift as well

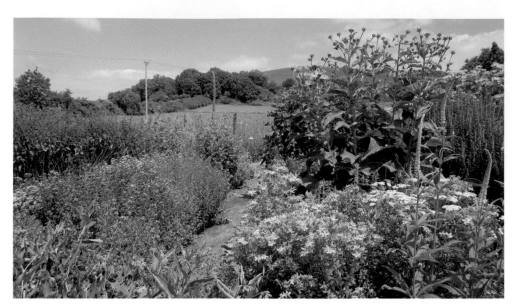

After five years I looked around me, and I could see that I had created a beautiful and productive herb garden.

as a challenging lesson. I had the experience of creating that herb garden, and I learnt so much from it, not just about the practicalities of herb-garden establishment, but also about myself. Working closely among the herbs in that field and harvesting them for use in my practice changed me and influenced me. It helped me to grow.

So, with the shortcomings of my herb garden establishment technique fresh in our minds, let me reassure you that there are various ways of making this initial weed-clearing process less daunting. It is quite possible to cultivate a plot in manageable sections, leaving some areas fallow until you are ready to clear them. You could cultivate the whole area first and then cover some parts of your plot with a light-excluding water-permeable geotextile, gradually bringing new areas into cultivation and cropping as you are ready. You could cultivate the whole area and plant an annual crop, such as potatoes, on part of the area for the first season. Potatoes allow intensive weed control between the rows when the crop is young and good weed control through shading once the crop is in full foliage. Harvesting the potatoes allows further cultivation of the land. While green-manure crops are an excellent way of increasing organic matter in the soil, do not be tempted to plant one in order to shade out perennial weeds. Green manure crops do not lend themselves to intensive weed control while they are growing, so any weeds that emerge alongside the crop will have a whole season to establish themselves. At the end of the season you will be ploughing them in, with their roots and their seeds, along with the goodness of the green manure. This especially problematic where you have weeds with spreading roots such as Nettle (*Urtica dioica*), Couch (*Agropyron repens*), and Ground Elder (*Aegopodium podagraria*).

It is not ideal to leave land bare for long periods, as it can result in nutrient losses and erosion. However, as a one-off management strategy, on a workable soil, a stale seed-bed system can be a good way of reducing the weed population. You will need patience, though. First, you need to dig out the worst of the persistent perennial weeds, to remove the roots. Then you dig or plough the land, followed by harrowing to break up the clods. Once the soil is friable and has the texture of a seed bed, you sit back and wait. As weed seeds from the soil are exposed to the light, they germinate. Very soon the soil will be covered with germinating weeds. You allow them to grow a little, waiting until they are around an inch long, and then hoe them or harrow them again. Provided that the soil is light enough to be worked, you can repeat this process several times. Each time there is a flush of new growth, fewer and fewer will sprout, as the numbers of weed seeds are reduced in the top layers of the soil. As the season progresses, you reduce the depth of the cultivations, so that you avoid bringing more and more weed seeds to the surface. You are aiming to keep the top 2.5–5 cm / 1–2 in of soil as low as possible in weed seeds. Once there is only minimal further germination, you can plant perennial herb crops, such as Peppermint (*Mentha piperita*) and Spearmint (*Mentha spicata*), which require a fairly weed-free start. Ironically, if you are growing Nettle (*Urtica dioica*) on your land, you will need that to be really weed-free too.

In some situations, going through the process of creating a stale seed bed will be a worthwhile investment of time and effort. You will be rewarded with a friable and relatively weed-free seed bed, which is ideal for establishing direct-sown crops. There are, however, some downsides to the stale seed-bed technique. If your soil is heavy, you run the risk of causing compaction by carrying out repeated cultivations on the same area. Additionally, the structure of the soil can be damaged by the disturbance, and nutrients can be washed away in wet weather due to the lack of a cover crop.

In practice, how you manage the task of reducing the initial weed burden in your herb garden will depend on how light your soil is and whether or not you are using machinery. As was the case with my own herb field, new herb gardens being established on pasture land with limited vehicle access may need to be mechanically cultivated in one pass and then fenced. Before assuming that a new herb garden should be ploughed or dug, consider whether a 'no-dig' system might be better.

No-dig system

There is much evidence to support the use of 'no-dig' systems. The principle is if the soil is left undisturbed, it maintains its own healthy structure, and weed seeds are not brought to the surface. There are different methods, one being to lay a cover of cardboard over the bed area and then pile well-rotted compost on top of it to a depth of at least 15 cm / 6 in. The cardboard excludes light and prevents further weed growth, eventually rotting away and adding to the organic matter in the soil. Instead of back-breaking digging, the worms and soil microflora do all of the hard work and bring the compost down in to the soil. The structure of the soil is not disturbed by 'catastrophic' digging. Although the soil may seem firm in texture, the minute air channels within it are not disturbed. This means that the soil remains well aerated and conserves water better than disturbed soil. Weed seeds are not brought to the surface, so that you are starting your cultivation with a clean slate. Of course, it is very important that the compost used does not contain weed seeds or pieces of viable root from perennial weeds. Animal manures tend to be relatively high in weed seeds, so try to find a source that has made the compost properly, or if you are making it yourself, ensure that it has reached a high enough temperature for any weed seeds to be destroyed. Peat and leaf mould are not really environmentally sustainable choices and are to be avoided, but you can use green manures or spent mushroom compost. Bear in mind that mushroom compost is alkaline in nature and is not suitable if you are intending to grow acid-loving herbs.

With years of experience of using different methods to start new herb gardens, 'no-dig' would be my first choice if I were ever to break in a new plot from pasture-land again. Although I would not pretend to be an authority on this method, cultivation at my herb field did morph into a 'no-dig' approach out of necessity. I had rows that were not trodden on or cultivated, and I used deep mulches of chopped hemp to suppress weeds and to build up organic matter. Within a few years, the soil was outstandingly rich, friable, relatively weed-free and healthy in these areas. It just goes to show that herb growing is a voyage of discovery and continued learning.

If you are drawn to discover more about 'no-dig' and the different ways to implement this, I thoroughly recommend looking at the excellent work carried out by Charles Dowding.

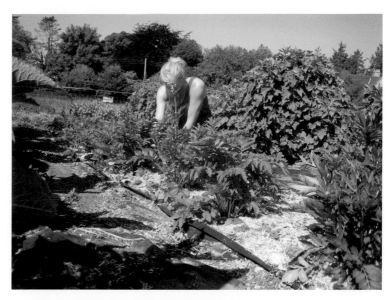

At my herb field I used deep mulches of chopped hemp to suppress weeds and to build up organic matter.

Fertility

It is a common myth that herbs grow best on poor soils; in fact, herbs will grow well on a wide range of soils. In the herb garden, we need to make sure that the fertility of the soil is adequately maintained. The cultivation of herbs leads to a steady depletion of the inherent fertility in the soil. This is due to a number of factors. Most herbs are shallow-rooted, so do not naturally provide large amounts of organic matter to be incorporated into the soil structure. Very few herbs are legumes, which fix nitrogen from the atmosphere and bring it into the soil. As areas of soil are left cultivated and weed-free between rows or between plants, the soil is vulnerable to atmospheric nutrient losses and further losses through the influence of irrigation washing nutrients down to deeper layers of the soil. On top of all of this, we are taking harvests of herbs and removing organic material from the garden, to be made into medicines. Fertility can be maintained by applications of organic matter in the form of well-rotted manure or compost or by growing and ploughing in crops of green manure. If you look around, there will be plenty of sources of organic matter available, depending on where you live. As well as maintaining

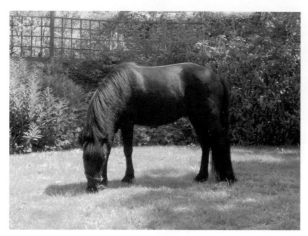

Bramble grew sleek and brave and cheeky.

fertility, soil with plenty of organic matter has a pH nearer to neutral, has a better structure and an improved drainage, and is easier to work.

I have been lucky enough to have free access to pony manure during most of my herb-growing life. While I was still a herbal student, I rescued a little black pony, whom I named Bramble. Bramble originally came from the semi-wild herds on Dartmoor. When I first met her, she was still a baby with a fluffy tail and was destined to be live-shipped to Italy for dog meat. I had heard about her through a friend and immediately contacted the livestock dealer and bought her for the princely sum of five pounds. A couple of days later, she was delivered – skinny, wide-eyed, and sweaty. She was terrified, completely unhandled, and totally mistrustful of human beings. From that first day, I spent every spare moment sitting on an upturned bucket in the corner of her stable, reading aloud from whichever book I happened to be reading at the time. I would like to tell you that it was Matthew Wood's 'Book of Herbal Wisdom',[1] but to be honest, I really cannot remember. Over time she grew sleek and brave and cheeky. We became really close friends. Bramble taught me about trust and unconditional love, and for many glorious years she provided me with plenty of manure for my herb garden.

When we had to move from Cattistock to Castle Cary, it was quite an upheaval. Many areas of the United Kingdom have waiting lists for allotments, but, amazingly, thanks to Lynn Johnston in the wonderful Bailey Hill Bookshop, I was able to take on a full-sized plot in Castle Cary before the formalities had been completed on the house that we were moving to. The allotment had been well tended and was left clear by the previous occupants. This was a huge blessing, as I did not have the time to break in a new herb garden while going through the stress and upheaval of moving to a new house. The soil on the allotment was quite heavy, and some areas had rushes and other typical wetland plants growing as weeds.

I knew that whatever I did, large applications of organic matter were going

---

[1] Matthew Wood, *Book of Herbal Wisdom*. Berkeley, VT: North Atlantic Books, 1997.

to be the most helpful thing on that plot of land to improve its texture and drainage. Now, at the beginning, it was a perfect opportunity to apply plenty of it to the bare ground before I started planting. Thanks to Bramble, I had access to large quantities of pony manure, and I spread the entire area with about 15 cm / 6 in of it. I left it for a few weeks and then started the herb transplanting process. That application of organic matter really did improve the texture, drainage, and workability of the soil on my allotment, and I have been blessed with a workable soil and abundant crops of medicines ever since then.

If you do not have access to livestock manure, making compost is an excellent way of recycling 'spare' organic matter from your herb-growing and medicine-making activities. Faded leaves or coarse stalks that are removed from herbs before they are dried, or the marc from tincture making, can be added respectfully to your compost. How can we honour and respect the herbs that we use for medicine if we just throw parts of them away without ceremony?

When Akong Rinpoché asked me to be part of his Tibetan herb-growing initiative, he invited a group of people to a meeting at Samye Ling Tibetan Centre. We gathered in the conference centre and shared ideas on how best to manifest his vision. He specifically asked me to give a presentation on how to make compost. I remember feeling embarrassed, because I felt there were others present who could have done this much better. I did ask him whether it would be better for one of the others to give the presentation, but he was quite clear that he wanted me to do it.

Good compost has a number of desirable features, the most important being that it is free of viable weed seeds or roots that can regrow. As compost is made, it heats up, and if it reaches a high-enough temperature, the weed seeds and roots will be inactivated. Good compost feeds the soil, not the plants, providing nutrition in the form of colloidal organic matter, which becomes available to plants through their interaction with the soil micro-organisms. It goes without saying that any compost you add to your garden should be free of toxic residues of pesticides or heavy metals. Organic certification bodies have guidelines on acceptable residue levels in their standards.

When making compost, it is preferable to use a good balance of different raw materials. You are aiming to promote natural biological breakdown of the material, and for this there needs to be an optimal carbon : nitrogen ratio. Woody material such as wood shavings or bark are highest in carbon and have very little nitrogen. Slurry or chicken manure is very high in nitrogen and low in carbon. Soil organisms need access to nitrogen in order to break down the carbon. If your compost materials are too high in carbon, any nitrogen present will be used up by the microbes as they break it down, leaving very little left to help improve the fertility of the soil. If there is too much nitrogen in your compost materials, much of it will be lost to the atmosphere in the form of ammonia. When this type of compost is added to the soil, it will provide too much soluble nitrogen, resulting in excessively lush growth, which can be prone to pests and diseases and will create less potent medicines.

Understanding of the effects of the carbon : nitrogen ratio on microorganisms enables you to vary the way in which you make your compost according to the materials that you have available to you. It also happens to be very helpful in pond management. Have you ever seen a pond that is choked by too much bright-green duckweed on the surface? This is not at all healthy for fish and is a sign that there is far too much nitrogen present in the water. The way to remedy this situation is to submerge straw bales in water. As straw is high in carbon and very low in nitrogen, the microbes will have plenty of carbon available to fix the excess nitrogen in the water.

The ideal ratio of carbon to nitrogen in finished compost is about 15:1. In order to create compost with this ratio, you want to start with a ratio of approximately 30:1. During the composting process carbon is broken down and is lost, leaving a final level of carbon that is much lower than the one that you started with. In his excellent book, *Herbal Harvest*[2], author Greg Whitten suggests some compost-making mixes in order to achieve this. One is 80% foraged grass, half green and half dead, mixed with 20% cow manure or tincture marc. You could also opt for 60% hay, 30% seaweed, and 10% wood shavings. These 'recipes' give you a guide to help you get good structure in the heap and the most helpful proportions of carbon and nitrogen. You can adapt them according to the materials that you have available. You will soon get a feel for the kind of mix that results in the best compost in your situation. You cannot make good compost from 100% kitchen vegetable peelings or lawn mowings: they are too high in nitrogen and will become a slimy, anaerobic mess. Likewise, you cannot make good compost from 100% wood shavings, as they are too high in carbon and will not rot down. As in all things, a

---

[2] G. Whitten, *Herbal Harvest*, Melbourne, Australia: Bloomings Books, 1999.

healthy balance is the key. A small proportion of wood shavings will provide useful structure and therefore aeration to the heap.

There are lots of different ways of building compost heaps, but these are all based on the same simple principles. You should aim to alternate layers of more carbon-rich materials, such as hay and straw, with moister materials, like seaweed and kitchen scraps. If you are going to incorporate wood shavings, add them in very thin layers. Some people like to add a thin layer of soil every now and then in order to help to inoculate the heap and absorb some of the liquid that can be generated. If you are working biodynamically, you will enjoy the magic of adding the special herbs and compost preparations to the heap.

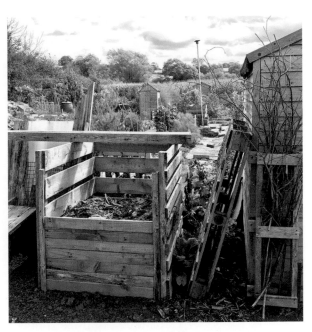

Compost bin at the Castle Cary allotments.

Successful composting relies on the heap getting quite warm and the heat being retained for long enough to complete the process. If it cools down too quickly, the compost will not be fully transformed. This is not ideal as you may end up with a lot of viable weed seeds remaining in it, and these will be spread back onto your herb garden when you apply the compost. In order to help retain the heat that is generated by the microorganisms, it is a good idea to find ways of insulating your heap. Some people use straw as a cover, others use old carpet or cardboard. Covering the heap also helps to reduce moisture losses through evaporation. An active compost heap is teeming with microbial life, and it needs moisture and air for that life to thrive.

The size of the heap will be based on the space you have available and the quantity of compost you wish to make; however, there are some general guidelines that should help you. If the heap is very small, there will be a large surface area that does not fully heat up, and the centre of the heap will be prone to cooling down before the weed seeds have been thoroughly killed. A very large heap will have a larger central area exposed to heat, but the lower layers may suffer with lack of aeration, as the weight of upper layers can cause compaction. The ideal heap is a balance between the two extremes

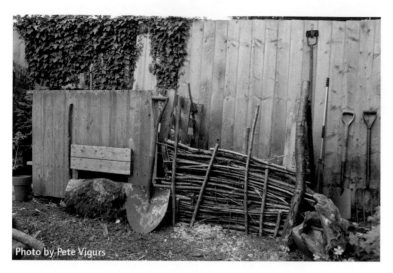

A compost-making area.

and is probably not more than 1.5 m / 60 in tall and approximately 1.75 m / 70 in wide. If you have the space, it is a good plan to set aside at least three bays for compost making. The idea is that you have one heap that you are building and turning, a second one that is curing, and a third that is being dug out and added back into the garden. If you need to make a very large volume of compost, you can make it in a series of long windrows. This is how commercial recycling centres usually organize their composting heaps. On a small garden scale, many people decide to use commercially available compost bins. These have the advantage of taking up minimal space but also have the disadvantage of being tall and thin, so the outside edges are prone to cooling down. It is quite difficult to turn the contents regularly too. However, if that is all you can manage, they are a very good way to keep your plot tidy.

Recently someone I bumped into at the allotments told me how much she disapproved of people taking their green waste to the municipal recycling centre rather than composting it themselves. She said that composting is easy, and everyone should do it. She had assumed that I always made my own compost and that I would automatically agree with her. Neither assumption was correct, but I was in a hurry to get back to my clinic with a basket of freshly harvested herbs, so I did not challenge her. I should really have said that although composting may be very straightforward, it does take up space, quite a lot of it in fact, if you are doing it properly. If you only have a very small amount of growing space available, you may find that it makes more sense to take your green waste to the recycling centre and use professionally made compost to add to the organic matter of your garden. Speaking as someone who moved my herb-growing operation from a half-acre herb field to a very small garden and an allotment, I know all about how precious growing space is. I would love to have a compost-making area with neat bays arranged by the stage they are at in the process, and I would love to have the capacity to make excellent compost using raw materials that have been gathered from my own plot. In practice, though, I make do with a couple of pre-made compost bins and regular trips to the very nearby recycling centre. Every situation is unique, and we all have our own reasons for our way of doing things. What matters is that we have weighed up the options and made our own decision mindfully.

If your compost heap has the perfect balance of raw materials and retains a good moisture content, you may find that turning it is unnecessary. Most people, however, need to aerate their heap by turning the material part-way through the composting process. Turning the heap also gives you the opportunity to monitor how it is doing. If it seems too dry, you can add a little water, and if it is too moist, you can add some absorbent material, like wood shavings or soil. Aim to turn the heap so that the material on the outside ends up in the middle and the material that was in the middle ends up on the outside. The turning process reinvigorates the decomposition, so that the temperature of the heap stays high. You know you are on the right track when the centre of the heap becomes too hot to leave your hand in, around 65°C / 150°F.

Green manures can be useful during the early stages of herb growing, when you are looking to improve the organic matter in the soil. Provided that your ground is relatively weed-free to start with, you can plant a crop that will grow for a season and then be incorporated into the soil. Green manuring involves ploughing or digging fresh green material into the soil as it breaks down, so it can lead to a temporary depletion of available nitrogen in the soil. Nitrogen fixing crops, such as Melilot (*Melilotus officinalis*), Alfalfa (*Medicago sativa*), and Red Clover (*Trifolium pratense*), will help to provide additional nitrogen in order to counteract this tendency. They also have the advantage of being herbal medicines in their own right.

Weeding

While uninvited wild medicines such as Dandelions (*Taraxacum officinale*) or Small-Flowered Willowherb (*Epilobium parviflorum*) can be viewed as serendipitous bonuses, too many 'weed' species or vigorous self-seeding from cultivated plants such as Motherwort (*Leonurus cardiaca*) will reduce the number of species that your herb garden supports. Couch (*Agropyron repens*),

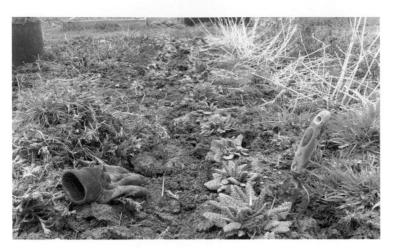

Weeding my Cowslips early in the season.

Dandelion, and Small-Flowered Willowherb are wonderfully valuable medicines, but we may be able to meet our needs for these by wild harvesting. If we are going to the effort of creating and maintaining a herb garden, we will want it to be filled with a range of different medicines that we can connect and work with. It is also worth noting here that harvesting is much more straightforward and efficient in a relatively weed-free crop. Take Peppermint (*Mentha piperita*) or Skullcap (*Scutellaria lateriflora*), for example: if you are working on a small scale, these are best harvested by gathering a handful together with one hand and cutting the stems with secateurs held in the other. If your crop is very weedy, you will need to cut each stem individually, and it will be a much more time-consuming process. This option is not available to you at all if you plan on harvesting using a scythe or a mower.

There is a school of thought that very dense planting is preferable in order to reduce weed build-up, due to the fact that the soil is shaded. This is not really accurate, as most herbs die back in the winter, and there are

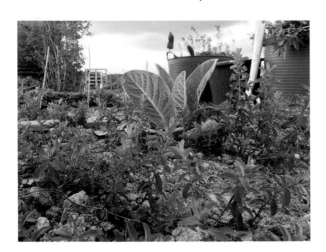

Weeding St John's Wort.

significant periods of the year when the soil is not covered and therefore prone to weed build-up. My herb garden is densely planted simply because I have so little space available. At the beginning of the season I can use a hoe in some areas, but once the plants come into full growth, all weed control has to be done by hand, up close and personal, with a hand trowel. It is the perfect method for me, as it enables me to tease out the roots of the weeds from my crops and carefully relocate earthworms and other invertebrates, as necessary. I love being there, crouching or kneeling among the crops, with my hands in the earth.

Not only does this method allow a 'minimal-harm' policy, but it also lets you find self-sown seedlings, so that you can pot them up or relocate them, as you see fit.

Pests and diseases / plant protection

Luckily, compared to other crops such as vegetables, herbs are generally quite resistant to most pests and diseases. If your herbs are tended well, have sufficient light, nutrients, and water, you will avoid most problems, especially fungal diseases and aphid infestation. This holistic approach is woven into organic and biodynamic growing techniques, as these emphasize crop health as a means of avoiding pests and diseases rather than the application of remedial chemical inputs. It is also worth noting that monocultures are more vulnerable, so the mixed planting of a self-sufficient herb garden is ideal to resist pest and disease problems. Having said that, even a carefully managed mixed planted herb garden can sometimes suffer from pest damage. Usually this is an indicator of a need to rotate the herb beds, or, if a particular herb is affected repeatedly, it is a sign that you should choose a different species. My advice is to walk your herb-growing area frequently. Notice everything. Just as we seek to understand why a patient has become ill by taking notice of factors other than the immediate symptoms, we should notice the effect of weather conditions, management practices and nearby species on the health of our herbs. We will soon learn what works best in our garden and in our location.

In the relatively high rainfall conditions of the South West of the United Kingdom, slugs and snails are my biggest obstacle, especially since I choose to avoid chemical applications and the taking of life in general. It always takes me much longer than my fellow allotmenteers to dig my herb garden, as I have to remove and relocate any earthworm or creature that finds its way into each spadeful of soil. With slugs and snails, I do a lot of picking off and relocating. I am pretty sure that they return. I try to cultivate the attitude that there will be enough for everybody, but it is hard to feel so accepting when precious seedlings or rare plants are at stake. My most precious herbs are grown in seed trays on a raised propagating area or pots on hard standing.

I have used coffee grounds, gravel, eggshells, and even copper strips as deterrents with some success, but the only real answer is unwavering vigilance. The more unusual and precious the herb is, the more voraciously the slugs and

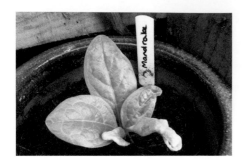

A precious young Mandrake plant.

snails seem to target it. I have lost Mandrake (*Mandragora officinarum*) seedlings, Beth Root (*Trillium erectum*), Black Cohosh (*Cimicifuga racemosa*), and Golden Seal (*Hydrastis canadensis*). This has usually happened when I have taken my eye off the ball, while travelling for a few days or simply prioritizing other commitments during very busy times in my clinic. Sometimes I have been so devastated by these losses that I have fleetingly questioned my nonviolent management attitudes, but I have never actually changed them. I will carry on doing my best using a combination of vigilance, deterrents, relocation, and a good dose of acceptance.

Some more rural areas are prone to animals – rabbits and deer, for example – browsing the herb garden. Large animals can be deterred by good fencing, perhaps electrified, and by the placing of scented deterrents. Human urine is considered to be especially effective against deer, and I have also heard of people successfully using the faeces of large cats. If you live near a zoo or a safari park, you may be able to get hold of some in order to experiment with this approach. If you have a large rabbit population, you may need to fence your plot with rabbit fencing, buried to a depth of at least 1 ft. Badgers can

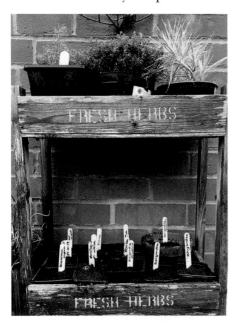

Nursery stack for seedlings vulnerable to slugs and snails.

be much more difficult to deter with fences, especially if your herb garden is in one of their established foraging areas. They will break through or dig under most fences, and in one garden I even had one that once broke its way into the hen house. The hen-house incident was terrible, but it took place during a prolonged drought, and I realized that the badgers must have been starving to go to those lengths. I immediately invested in a much more heavily fortified hen house, and the surviving hens lived happily to a very ripe old age. On a much less serious note, the resident badgers seemed to be particularly partial to Parsley (*Petroselinum crispum*). As a result, I was completely unable to grow it in that garden. They would leave all of my herbs alone except the Parsley, which would be uprooted and eaten as soon as it had formed decent roots. I have to say that, apart from the hen-house incident, I never had a problem with the badgers going about their business. I hope that they enjoyed their Parsley.

Propagation

Being able to propagate our own herbs is a very useful skill. It enables us to establish a new herb garden at a fraction of the cost of buying in everything as established pot-grown plants. It gives us the capacity to spread the herbal love by giving excess plants to friends and colleagues, and it allows us to build up a population of herbs that are especially suited to our unique growing conditions. Perhaps most important from my perspective is that it allows us to increase and share stock of scarce or endangered herbs. Let us review the main methods of propagation.

Seeds

Seeds are a fabulous way to increase stock. They are more easily transportable than plants and are not as costly to buy. Plants grown from seed are usually healthier and less prone to disease than those grown from cuttings or by root division or layering, because seed-grown plants have their own genetic make-up, whereas plants produced from vegetative propagation are clones of the parent plant. If you are growing rare or scarce plants, gathering seed and distributing it to other growers is a very valuable way of conserving them.

I was very fortunate a few years ago to be able to grow some unusual Tibetan medicinal plants, thanks to the then seed exchange programme of the Himalayan Plant Association, which was based in the United Kingdom. Sharing of seeds is much easier than the sharing of living plant material, at least within your own country. If you intend to share seeds beyond the borders of your country, you will need to check customs regulations. Plant health teams work very hard to protect their country from exotic pests and diseases, so it is understandable that, if the seeds are found to contravene the regulations in some way, they will be confiscated and destroyed. I once tried to import fresh Mandrake seeds from the United States without doing proper research. They were destroyed at Heathrow.

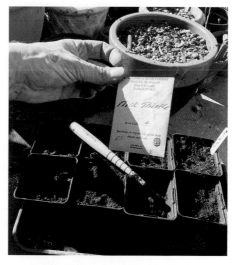

Planting Milk Thistle seeds.

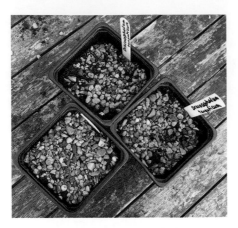

Propagating *Dracocephalum tanguticum*, a Tibetan medicinal plant, by seed.

Seeds are living, even though they are dormant, so they should be stored appropriately in order to safeguard their quality and a good germination rate. Do not allow your seeds to be exposed to dry heat or to dampness. Some seeds need to be planted very soon after they have ripened, and others stay viable for several years.

If you are new to growing plants from seed, please do not be daunted by the different instructions about how to prepare the soil and plant the seeds. Differences in cultivation techniques and choice of growth medium increase your chances of success, because they are tailored to the individual type of seed. When you buy seeds, they will usually come with instructions as to when to plant and what sort of growth medium and care they will require. If all you have is a seed head from a friend's garden, you will need to do a little research to find out the best way of being successful with that particular species. In the end, though, with seed planting, no matter how much research you do and how carefully you choose the growth medium and plant the seeds, there will always be some seeds that fail to germinate, and others that germinate well but then, for some reason, fail to thrive. That is the nature of growing. We learn from our experiences each season. The important thing is not to give up but to resolve to try again.

There are different types of seeds, and each type needs to be treated slightly differently. Herbs such as Lobelia (*Lobelia inflata*) have tiny dust-like seeds. Tiny seeds should be sown thinly on the surface of firm, even soil. To make it easier to distribute the seeds evenly on the surface, try mixing them with a small quantity of dry sand or seed compost before sprinkling. Do not attempt to do this outside on a breezy day, as I once did! Once the seed is scattered over the surface of the seed tray or pot, sprinkle with a very, very thin layer of fine sand or soil, but you can also just leave the seeds on the surface. Cover the planting receptacle with a pane of glass to preserve the moisture. Lobelia needs light to germinate, so leave it with just glass, but if you are planting seeds that germinate in the dark, then you can cover the glass with a sheet of paper to exclude the light.

Fleshy seeds, such as Mandrake (*Mandragora officinarum*), can develop a hard coat if they are stored for any length of time. Better germination will be achieved if you soak them in tepid water for a day to soften the coat before sowing.

Nuts such as Hazelnut (*Corylus avellana*) and the acorns of the Oak (*Quercus robur* or *Quercus petraea*) have a very hard coat, and it can be helpful to chip the outer hard casing with a knife or rub them a little with rough sand-

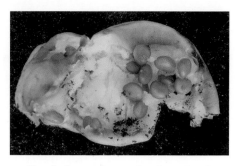

Mandrake seeds can develop a hard coat if they are stored for any length of time.

paper. This helps moisture to penetrate the casing and breaks the dormancy more quickly than if you just plant them as they are. The filing or chipping should be done at the opposite side from the 'eye' of each seed, in order to avoid damaging the embryo. On most seeds, you can see fairly easily where the 'eye' is. It is the point where the seed was attached to the mother plant. If you are planting nuts that are surrounded by pith, such as Ginkgo (*Ginkgo biloba*), remove the pith first.

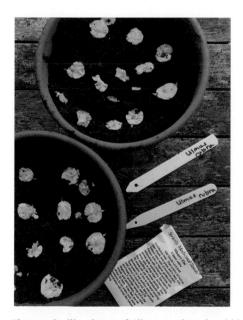 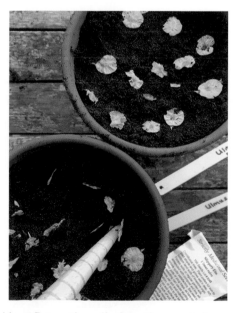

Flat seeds, like those of Slippery Elm, should be laid out flat on the soil where they are to be planted and then pushed gently onto their sides using a pencil or a pointed stick.

Flat seeds, like those of Hollyhock (*Alcea rosea*) and Slippery Elm (*Ulmus fulva*), should be laid out flat on the soil where they are to be planted and then pushed gently onto their sides using a pencil or a pointed stick. This will result in a much better germination rate than if they were left lying flat.

Seeds of the Carrot family are oily in nature and do not stay viable for very long. If you are growing Parsley (*Petroselinum crispum*), which is a member of this family, from seed, you will need to use seed that has not been stored for more than one year.

Seeds within fleshy fruits, such as Hawthorn (*Crataegus monogyna*) and Rosehip (*Rosa* spp.), will be easier to handle and more likely to germinate if the fleshy covering is removed from the seeds and the inner seeds are exposed to frost before planting. The best way to do this is to store the seeds in layers inside a box of sand and to leave it outside, exposed to frost.

In general, when sowing seeds, you need to plant them in soil that is not too loose. The soil should consist of a fine tilth and not contain large air gaps. If you are sowing in the garden, it is a good idea to firm the seed bed before planting by treading or rolling, or, if it is in a container, by firming it gently with your hands. Aim to cover seeds with a layer of soil or seed compost that is equivalent in depth to their own size; an exception to this is leguminous seeds, which tend to push themselves out of the soil as they grow. Try not to plant the seeds too thickly. As they grow, they will compete for light and nutrients, becoming overcrowded and spindly. It can be difficult to thin them out, and the process of removing seedlings can damage the root systems of their neighbours. Spindly seedlings are prone to damping off, a fungal disease that spreads rapidly over the surface of the soil and infects the base of the stems, causing the young plants to collapse and rot.

Once you have sown your seeds, watch carefully for signs of germination. If you have sown them in pots covered with glass and paper, this should be removed as soon as the first sprouts appear. When the seedlings develop their first true leaves – as opposed to the cotyledons, which are their baby leaves – they can be transplanted. This process is known as 'pricking out'. This has to be done very carefully, as the young seedlings are very prone to damage at this stage. Use a small pointed stick or a dibber to make a hole in the soil to loosen the soil next to a seedling, and then pick it up very gently by its true leaf; do not, under any circumstances, handle the stem. Immediately transfer the seedling to a moist container of freely drained seed compost, and firm it in very gently.

If you are growing plants from seed indoors and they are intended to be planted outside in the garden, you will need to harden them off before they are planted out. Place the containers outside for gradually increasing periods so that the plants can get used to the cooler temperatures and the effect of wind on their stems and of rain on their leaves. At first you will bring them inside at night; as they get hardier, you can leave them out with a cover and then, finally, leave them uncovered, in a sheltered place. Once they are strong enough to plant out, keep an eye on them to make sure they have enough water and not too much competition from weeds.

The time that you need to sow each seed will vary according to the species and where your garden is located. If your crop needs to be sown in the spring, wait until the soil has warmed up. Autumn-sown herbs may need to be exposed to a period of cold. Some Himalayan plants, such as Himalayan Blue Poppy (*Meconopsis* spp.), have very exacting requirements involving time spent in the freezer before they will germinate. The few times that I have grown Meconopsis, I felt that all the effort was well worth it as soon as I saw the iconic blue flowers.

If the ground is very dry, water the seed-sowing area before you plant the seeds, rather than afterwards. The seed beds of some crops that are slow to germinate, such as Parsley (*Petroselinum crispum*), are traditionally treated with hot water before planting, as this is believed to speed up the process. Parsley can take 6–8 weeks to germinate, so be patient. It is said to 'go to the Devil and back six times' before emerging.

Growing herb plants from seed is deeply rewarding. If you are anything like me, you will make plenty of mistakes and have losses, but these will be more than compensated for by the times that you get it right.

Before moving on to other forms of propagation, I would like to highlight the technique of encouraging herb plants to self-seed into the garden directly. This can only happen if you leave the seed heads over the autumn and winter to disperse naturally. When using this propagation technique, you have to be very careful with your spring weeding, so that you do not remove new useful seedlings accidentally. Any self-seeded herbs that you want to keep can either be can be thinned out *in situ* or be transplanted. This is a really excellent way of increasing your herb stock naturally. I have built up popula-

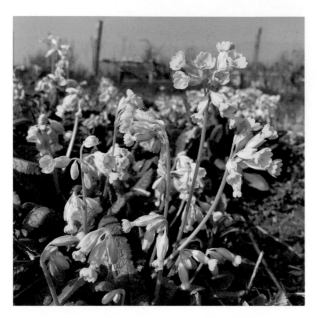

Now that my Cowslip colony is well established I have enough flowers for my own needs and I am able to share seedlings with my allotment neighbours.

tions of many herbs using this method. One example is my Cowslip (*Primula veris*) colony.

In general, Cowslips are not particularly abundant and should not really be foraged from wild populations. There are some isolated areas where Cowslips are plentiful, but I think it is much better that they are left to their own devices and that as herbalists we grow our own. I started with two Cowslip plants that were given to me by a friend. I planted them in a flower bed in my West Dorset garden, and they thrived. Each year the original plants grew bigger, and they self-seeded prolifically – not, as it turns out, into the flower bed, but into the neighbouring lawn. For several years I painstakingly removed the tiny seedlings from the lawn and transplanted them back into the flower bed. I did this until we had to relocate to Castle Cary. At that point, I carefully potted up every single plant and brought them all with me to my allotment. They seed prolifically there, and now that my colony is so well established that I have enough flowers each spring for my own needs, I am able to share seedlings with my allotment

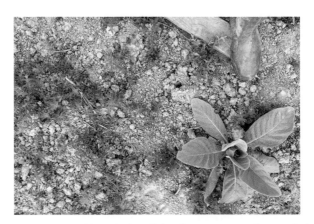

A carefully preserved self-seeded Mullein plant amongst the St John's Wort.

neighbours. I have done a similar thing with my beloved Agrimony (*Agrimonia eupatoria*) patch – or, in fact, patches. I love that herb so much I have increased my growing area considerably over the years through its abundant self-seeding when left to its own devices. I started with one Agrimony plant and now, years later, I have a large and thriving colony.

Cuttings

Cuttings are an easy and low-cost way to propagate plants. The idea is that you take a piece of a growing plant and encourage it to produce roots, thereby forming a new plant. Plants produced from cuttings will be exactly the same as the parent plant, and this is an advantage when preserving special characteristics that may have developed within a certain plant population. If you have noticed that one of your plants has particularly desirable characteristics, such as a long flowering period or a stronger aroma, you can increase your stock by taking cuttings. However, the lack of genetic variability that results can be a disadvantage. If you have many plants with exactly the same genetic make-up, they will all behave in the same way when faced with an environmental or pest challenge. If one plant is vulnerable, the chances are that they all will be.

The most common type of cutting used to propagate medicinal herbs are stem cuttings. Stem cuttings are taken from the aerial parts of a parent plant, pieces being removed with a sharp knife or secateurs. They can consist of soft-wood, half-ripened wood or hardwood (sometimes referred to as ripe wood). Soft wood cuttings are taken from young tender growth of the current season, half-ripened wood cuttings are taken around mid-summer when the stems have been growing long enough to start to harden up, and hardwood cuttings are taken from mature stems at the end of the growing season. All stem cuttings are prepared in the same way. First, you remove the lower leaves from the piece that you have cut from the parent plant. You then trim the bottom of the cutting by making a cut in the stem just below a dormant bud on a joint or node. The cuttings should be about 7.5 cm / 3 in long. Cuttings taken from hardwood are often used to propagate trees and shrubs. These can be larger, around 25 cm / 10 in long. Sometimes with hardwood cuttings it can be helpful to leave a heel of old wood at the base rather than trimming the stem with a flat cut.

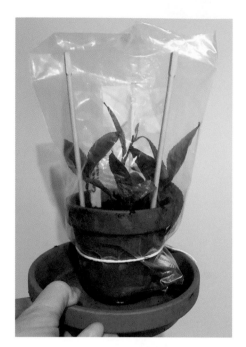

When using a recycled plastic bag to cover new cuttings, support it with a frame of chopsticks or bent wires.

Once the cuttings have been prepared, they should be inserted into a rooting medium, using a dibber to make a hole, and then they should be firmed in. I usually put cuttings around the edge of a pot. The cuttings should be inserted to a depth of about one inch, unless they are larger ripe-wood cuttings, in which case insert them to about half of their length. Use a free-draining compost, but do not be tempted to add too much additional sand, as this can mean that there will be too much air around the base of the cutting, and this can inhibit root growth. Water with a watering can fitted with a fine rose to settle the cuttings in, and then cover the pot with an impermeable layer to keep humidity levels high. For this you can use a large glass jar or the cut end of a recycled large plastic bottle. You can also use a recycled clear plastic bag. It is important that the cuttings are kept moist but not too moist and that they are exposed to the light. If you are using a plastic bag, keep it from sagging onto the cuttings themselves by supporting it with a frame of chopsticks or bent wires. Remove the covering once the cuttings are showing signs of growth. Do not be tempted to investigate to see whether any roots are developing. You will see the signs as the cuttings start to grow.

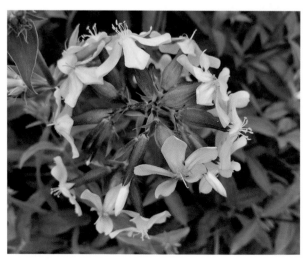

Soapwort (*Saponaria officinalis*).

Ripe wood or hardwood cuttings can be placed into a designated outdoor bed and left for a year to root before being transplanted. The same principles apply regarding properly firming in the cuttings and ensuring that the soil is free-draining but not too sandy.

Herbs can also be propagated using root cuttings. These are sections of root containing a growth bud, and they are planted below the surface of the soil with the bud facing upwards. Herbs such as Horseradish (*Armoracia rusticana*), Elecampane (*Inula helenium*), and Soapwort (*Saponaria officinalis*) are especially well suited to this form of propagation.

With cuttings, it is important not to delay the move to larger individual pots or more bed space. Overcrowded cuttings will not transplant well. As soon as the cuttings are established and starting to grow roots, separate them very carefully and transplant them, ensuring that you disturb the roots as little as possible. Cuttings do not always take, for various reasons: if the cuttings are not firmed in enough in the soil, excessive callous may form at the base because of excessive aeration; if the soil is not free-draining enough and the cuttings have been over-watered, the bases may rot; if the cuttings are from plants with pithy wood, they may have failed because you did not leave a heel with mature wood attached to the base

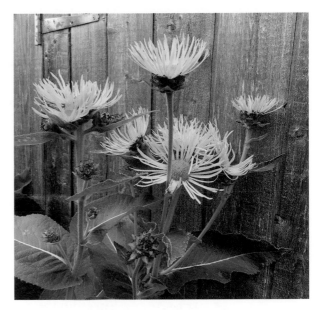

Elecampane (*Inula helenium*).

of the cutting. Do not be daunted by the ins and outs of taking cuttings. If you do not succeed at first, try again but try varying the growing conditions. Experience is a great teacher.

Division

This is a very simple method of vegetative propagation that is suitable for plants with multiple stems arising from a root system. The plant is pulled apart, and pieces are cut or severed so that each piece has some roots and either a piece of stem or a stem bud. These pieces can be planted and will form new plants. Plants with a fibrous root system, such as Goldenrod (*Solidago virgaurea*) or Lady's Mantle (*Alchemilla mollis*), are ideal subjects for increasing by division. You can also separate large clumps of Marshmallow (*Althaea officinalis*), Lemon Balm (*Melissa officinalis*), or St John's Wort (*Hypericum perforatum*). Division is best done during the dormant season, because the new plant does not have to support the demands of mature foliage while it has, temporarily, a depleted root system. If you do have to try this during the growing season (something that can happen if you are making a visit to a green-fingered friend and they offer you a piece of one of their established plants), then minimize the stress on the new plant by trimming the aerial parts right back. It will establish much better, and you will be able to enjoy the beauty of the flowers and foliage the following year. With any propagation by division, make sure that each section of plant that you are choosing to replant has both roots and a healthy stem or bud. Give the new plants plenty of care and attention until they are established.

Layering

Layering is a good way of propagating herbs *in situ*. It is well suited to plants like Rosemary (*Rosmarinus officinalis*), Sage (*Salvia officinalis*), and Bay (*Laurus nobilis*). With this method, the new plant is nourished by the parent plant until it is ready to grow independently. Choose low-growing, vigorous stems, and bend them down to see which point on the stem would naturally rest on the soil. You will need to choose a branch long enough to leave a section at least 5 cm / 2 in from the end to stay free of the soil. This will form the aerial parts of the new plant. Trim the leaves and side shoots off the section nearest to the parent plant. The length of the section that you trim will depend on the size of the plant and the size of the branch you are layering. Roughen the underside of the stem a little at the point that it would naturally touch the ground, and then peg it down, so that the treated area is in contact with the soil. Make sure that the soil at this point is weed-free, pliable, and free-draining, so that it encourages the plant to form roots at this point. Bend the section of the stem beyond the rooting area upward, so that it is vertical. You may find it helpful to secure the end by supporting it with a bamboo stake. The vertical orientation of the end of the stem is very important, because it encourages the formation of roots at the lowest point. Do not be tempted to leave the natural arching growth of the lower branches, since this would create an angle that is nearer 45° with the soil rather than 90°, and a more acute angle such as this does not encourage such effective rooting. Keep the rooting point moist and free from weeds for a growing season. Once the layer has developed roots, you can sever it from the parent plant with a sharp knife and transplant it.

You can also use this technique to reinvigorate plants such as Sage (*Salvia officinalis*) and Thyme (*Thymus vulgaris*), which have spread out and end up with an 'empty' centre and leggy growing branches falling outwards around the outside. To do this, you mound soil over the centre of the plant in the spring. Keep this soil mound firmed down and moist during the growing season. It can be a good idea to peg down the growing branches to stop them disturbing the soil as they are moved by the wind. By the autumn, many of the growing branches will have formed roots themselves and can be separated from the parent plant. Once you have harvested your new plants, you can remove the old plant from your garden, knowing that it is living on via its new offspring.

Records and labelling

It is essential to label pots and seed trays as they are planted with the species and, if applicable, the variety. It is very easy to lose track of what you have planted where. I would also recommend recording the date that you planted each batch, so that you can easily see how long it takes for each sowing to emerge or each batch of cuttings to form roots. You may find it helpful to have a garden record book, if you are that way inclined. Over time, recording information such as date planted, how long it took for the seeds to emerge and other factors that may seem noteworthy will deepen your knowledge of growing from seed in your unique environmental circumstances, and the variations that can be predicted in different years. Also, when growing rare or endangered plants such as Slippery Elm (*Ulmus fulva*) or Bloodroot (*Sanguinaria canadensis*), it is quite possible that germination can be spread out over a couple of subsequent springs. By recording the date of sowing alongside the species, you can check apparently unsuccessful batches for a further year or two, knowing that there may be further germination in the future. The knowledge and experience that you build-up can add to our collective knowledge about cultivating these plants in different locations and can help others to be more successful with growing them. The more people succeed in cultivating rare and endangered plants, the more will the pressure on wild populations be alleviated.

When my spiritual teacher, Akong Tulku Rinpoché, asked me to start growing Tibetan medicinal herbs, the

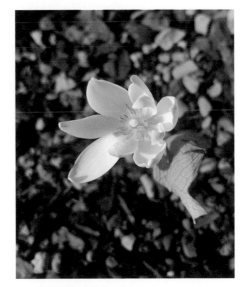

Bloodroot (*Sanguinaria canadensis*).

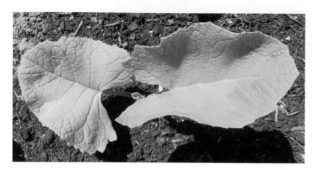

Himalayan Burdock, also known as Costus or Ruta
(*Saussurea lappa*), is officially extinct in the wild.

idea was to learn how to grow them here in the West and, eventually, to help to establish a sustainable supply chain to help take the pressure of wild populations. As part of this mission, I regularly attempt to grow plants that may not naturally grow in this country. I have learned a lot from this process and am still working on it. I do believe that many important Tibetan medicinal plants can be cultivated successfully in this country. Although I may not be in a position to produce crops on a commercial scale, I can learn how to cultivate the plants and propagate them so that others can grow them too. One of the plants that I cultivate, Himalayan Burdock, also known as Costus or Ruta (*Saussurea lappa*), is extinct in the wild. Other species may follow. To have viable populations in cultivation is a crucial back-up. Growing rare plants matters.

Many of the scarcer herbal medicines that we use in the West originate from the United States. It is inspiring to see the groundswell of people growing rare plants both in traditional cultivation and in wild locations. There is definitely room for more of this. If you would like to know more about growing endangered and scarce medicinal herbs native to the United States, I wholeheartedly recommend Rico Cech's book, *Growing At-Risk Medicinal Herbs*.[3]

If you are new to gardening or have not grown medicinal herbs before, I hope that you will feel inspired to make a start. Please try not to worry too much about whether or not you will 'get it right'. The reality is that sometimes you will be successful, and other times you will experience what can only be described as 'botanical setbacks'. I have had plenty of those during my life, and, to be honest, they show no sign of letting up. My work with conserving Tibetan medicinal plants means that I am constantly investigating what will work in this climate and what will not. It is a process of trial and error. In some ways, the setbacks are as important as the successes, although it usually does not seem like that at the time. Luckily, as growers, we are sustained by

---

[3] R. Cech, *Growing At-Risk Medicinal Herbs, Cultivation, Conservation and Ecology*, Herbal Reads LLC, 2002, 2017.

great joys to counterbalance our setbacks. It is always thrilling to see the emergence of new seedlings or the first flush of growth from a batch of cuttings that have rooted. I still get ridiculously excited when I see a species flowering for the first time in my herb garden.

Apart from all the many practical benefits of growing herbs, it is a truly great way to cultivate acceptance. We learn that obstacles can actually be helpful, keeping us on track and helping us to learn how to do things better. Working in the soil with our hands helps us to feel grounded and connected to the bigger picture, whatever that may be for us. When we grow herbs for medicine, we have the motivation that our harvests will bring benefit to others, and this is, in itself, deeply balancing, helping us to step away from our own habitual inner narratives and to form

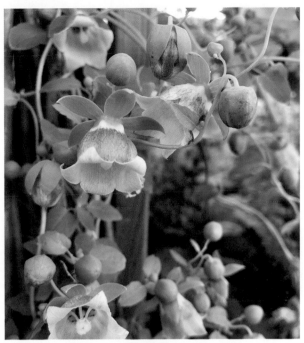

Dang shen (*Codonopsis pilosula*).

new ones. Growing herbs is so much more than just growing herbs. Once we start a herb garden, we cannot help but find ourselves growing alongside our medicines.

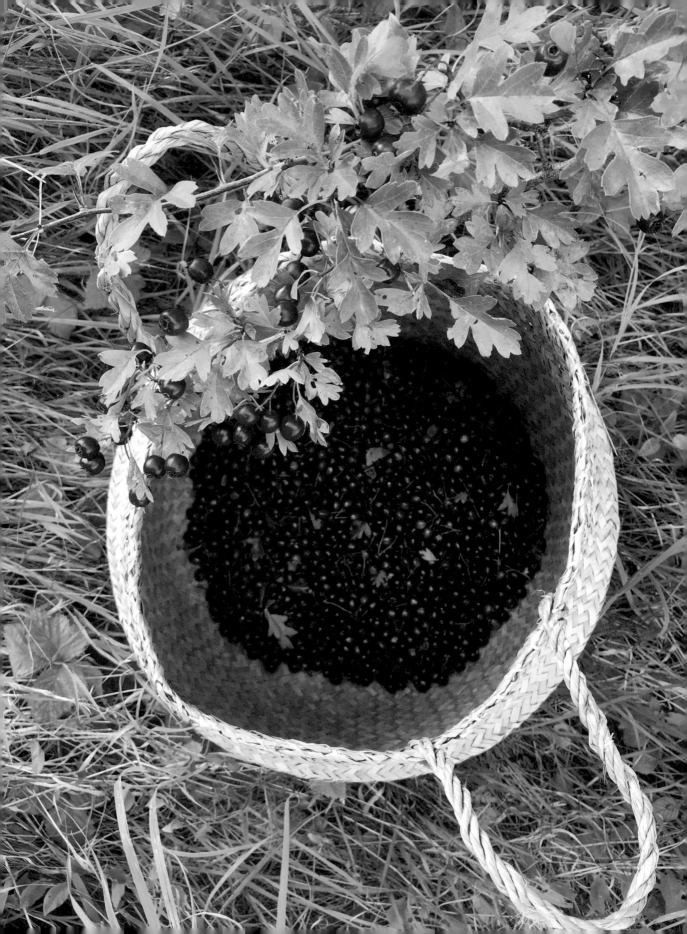

9

Harvesting

Harvesting is the culmination of our growing efforts and represents the beginning of the transition from a growing herb to medicine. Many, many gardeners are drawn to creating and maintaining beautiful medicinal herb gardens, but often the herbs are left unharvested, enjoyed for their beauty and scent but not fulfilling their full potential as agents of healing. It seems that as human beings we are deeply drawn to growing and working with herbs, but we have somehow lost the day-to-day knowledge of how to move beyond the growing part of the process. There is no doubt that herb gardens are beautiful and healing in their own right, but to me it feels so much more 'complete' to harvest at least some of them in order to capture their healing properties for ourselves and for others.

I used to think that every herbal student was taught 'hands-on' plant-based aspects of herbal medicine, but this is by no means the case. All too often practitioners tell me that they 'never learnt this stuff'. It is all very well for herbal educators to teach students about 'herbs and how herbs work', but if we lose the knowledge of how to grow and harvest them, we become vulnerable to losing access to the very herbs that we wish to work with.

In one sense harvesting herbs is one of the simplest and most natural things that we could do, but the way that we harvest them can have a very significant influence on their quality as medicines. By paying attention to when we harvest, how we harvest, and how we treat the crop once we take it back to our processing place, we can make quite a difference to the final quality of our herbs. The adjustments that we need to make at each step of the harvesting process are very straightforward and easy to implement, once you consider them. My aim in this chapter is to empower everyone, whether they are seasoned or new herbal harvesters, to produce the best possible medicines from herbs and to understand how this has been achieved. The main factors that influence the final quality of herbs and herbal medicine at harvest are the timing of harvest, the weather conditions, the actual harvesting technique, the containers into which the harvested herbs are put, the time lapse before they are processed or dried, and our mental attitude while harvesting.

Time to harvest

Each herb has an optimum growth stage and time of the year for harvest. Traditional times of harvest, recorded in old herbals, tend to have been specified because they coincide with when the medicinal constituents are at their peak. The best time to harvest depends on the type of medicine and plant part that is being harvested. In practice, your harvest timing may also be influenced by the prevailing land management of the place where you are harvesting. You may need to time your harvest to gather herbs before they have been mown down or ploughed up.

Above-ground parts, known as aerial parts, are usually best harvested when the plants are just about to flower. There are exceptions, though. Many herbs produce a mass of foliage early on in the season, but at the time of flower-

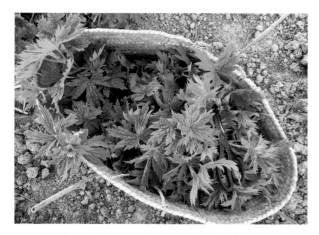

Motherwort is harvested before flowering when destined for herbal infusions.

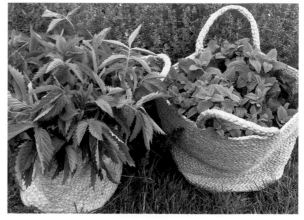

Lemon Balm and Agrimony foliage harvested before flowering.

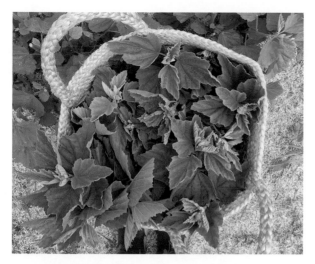

Marshmallow foliage, harvested early in the season.

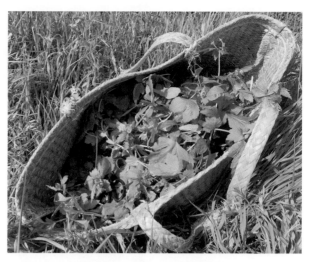

Foraged Wood Avens foliage.

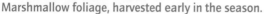

ing the foliage becomes rather sparse and not in such a good condition. The herbs I am thinking of here include herbs like Motherwort (*Leonurus cardiaca*), Agrimony (*Agrimonia eupatoria*), Marshmallow (*Althaea officinalis*) leaf – as opposed to the root – and Wood Avens (*Geum urbanum*). These herbs are usually gathered both for their leaves and for their flowering stalks. How-

ever, for these particular herbs I prefer to maximize the yield of leaves, especially if I intend to use them for herbal infusions. To achieve this, I aim to harvest earlier in the season, before flowering starts. I try to time it for when the leaves are vibrant and mature but have not started to die back at the base of the plant. Once the leaves start to die back at the base, they become less vibrant, as the plant concentrates its energy into the flowering stem. If I time my harvests right, I get an abundance of leaves, which are much more suitable for infusions, especially since I store my herbs whole and then cut them by hand once they are prescribed. If you have ever tried to cut by hand a large quantity of dried Motherwort stems with their very prickly seed heads, you will know that this can be a difficult and somewhat uncomfortable task. It is also worth pointing out that plants like Motherwort and Wood Avens seed

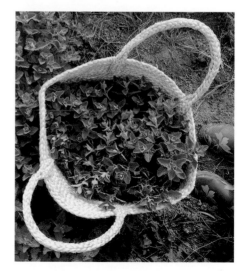

An early harvest of Catmint foliage for infusions.

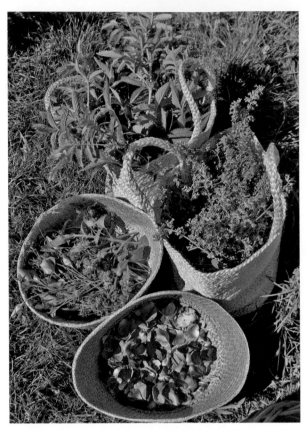

A later harvest showing Catmint in flower, also Agrimony, Borage, Eschscholzia, and Rose petals.

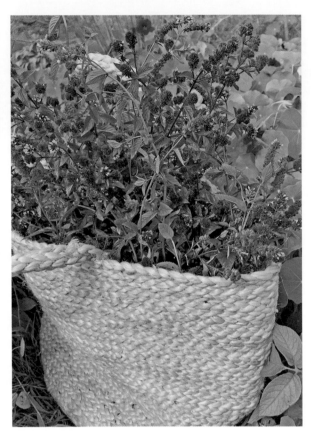

A harvest of flowering Peppermint; Nasturtium in flower behind.

very prolifically in the herb garden, and if you let them seed, you will end up with a mass of seedlings that need to be weeded out from in between your other crops. In the last few years I have started to cut all of my cultivated Motherwort and Wood Avens early in the season, in order to avoid this problem. This issue does not arise when wild harvesting, but I still recommend an early harvest of Wood Avens in order to get the best yield from your foraging efforts. Some plants are best left until flowering, as there is such a difference in the level of medicinal constituents. Peppermint (*Mentha piperita*), for example, has a much higher yield of essential oils at flowering, even though at this stage the leaf yield will be reduced. For the mints, I prefer to take some early harvests and some later ones, once the plants are flowering; I mix the batches together so that I get a good balance between the additional volume of vibrant leaves and the more potent flowering stems in the herb store.

Flowers

When taking harvests of flowers, the best growth stage to choose is when they have just fully opened. Your choice of timing will also be somewhat influenced by the land management of the area where the flowers are growing. It is worth getting to know this. For example, in the spring you may have access to meadows filled with Dandelion (*Taraxacum officinale*) flowers, and it is best to pick these before the first cut of silage is made. It is also better to gather at that very early stage when all of the flowers are yet to go to seed, because you can work through the crop, picking, knowing that every flower that you pick will be suitable. If you are harvesting Red Clover (*Trifolium pratense*) flowers, you need to examine each flower before picking, as they tend to mature over a wider time period. In practice, it is best to find an area where they are abundant and to pick them regularly until the area is either mown or the flowers go over. I like to walk through the same meadow every couple of days during the Red Clover season, gathering a small harvest each time. Over the season, the harvest mounts up in the herb store. Likewise, Daisies (*Bellis perennis*) bloom over an extended period, depending on the management of the place where they are growing. I usually gather my Daisies from a wide grass verge at the edge of a quiet country road near where I live. This verge is kept mown, and this management strategy has encouraged a proliferation of Daisies, which all flower at once during the spring. It is a fabulous sight to see such a large number of Daisies flowering *en masse*, and it makes it much easier to fill your basket if you find a concentrated source such as this. Knowing that the area is kept mown, I drop everything in order to make my harvest as soon as I see that the Daisies are blooming. This is not so much because of the growth stage that the Daisies are at, but because I know that if I delay, I risk losing the chance of harvesting clean vibrant Daisies uncontaminated by short pieces of mown grass and the tyre tracks of a ride-on mower. Last year I picked my fill of Daisies from this particular place on a sunny Sunday afternoon. The

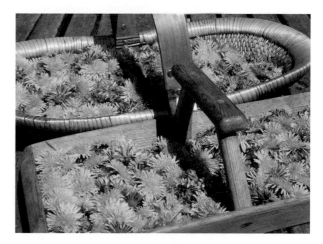

Dandelion flowers.

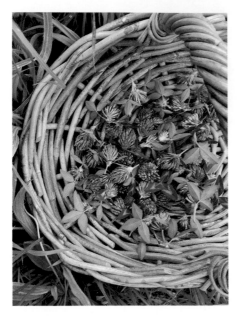

A small harvest of Red Clover flowers.

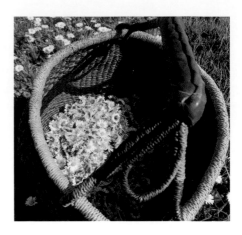

Daisy flower harvest.

very next afternoon I saw that the area had been mown. It is hard not to feel sad when you see muddy tyre tracks and the clumps of grass cuttings where the previous day there had been a swathe of white and pink, but I took comfort in knowing that at least some of those Daisies had found their way into herbal medicine.

When harvesting cultivated flower crops, I find it easier to make regular harvests of my flower crops by cutting every single flower that is open. At the same time, I can deadhead any flowers that have gone over. If you do this, your basket will be filled with flowers that range from just first opening to those that are fully open. You can also include those that are older but still in good condition. If you are able to maintain regular harvests every two or three days throughout the flowering season, you will find that deadheading will not be necessary. I like to harvest my Calendula (*Calendula officinalis*) crop daily throughout the flowering season, provided that weather conditions allow.

Seeds

The timing for harvesting seeds is much more critical than is the case with other plant parts. Once a plant has produced seeds, those seeds are designed to be dispersed, so that they can produce new plants. You need to harvest just at the right moment, when the seeds are ripe but have not yet dropped from the plant. There are two main seed-harvesting strategies. The first is to wait for the seed to ripen on the growing plant, and the second is to cut the plant and allow the seed to ripen afterwards. On a large scale these two options are described as 'field ripening' and 'stook ripening'. If you allow the seed to ripen on the plant, you need to wait until the seed is plumped out and hard, showing that it has been fertilized and has matured fully. It is likely that when most of the seeds on the head are ready, some will have started to fall. It is a juggling act to wait until the seeds are ripe but to catch them before they either fall to the ground or are eaten by the birds, although I like to think that there should be enough for everyone. Taking all of these factors into account, you need to try to judge it so that when you harvest, you will get the best yield of good-quality seed. You will need to inspect your crops very regularly at the time when the seeds are ripening. Usually, as soon as you notice the seeds changing colour, you need to harvest. The second option of stook ripening can lead to a higher yield of seed, but it takes practice to get the timing right. You aim to cut the stalks about two weeks before the seed is fully ripe. The seed is softer at this

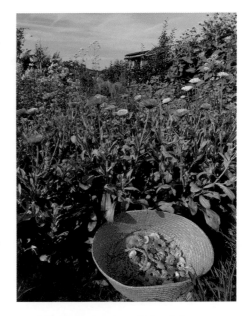

I like to harvest my Calendula crop daily throughout the flowering season.

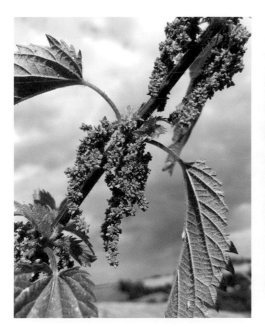

Nettle seeds at the perfect stage for harvesting.

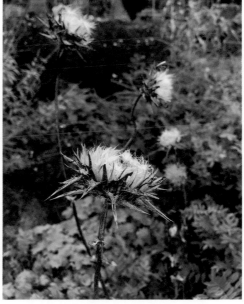

Milk Thistle seed heads ready for harvest.

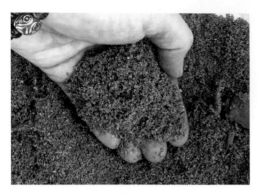

Nettle seeds once removed from the stems.

stage and can be described as being 'doughy'. The cut stems can be gathered together into sheaves and stacked in little stacks, called stooks, which keep the seed heads off the ground; on a smaller scale, you can lay your cut stems out onto drying trays indoors and let them ripen, away from adverse weather and birds. It is worth noting here that some seeds are deliberately harvested at an even earlier stage. Wild Oats (*Avena sativa*) are gathered when they are immature, and Nettle seeds are harvested when they are green and plump, before they change colour.

Roots

Roots are usually dug when the plant is dormant; in theory, this can be at any time between autumn and early spring. The traditional time to harvest roots is during the autumn, and you will read this recommendation in most herbals. In the autumn, the aerial parts of the plants generally die down, and all of the plant's energy is concentrated in the roots. Part of the rationale for

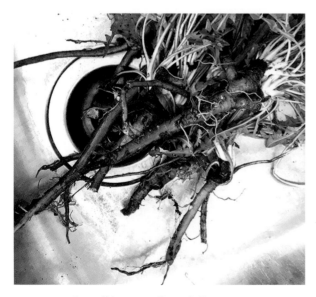

A small harvest of Dandelion roots.

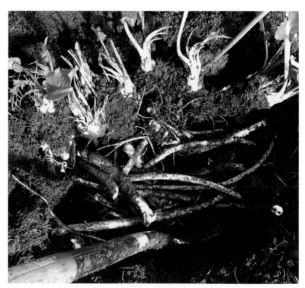

Harvesting Horseradish roots.

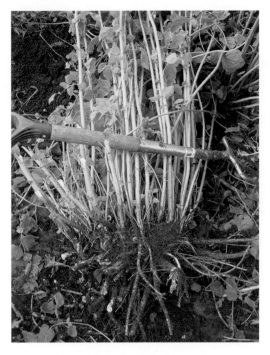

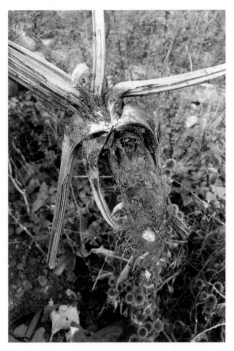

Harvesting Marshmallow roots.

A large Burdock root dug in autumn.

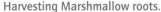

autumn harvesting is that in the autumn it is often easier to gain access to the soil and dig the crop without causing compaction. At the end of the summer the soil is friable and not too waterlogged, making the roots easier to dig out and to clean. Another consideration is that digging roots at this time will enable the most successful replanting of root cuttings. However, the balance of constituents of roots does change between autumn and spring. Roots dug in autumn have higher levels of inulin, making them more palatable and especially suitable as a prebiotic mineral-rich tonic. If your main intention is to use Dandelion (*Taraxacum officinale*) root as a digestive stimulant, you will be looking to maximize the bitterness of your harvest, and to do this I recommend harvesting in the spring. I was taught to harvest Dandelion and other bitter roots in the spring.

If you have very heavy clay soil, however, and digging in the spring is not practical in your situation, digging them in the autumn may be the best strategy. When you come to use your own Dandelion roots as medicine, you can bear in mind that they may not be as bitter as they might be. If you feel that it would be helpful, in certa*in situ*ations you can adjust your prescribing

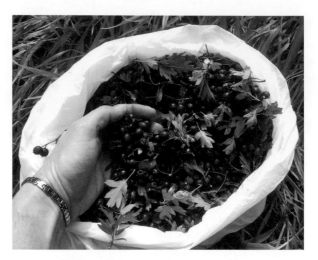

A harvest of Hawthorn berries.

by combining the Dandelion root with other bitters. The medicine that you make from your own roots is for you to get to know and to work with. Working with living, variable plants and the environment that they grow in encourages us to be flexible in our approach, to make adjustments, as needed and not feel that there is only one right way of doing things. What matters is that we understand why we have chosen to do it the way that we have done, and that we have connected with the herb in our own way.

Fruit

Fruit is harvested when available and ripe. The best-quality fruit is usually gathered when it is not over-ripe, although if you have fruit that is very ripe and you intend to process it immediately, it is not such a problem. An exception to this is the harvesting of Chaste Berry (*Vitex agnus-castus*), which is best left on the plant to mature and harvested once the leaves have fallen. Rose-hips (*Rosa* spp.) are considered to be sweeter after the first frost, but you will find that they have a tendency to be affected by surface moulds at this stage. This may not matter if you intend to process them straight away, into syrup, for example, but for your dispensary I recommend harvesting them in the autumn, when they are in the best condition.

Bark

Bark is harvested when the plant is dormant; harvesting it can be combined with pruning or coppicing. You should not harvest bark from a growing tree, as you might damage it. If bark is removed from all the way around a growing tree, it will be 'ring barked' and will die. This is why traditional old parkland trees in grazed areas are usually protected with mini fenced enclosure areas and why the young trees in newly established woodlands are usually protected by grow tubes or spiral stem guards. If you are planning to harvest bark from your own plants, it is best to coppice them, removing stems from the base once every four years. The medicinal constituents tend to be highest in the spring and when the sap starts to rise, so this is a good reason to choose the spring for your harvest of coppiced stems or branches. It is also much easier

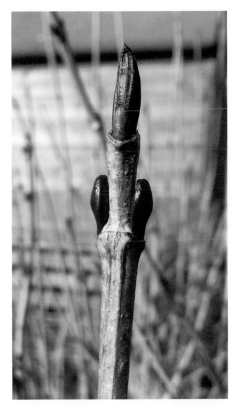
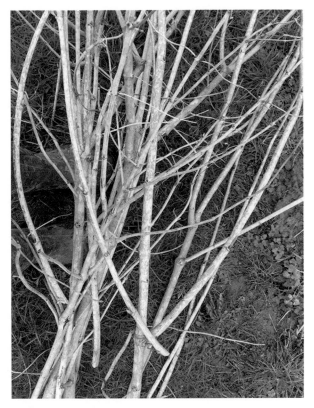

Cramp Bark is traditionally harvested in early spring, just before the buds burst. On the right is a harvest of Cramp Bark stems from a coppiced plant.

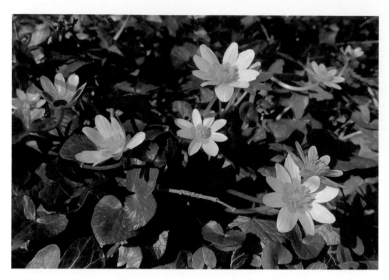

Pilewort plants are harvested while they are flowering in early spring.

to strip the bark from branches or stems that have been freshly cut in the spring. Do not be tempted to make a large harvest of branches and then gradually strip the bark from them over the next few weeks. Believe me, the difference between stripping moist bark in the spring and dried bark from older branches or summer wind-falls is enormous.

Cramp Bark (*Viburnum opulus*) and White Willow (*Salix alba*) bark are traditionally harvested in early spring, just before the buds burst. Oak bark is harvested a little later, in May. Having said this, you may need to harvest bark at other times, when faced with the opportunity to make use of a fallen branch or tree. If the bark is in good condition and you are able to strip it, then take a harvest. Provided the bark has the characteristic scent of the medicine in question, it is better to take the harvest at the 'wrong time' than to let it go to waste.

Whole plants

Whole plants should be harvested when they are in flower. In my practice, Pilewort (*Ranunculus ficaria*) is the only herb that I regularly harvest as a whole plant. This is one of the earliest harvests of the year, as Pilewort flowers in early spring.

Seaweed

I harvest seaweed in the summer from select beaches with very clean water. I always gather seaweed from the sea where it has been submerged in clean sea water rather than being washed up and exposed to unknown polluting agents, including dog waste, on the beach. My favourite seaweed-gathering place is a beach in West Dorset, where my family had spent every summer holiday while I was growing up. My cousin and I used to explore the Black-thorn (*Prunus spinosa*) thickets on the undercliff and clamber about on the cliff tops. We regularly walked along the secret smugglers path that led from the sea to the cliff top, but we chose to walk it downhill, as it was much easier that way. It must have been really gruelling to climb up there in the dead of night with a barrel of French brandy on your back. I still know every inch of that beach and the land surrounding it. Whenever I walk there now, I am completely filled with happy memories of collecting glass stones, hag stones, and, of course, seaweed.

Strictly speaking, the ideal time to harvest seaweed is in the spring when it is growing most vibrantly, but sea temperatures here are bracing at the best of times, so I prefer to wait until late summer. At my gathering spot the water is very clear, and it is easy to see the best areas of growing seaweed. Once the tide is out, I wade into the water and dive down to pick the best and most vibrant fronds of Kelp (*Laminaria digitata* and other species) and Sea Lettuce (*Ulva lactuca*), placing them each into their own gathering bag. Once I have gathered enough, I store the bags of wet seaweed in the shade until I am ready to return home. Sometimes I set up a temporary drying line on the beach to start the process of drying and make the bags lighter to carry at the end of the day.

Recently I ran out of Kelp early in the year and needed some urgently, so I braved the water on a sunny day in late spring. To say it was absolutely freezing was an understatement, but I did man-age to gather enough to fulfil a much-needed prescription. It is not something that I relish repeat-ing, so I heartily recommend that you gather what you need during the summer.

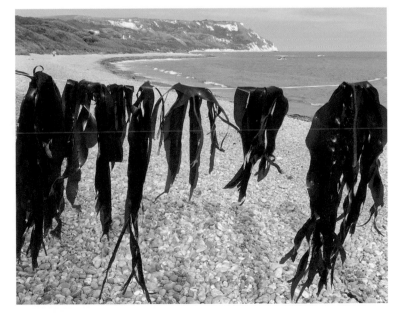

Sometimes I set up a temporary drying line on the beach to start the drying process.

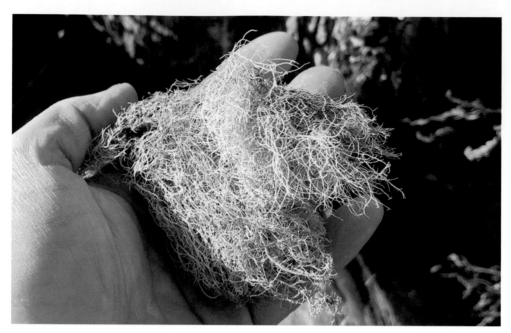

Gathering Beard Lichen in the Scottish borders.

Lichens

Lichens are best harvested from fallen branches, as they are so slow-growing and this helps to conserve the stocks on growing trees. If medicinal lichens, such as Beard Lichen (*Usnea* spp.), grow abundantly in your home gathering area, then I suggest that you go out after high winds and look for fallen branches of Birch (*Betula pendula* or *Betula pubescens*) or conifers that are covered in *Usnea*. If, like me, you do not live near abundant sources of *Usnea*, you may need to gather it sparingly whenever you visit the area, again focusing on fallen branches where possible.

Mushrooms

Medicinal mushrooms are gathered in autumn and winter. It is a joyous thing to find an abundance of Turkey Tail (*Trametes versicolor*) growing on an old hardwood log or to come around a bend in a track and see a colony of beautiful Fly Agaric (*Amanita muscaria*) among a stand of pine or spruce.

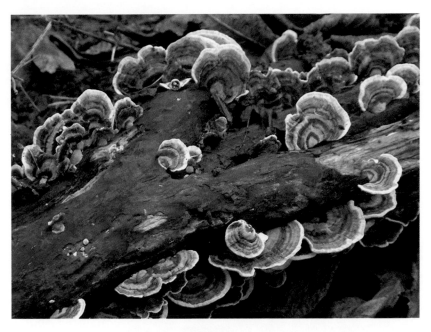

An abundance of Turkey Tail growing on an old hardwood log.

Weather conditions at harvest

When harvesting herbs, it is important to consider the weather conditions. There are some herbal harvests that require good weather conditions, and others that can pretty much be harvested in any weather. Roots and whole

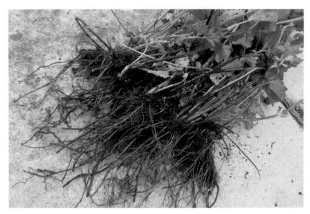

A harvest of Wood Avens roots with most of the soil shaken off.

plants that will need to be washed before processing can be harvested during most weather conditions, provided that you can dig the soil without causing damage. Water-logged conditions are best avoided, because of the risk of causing soil compaction; in hard frosts, it becomes impossible to dig. The best time to harvest roots is when the soil is friable and easily dug. At this time, most of the soil can be shaken off the roots before the washing process begins, making it much easier.

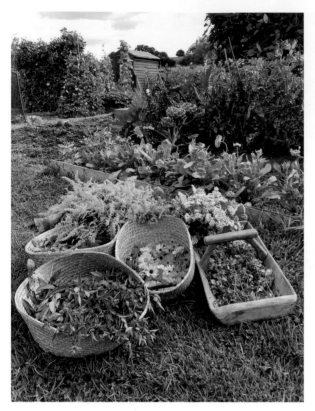

Aerial parts of herbs should be harvested when they
are dry to the touch.

Aerial parts of herbs should be harvested when they are dry to the touch, so it is the perfect excuse to be a 'fair-weather' herbalist. If you enjoy reading old traditional herbals, you will see repeated references to harvesting once the dew has dried. Whether surface moisture is due to dew or rain, you need to avoid it. Wet herbs are more prone to damage through compaction and dry more slowly. If you intend to process your fresh herbs and skip the need for drying, you should be aware that processing wet herbs will lead to a much lower-quality product. So, rainy days or early mornings are generally not suitable for herbal harvesting. Likewise, if you are growing in an area that requires irrigation, make sure you avoid overhead irrigation just prior to harvest. The advantage of starting with dry herbs is that it is best to harvest clean herbs whenever possible, as this removes the need for washing.

In the spring and summer, when it is the main time for harvesting flowers and above-ground parts, I always take a keen interest in the weather forecast. I want to make the most of dry periods, when the herbs will be properly dry on the surface. I often dash out to harvest a basket of something before a predicted rainstorm or spell of wet weather. If the wet weather is prolonged, it can become a bigger issue. I remember some very wet springs and summers that seriously hampered my ability to harvest the herbs that I needed. One year it seemed to rain continuously throughout July and August, and there was widespread flooding in the South West of the United Kingdom. It was worrying to think that I might not be able to harvest the herbs that I needed that season. Every day it poured and poured, and my angst over the lack of opportunities to harvest was compounded by the frustration of my kids, who wanted to be outside during their summer holiday break from school. Finally, there was a break in the weather, and we were all mightily

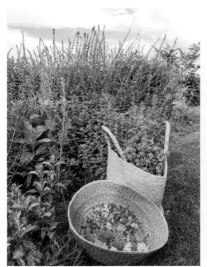
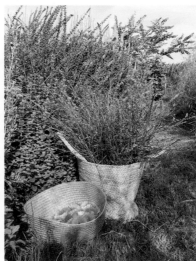
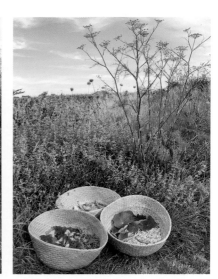

Fair-weather harvesting. *Left*: Motherwort, Horehound, Yarrow, and Calendula. *Centre*: Vervain and Calendula. *Right*: Nasturtium flowers and leaves, with Borage, Mullein flowers, and Calendula.

relieved. Experiences like that, although they do lead to some stress at the time, are really a lesson in acceptance and in not taking the gathering of herbs for granted. As time has gone on, I have learnt to be more in tune with external circumstances. I try to accept that if the weather is adverse, I just have to be patient.

With bark, I prefer to harvest when the bark is dry, but this is less critical, as bark is more resilient to handling and it dries quite quickly anyway. Like-wise, mushrooms and lichens can be harvested in any weather conditions, although always aim to let them surface-dry before processing. Fruit is best harvested when dry, but again, provided it is not over-ripe, you do have some leeway with weather conditions, since you can leave fruit to air-dry for a little before processing. If you are harvesting seeds, they must be totally dry, so choose a sunny day. As already described, the harvesting of seaweed is best done on a sunny, warm day, but if you are hardy or have a wetsuit, it can be done whenever you like.

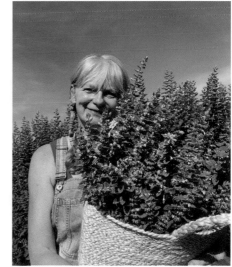

Gathering Lemon Balm on a hot, dry day.

Purity of harvest

When harvesting, it is essential to get a crop that is not contaminated by other species. If you end up with a harvest that contains a high proportion of non-crop species, it will be, at best, less effective than it should be, and, at worst, it may be harmful. These pitfalls are avoided by proper identification of the plants being foraged as well as careful and mindful harvests of cultivated crops to ensure that weed species are not included. It is definitely worth spending extra time in the field and ensuring that you are picking only the target species. Sorting out the odd stray weed that has found its way into the basket is much easier to do at the time of cutting. Once the plant material is back at your processing area and may be beginning to wilt slightly, it is more difficult to spot and remove weeds. If you have gathered a very weedy harvest basket, it really slows down the flow of the processing work – and if processing takes longer, there is more scope for deterioration of the harvested herbs.

Containers for harvesting

You will need suitable containers or receptacles for your harvested herbs. For me this is an excuse to have a large collection of baskets and trugs (trough-shaped, shallow baskets) of all different shapes and sizes. To be honest, this is not strictly necessary. In brazenly admitting this, I am hoping that my husband skims through this chapter and does not notice what I have just said. Baskets and trugs are beautiful and practical, but you can also use canvas shopping bags, trays or even cotton pillowcases or bed sheets. In general, I recommend that you aim to use containers or bags made of natural materials, since they allow the harvested plant material to breathe. The exception to this is when harvesting roots or whole plants. Tubs or buckets are most suitable for these, since they can also be used to do the first couple of rinses and are easily cleaned afterwards.

One of the main principles of successfully harvesting aerial parts is that compaction should be avoided in order to prevent bruising. Flowers such as Chamomile (*Matricaria recutita*) and Calendula (*Calendula officinalis*) are best harvested into rigid, flattish receptacles that allow the harvested flowers to

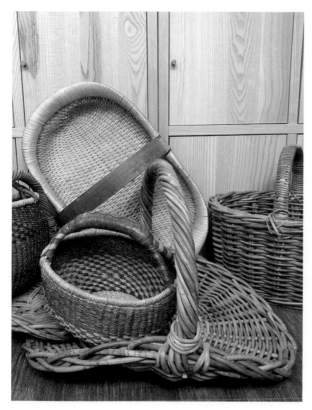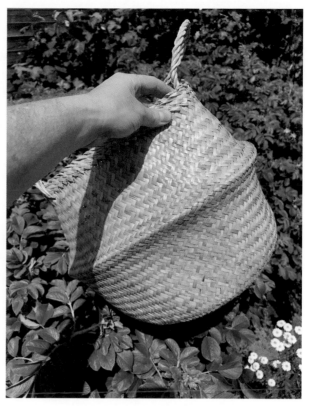

Baskets and trugs are beautiful and practical, but you can also use canvas shopping bags, trays, or even cotton pillowcases. High-sided baskets are useful when harvesting light plant material in windy conditions.

be placed in a single layer, or at least a very shallow one. The problem with using a canvas bag or a bed sheet is that when you gather your harvest up, the flowers are pushed against each other and are likely to become compressed and bruised, even on a short journey back to your processing area. If you do not have a herb basket or trug, use a tray for this job, or spread a canvas bag wide open on a tray, so that your harvest can be transported without causing compression of the contents. In practice, when working on a self-sufficient scale, flowers such as Calendula and Chamomile are harvested little and often throughout the growing season, making it easier to avoid bruising.

Leafy herbs, such as Nettle (*Urtica dioica*), Cleavers (*Galium aparine*), Agrimony (*Agrimonia eupatoria*), Lady's Mantle (*Alchemilla mollis*), and Raspberry (*Rubus idaeus*), are more resilient and can be collected into larger and deeper containers. Even so, bruising needs to be carefully avoided by speedy process-

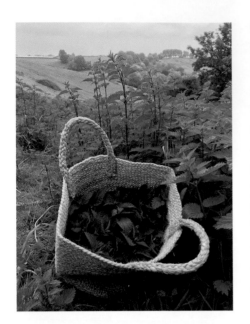

A basket of Nettles. When harvesting stems, I like to place them into my baskets so that they are all lying the same way.

ing and careful placement into the harvesting container. I have several large flexible baskets that, as well as being well suited to the job in hand, serve as a useful measure of the quantity I need to harvest. For example, I know that each year I need to harvest at least six large baskets of Nettle. I also know that one basket will probably fill two of my dehydrators once the leaves are plucked from the stems. Knowing my baskets and their capacity helps me to pace my harvesting in tandem with dehydrator availability. When harvesting stems, I like to place them into my baskets so that they are all lying the same way. This helps to reduce the risk of contaminating clean upper leaves with lower leaves that may have soil splash. It also considerably simplifies the process of trimming and laying out the herbs when you get back to your processing area. By laying the herbs in the same direction, you can remove them from the basket without pulling them through each other – something that can result in damage and bruising.

If I were to distil my basket recommendations to two type of baskets, I would suggest that you start with one large woven basket and one smaller, wider and flatter trug. The large woven basket will be light to carry when out foraging but has enough rigidity to minimize damage to the herbs and make it easier to orientate the stems while you are cutting them. The trug will be more suitable for harvests of flowers. If you are a basket addict, then I recommend that you consider adding a deeper, heavier basket to your collection to use when harvesting light plant material, such as Rose (*Rosa* spp.) petals, Lime (*Tilia* spp.) flowers, or Dandelion (*Taraxacum officinalis*) leaves, in windy conditions. I have a heavy potato basket for this purpose, and it has served me very well for many years.

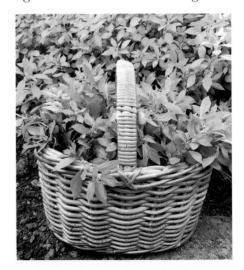

A heavy potato basket full of freshly harvested Pellitory-of-the-Wall.

Time lapse before processing or drying

It is essential to minimize the time lapse between harvest and processing or drying. As soon as plant material is cut, it begins to heat up, and the constituents start to deteriorate. Anyone familiar with the process of hay-making will know how much effort is made to cut the hay when the weather forecast predicts a good few days of dry, hot weather. If you have never thought about hay-making then think about what happens when you mow a lawn and heap up the grass cuttings. They heat up quite quickly, as micro-organisms start to break down the plant material. When making hay, the farmer aims to get the moisture content of the cut grass down as quickly as possible by turning it regularly, exposing each part of the crop to the sunshine and the drying breeze. Hay that lies in the field too long, reabsorbing moisture each evening and then drying again the next day, rapidly reduces in quality. If the hay crop is fully rehydrated in a rain storm, it will lose even more quality. In a worst-case scenario, the entire hay crop is completely spoiled and cannot be used. Hay-making may seem like an idyllic and gentle part of rural life, but it is actually an exacting art, and much of the economic viability of the farm's year ahead depends on the crop being preserved well. No wonder everyone feels happy relief once the crop has been safely gathered in. My own experiences of making hay in the past taught me a lot about how to treat herbs when they are harvested and dried.

When drying herbs, then, it is essential to avoid a long delay between harvest and drying. The longer the herbs sit around, the more they will deteriorate. A self-sufficient herbalist has an advantage in that quantities harvested will be smaller and more manageable than those harvested by large-scale

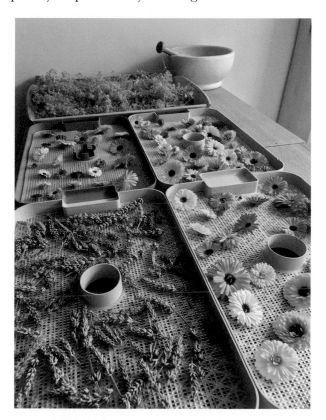

With flowers it is important to harvest only the quantity that can be laid out or processed within an hour of picking. Pictured are trays of Lavender, Calendula, and Lady's Mantle flowers laid out at my clinic straight after harvesting.

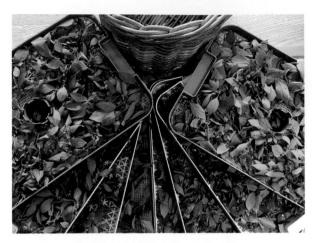

Pellitory-of-the-Wall laid out on trays.

commercial herb growers. Each batch needs to be laid out, processed or placed in your drying system, as soon as possible. This is especially important for flowers, leaves, and aerial parts in general. A good rule of thumb is to harvest only the quantity that can be laid out or processed within an hour of picking. Roots are usually more resilient and can withstand a longer holding time. If you do need to gather large quantities of certain herbs, it is preferable to make several smaller harvests over a period of consecutive days or look into increasing your drying capacity.

Mental attitude when harvesting

It is important to have a good mental attitude, or at the very least to avoid a negative state of mind, while harvesting herbs. Since everything is interconnected, our state of mind will have an influence on the medicine that we are harvesting and making. Tibetan medicine teaches that as we harvest medicinal plants, we should maintain the attitude that we wish these plants to be of benefit to those that need them. I like to repeat mantras and do healing visualizations. Whatever spiritual framework you feel most comfortable connecting with, I recommend that you set a positive healing intention before harvesting. If you are feeling emotionally unstable or out of sorts, then by all means go and sit with your herbs but save any harvesting for a better day.

Harvesting techniques

Aerial parts

For herbs that are harvested by cutting leafy stems, I cut each stem individually, using a pair of sharp secateurs or heavy-duty scissors. That way I can choose how low down the stem I cut, avoiding discoloured or damaged leaves.

I can also make sure that unwanted plant species do not find their way into the basket. This technique allows me to have more control over where I make each cut. With plants such as Agrimony (*Agrimonia eupatoria*) or Wormwood (*Artemisia absinthum*), I aim to cut the plant just above a node, so that it will branch out again and offer more stems for a late harvest. The line between harvesting and pruning can be blurred, especially with shrubs such as Rosemary (*Rosmarinus officinalis*) and Bay (*Laurus nobilis*).

Flowers

Flowers are delicate and deteriorate quickly, so the most important principle when harvesting them is to minimize the time lapse between harvest and processing. Avoid compressing the crop by piling it too high in the harvesting containers, as it will start to heat up very quickly. Inevitably you will find that bugs and insects will be attracted to your basket and will find their way into it on the flowers that you are harvesting. Gently shake each flower to dislodge the bugs before you place it into the basket. Some flowers, such as Dandelion (*Taraxacum officinale*) and Meadowsweet (*Filipendula ulmaria*), are especially prone to being filled with little black bugs. When harvesting these, try covering your basket with a thick white cloth and leaving it for an hour in a shady place before taking it back to your processing area. The bugs are attracted to the light, and many congregate on the under surface of the cloth. Carefully remove the cloth, and take it away from the basket to shake the bugs off. You can also try harvesting these flowers on a cloudy day, as the bug load seems less. Once you get back to your processing area, lay out your flower harvest on trays, and open the windows, so that any remaining bugs can find their way out. I spend a lot of time gathering up and releasing bugs from the windows of my clinic.

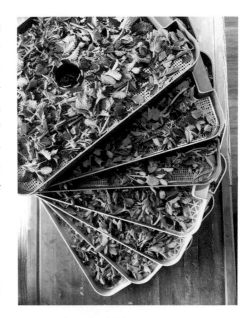

Catmint laid out on trays.

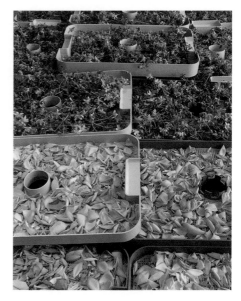

Rose petals and St John's Wort flowers laid out on trays.

Bark

I usually harvest my bark medicines by coppicing. Use a pruning saw to cut the base of the chosen stem with a cut that slopes away from the centre of the coppice stool. The purpose of the sloping cut is to angle rainwater away from the centre of the plant. Cut each stem carefully and support the weight of the stem as you get nearly all the way through its base. You want to avoid the cut stem tearing a piece of bark away from the remaining part of the plant as it falls. Be careful not to damage adjacent stems when using the pruning saw. Sometimes this is difficult to achieve, and in practice it is a good idea to harvest all the stems on a coppice at a time. Once you have cut your coppice stems, trim off and discard the small end twigs before transporting the main stems to your processing place to strip off the bark.

Roots

Root digging is best done with a fork, since this minimizes mechanical damage to your harvest. Start a reasonable distance from the plant and work gently, freeing each root with a small hand fork and your hands as you get closer the unearthing the plant. Some roots such as Burdock (*Arctium lappa*) and Liquorice (*Glycyrrhiza glabra*) grow very deep, and it is quite a marathon job to harvest them. For these you will need a narrow spade. Large plants like Elecampane (*Inula helenium*) and Comfrey (*Symphytum officinale*) can have very large and heavy root systems. These can cause all but the strongest of garden forks to break if you are not careful. It can be a good idea to enlist the help of a friend, so that you can apply leverage from opposite

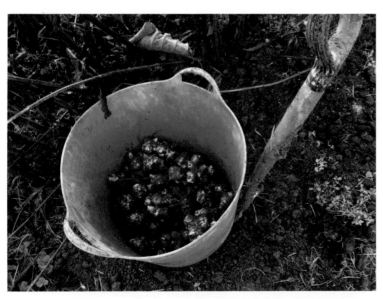

Jerusalem Artichoke tubers harvested into a tub, ready for on-site washing.

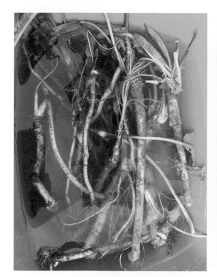
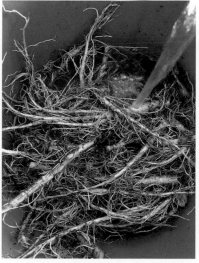
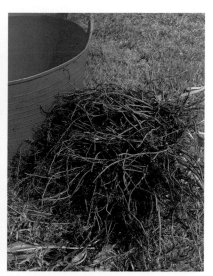

Washing Horseradish (*left*) and Teasel (*centre*) roots. *Right:* Washing Culver's Root on site.

sides of the plant simultaneously. Take your time. Try to minimize broken and damaged roots and also, for that matter, broken tools.

When digging roots, it is the ideal time to divide large plants. Parts that are surplus to requirements or are unsuitable for medicine can be replanted into the newly dug earth. Culver's Root (*Veronicastrum virginicum*), for example, develops a very dense root crown with a central area that is difficult to clean and process for medicine, whereas it has side roots that are long and straight and easy to clean. With plants such as these, it makes sense to snip off the side roots and replant the central crown, so that you can take another harvest in two or three years.

Roots will need to be washed. Separate the aerial parts from the roots and add them to your compost heap or return them to the soil. Place the harvested roots into a bucket or tub, and, if possible, rinse them two or three times

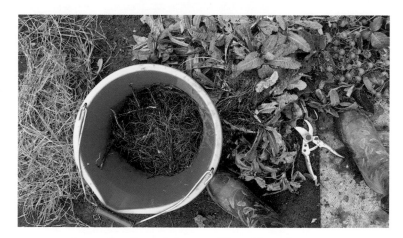

Separating the aerial parts of Teasel from the roots.

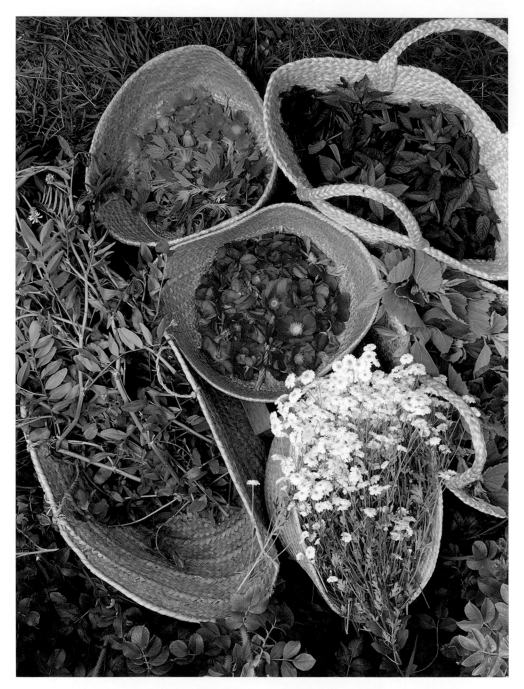

A summer harvest: from top left clockwise: Calendula and Motherwort, Peppermint, Marshmallow leaves, Feverfew flowers, Goat's Rue, and Rose petals (*middle*).

on site, using your fingers to tease the soil away from the root system and rubbing the larger roots to remove most of the soil. Return the water and the soil to the growing area. Once most of the soil has been washed from the roots, you can take them back to your processing area for scrubbing.

Fruit

Fruit is harvested by hand when ripe, but not over-ripe. Pick fruit by hand or snip clusters of fruit and place them carefully into your basket. If you are harvesting them before the first frost, they will be quite resilient to handling and storage. Fruit harvested after a frost will need to be processed immediately.

Seeds

Seeds are usually cut in seed heads, and the individual seeds are separated from their pods back in your processing area. Seeds are very resilient, so you can take your time over this task, and possibly postpone it to a spell of wet weather.

Seaweeds

Pick individual fronds directly from where they are growing under the water. Take care to positively identify each species, and place them into separate gathering containers, as they are more difficult to separate later. Once back home, hang them up to drip dry for a while before taking them to your processing place. I always hang mine on the washing line.

Summary

Attention to detail during harvesting makes a big difference to the final quality of the crop. If we carry out each step of the process in a positive, mindful, conscientious manner, we will end up with much higher-quality medicine than herbs that have been harvested in bulk with the attitude that it is a chore. Whether we are wildcrafting or cultivating our herbs, it is deeply satisfying to harvest them in tune with the seasons and with positive healing intention.

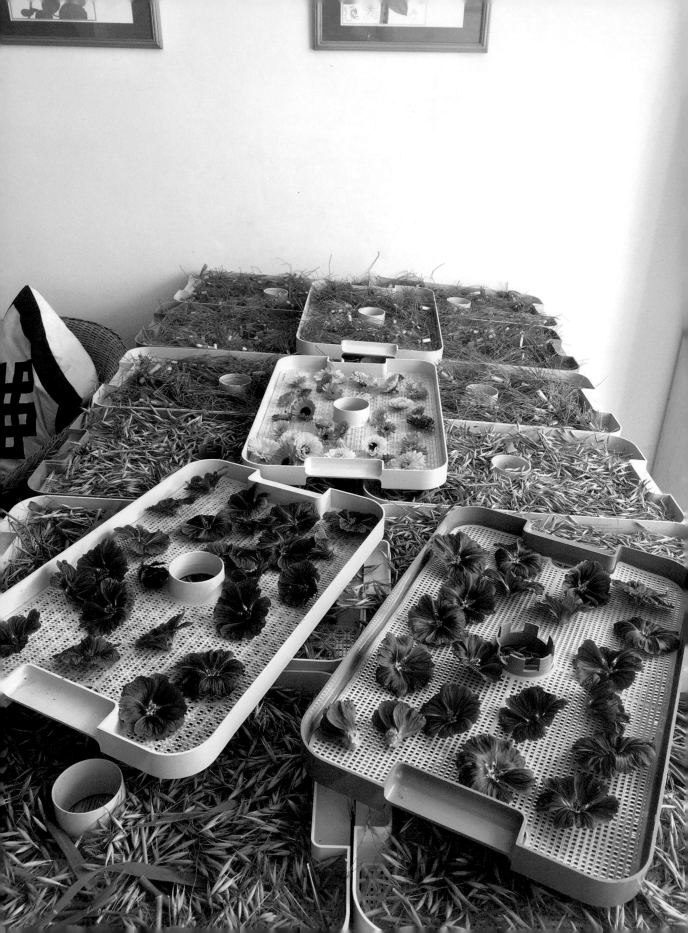

10

Drying

Before I describe the various techniques for drying herbs and the principles involved in preserving maximum therapeutic quality, I would like to tackle the whole issue of why it can be a good idea to dry herbs in the first place. I have always dried my own herbs. My Western herbal mentors, Edith, Barbara, and Ifanca, taught me to work with dried herbs, and in Tibetan medicine we are taught that it is normal practice to use dried herbs. Drying herbs suits my way and scale of working very well, but I often meet people who feel that drying herbs in order to make herbal medicines is a terrible thing to do. I agree that there is nothing better than making a pot of herbal tea or a decoction using herbs just picked from one's own apothecary garden. It is also lovely to make tinctures and infused oils from fresh herbs, provided that adjustments are made to compensate for the extra water content. I am certainly not against using fresh herbs for medicine, it is just that drying herbs brings a number of advantages for certain types of herbal practices, especially if those dried herbs are of outstanding vibrancy and quality. Let me explain.

First, if we are using herbs to treat patients and only ever make tinctures from fresh herbs, we need to make enough to last for the entire year during the time when each plant is at the optimal stage for harvesting. This may be a great solution if we need only enough to treat a few patients, but if we find ourselves treating many patients and needing to make quite large volumes of tincture, it becomes logistically more difficult to use only fresh herbs. Each year in my practice I need to make 2–20 litres / 3.5–35 pints of each type of

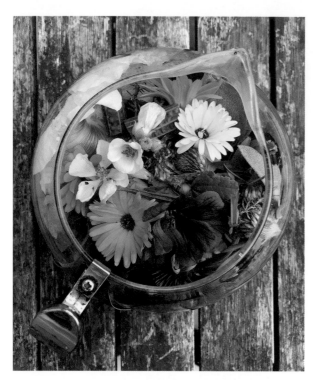

There is nothing better than making a pot of herbal tea using herbs just picked from one's own apothecary garden.

herbal tincture that I need. I work with several hundred herbs in tincture form, and while not every single one will require new batches to be made each year, most do, and it is quite a lot of tincture to make all in one go.

If we have an enterprise that specializes in making herbal products for retail sale, as opposed to treating patients individually, we may be able to quite happily use fresh herbs to make our products and accept that some of those products may run out before the following harvest season. However, in a patient-centred herbal practice we cannot realistically work with a 'when it is gone, it is gone' system. We need to strive to maintain continuity of treatment for our patients. If we have a stock of our own carefully dried herbs, we can easily make more medicine if we need it.

It is also a consideration that making small batches of medicine throughout the year requires less working capital than does a business that makes in one go all of its processed medicine for the year ahead. If we are making tinctures, we can space out orders for alcohol and storage bottles rather than placing one huge order before the season starts. Overall, we need to purchase less alcohol each year, since making tinctures with dried herbs requires lower concentrations than does making them with fresh herbs. Alcohol is a relatively expensive input. If we decide to make all of our tinctures from fresh herbs, we may have to charge our patients more for them in order to remain economically viable.

By drying our herbs, we do not need as much processing and storage space in our premises. We can store dried herbs more efficiently than storing tinctures in bottles. We also have the flexibility to decide in what form we are going to deliver herbal medicine to our patients. We may decide that it is more appropriate to prescribe herbal teas or capsules, or we may wish to make an infused oil for a specific topical treatment. Overall, I suggest that if we plan to treat patients with our own herbs, we sooner or later come to the conclusion that drying them is a good idea.

People have questioned my use of dried herbs many times, and I have suspected that they assumed that dried herbs are inherently of lower quality than are fresh herbs. It is completely understandable that if your only experience of dried herbs is of 'badly' dried herbs, you would conclude that using dried herbs is not a good idea. I hope that in this chapter I can persuade you that carefully dried herbs are totally different from poorly dried herbs, and that the use of dried herbs, as an option, is a very helpful and appropriate part of self-sufficient herbal practice. A well-stocked herb store filled with beautifully dried home-grown and wild-harvested herbs is an absolute joy to behold. My herb store is the heart of my practice.

So, what do we need to know about drying herbs? When we dry a crop, the aim is to remove nearly all the water from the herbs, so that they

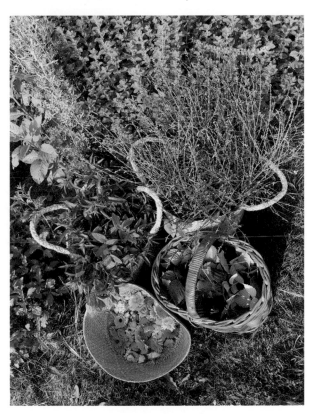

remain in a stable condition until they are rehydrated by infusing, decocting, or tincturing, or by the gastric juices inside our digestive tracts. However, if we only focus on the removal of water content and lose sight of the preservation of therapeutic constituents, we could end up with a batch of perfectly dried but pretty low-quality herbs. There are a great many ways in which we can preserve the best possible medicinal qualities in our dried herbs, and these depend on certain logical principles. Once we understand these principles, we can understand how to get the best out of whichever drying system – passive (air-drying) or active (using equipment such as a dehydrator) – we are working with. We can even understand how best to approach the drying of a herb that we may never have worked with before. Before we talk about the different options for drying herbs, let us look at these principles.

A summer harvest.

Preparation for drying

It is important to minimize handling of herbs once they are beginning to wilt, so it is best practice to lay out herbs in their final drying position as soon as possible after harvesting. Once they have been laid out, it is preferable for the individual stems, leaves, or flowers not to be moved or disturbed until the drying process is complete. They should be laid out in a single layer, so that the bottom layers do not heat up and begin to deteriorate. In my practice, especially in spring and summer, I plan my harvests around the availability of laying-out and drying capacity.

With passive drying systems, it is important to allow more space between flowers or stems than you would with an active drying system. Individual flowers, such as Calendula (*Calendula officinalis*), should be laid out in an even

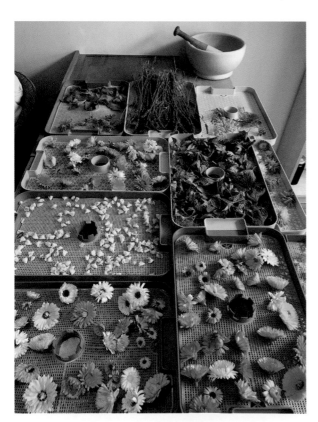

I plan my harvests around the availability of laying-out and drying capacity.

layer one flower thick, with space between the flowers to allow air flow. Plants with soft stems can be cut into even-sized lengths and spread out onto the trays. It is advisable to avoid finely chopping the herb at this stage. This would result in far greater losses of constituents through the exposure of a larger cut-surface area, not only during drying, but also subsequently, in storage. It is better to strip the leaves from plants with tough stems, especially if they are harvested later in the season. Agrimony (*Agrimonia eupatoria*) is a good example of this. The idea is that the material on the drying trays or racks should dry evenly in the minimum time possible. If the stalks take much longer to dry than the foliage, there is a risk of deterioration through over-drying of the latter. If you want to include the stalks in your medicine, dry them separately and add them back to the leaves later. Likewise, if you are drying leaves with large, fleshy midribs, it is often preferable to remove them and dry them separately. Roots should be cut into evenly sized pieces, preferably matchstick-shaped rather than slices, but in practice it depends on the roots and what seems easiest at the time. Smaller roots, such as Valerian, can be left whole. The aim is to get the root pieces to be of even width and size, so that they all dry at the same rate. Bark will tend to be of a more-or-less constant width so will dry at the same rate, regardless of the length of the pieces. Fruits need to be prepared according to their shape. I slice Pomegranate (*Punica granatum*) and Karela (*Momordica charantia*), but I dry small fruit such as Goji berries (*Lycium barbarum*) and Hawthorn berries (*Crataegus monogyna*) whole.

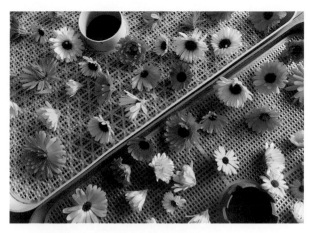

Calendula should be laid out in an even layer one flower thick, with space between the flowers to allow air flow.

Horse Chestnuts (*Aesculus hippocastanum*) are best broken into even-sized pieces in a pestle and mortar before drying.

When drying leafy herbs hanging in bunches, it is necessary to retain the stems as a framework for drying the leaves. The stalks will shrink as the herbs dry, so a tying method that remains secure throughout the process needs to be used. If you soak the string in water before tying the bundles, it will shrink and tighten as the herbs dry. Each bunch needs

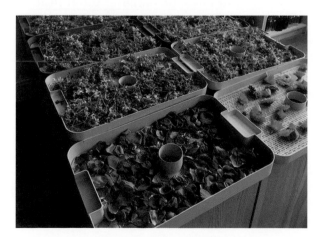

Rose, Calendula and St John's Wort flowers laid out straight after harvesting.

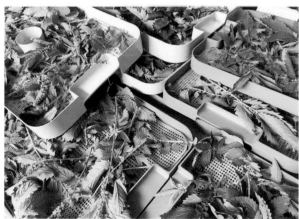

Strip the leaves from plants with tough stems. Agrimony is a good example of this.

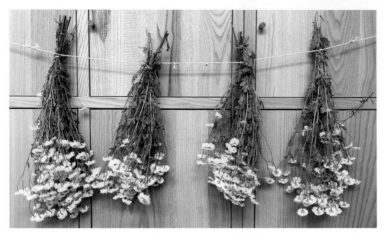

Feverfew bunches ready for drying.

to be small enough so that all parts experience good air flow. When hanging space is limited, it is tempting to make larger bunches, but bunches that are too large have a tendency to stay moist on the inside. This gives rise to pockets of deterioration and mould. Reorganizing the bunches part-way through drying is best avoided, as it can cause bruising.

Bruising

Bruising of freshly harvested aerial parts is a common fault in dried herb batches. Herbs are very prone to bruising once they begin to wilt. If bruised, the herbs turn dark due to fermentation. This is the principle that is used to positive effect in the process of making black tea, but for therapeutic herbs it is not desirable. Bruising of herbs is avoided by handling them very carefully during harvest and laying them out in a thin layer, or hanging them in individual stems or small bunches, as soon as possible after they have been picked. Once the herbs are laid out or hung up, you should leave them untouched until they are completely dry.

Temperature

During drying the temperature should be low enough to avoid altering the constituents of the herbal medicines, but warm enough to ensure efficient and quick drying. Drying herbs hanging over a stove such as an Aga, or in the bottom warming oven, usually subjects them to too high a temperature. Volatile constituents, such as essential oils, are lost more rapidly during the drying process at higher temperatures. Aromatic herbs should be dried at temperatures under 33°C / 92°F; non-aromatics, which are more robust, can be dried at temperatures of up to 45°C / 113°F.

Although low temperatures may at first seem like the best choice, there is a balance between the drying temperature and the speed of drying. The longer the drying time, the greater the potential for deterioration, so lower temperatures are not always best. This is especially the case if ambient humidity is high and plant material may reabsorb moisture over-night. When ambient humidity is very high or plant material is especially high in water content, it is best to use a slightly higher temperature, at least for short time periods. It is a juggling act. If you choose too high a temperature, you risk reducing quality through the loss of some aromatic constituents and changing the nature of others. If you choose too low a temperature, you risk herbs deteriorating due to longer drying times and the reabsorption of moisture when temperatures are cooler, for example during the night. The best way to learn is to start and then adapt what you do in the light of experience. In the end, you will learn what works best with your crops and in your situation.

It is worth noting that in large-scale drying operations, there may be a great deal of pressure to free up the dryer between batches as quickly as possible. In such circumstances, there is a temptation to increase drying temperatures to speed up throughput. This results in lower-quality batches, though the batches may be considered to be of an acceptable quality for sale. A self-sufficient herbalist producing high-quality herbs for use within their own practice will see that this is a false economy.

Light

Harvested plant material deteriorates when exposed to light, so drying herbs in sunlight results in a significant deterioration in quality. It is much better to dry herbs in darkness, but if you cannot provide total darkness, then at least aim to avoid direct sunlight. If you have never seen the difference that light exposure makes, try drying some herbs from the same batch in the light and some in the dark. You will see that even just one day's exposure to light will result in noticeable deterioration of colour and aroma. Usually roots are much more resilient than aerial parts to light exposure.

Airflow

Adequate airflow is essential to produce good dried herbs. Ideally the air should be constantly moving. If moisture-laden air is removed immediately from the proximity of the plant material, a good air-drying gradient will be maintained, and more efficient drying will be achieved. Good airflow can be achieved by proper spacing between herbs in whichever drying system is used, together with well-placed ventilation points or a fan. It is important that the airflow is gentle and steady: you do not want all of your herbs blowing away in the breeze when they are nearly dry.

Relative humidity

The relative humidity of the air around the drying herbs will affect the process of drying if it is being done purely in ambient conditions. In conditions of high humidity, say 80–100%, there will be no drying at all. If relative humidity is greater than 40%, it is not possible to complete the drying process without the addition of extra heat. Herbs need to be brought down to a moisture content of 10% for safe long-term storage. There is no need to invest in a moisture meter, though. You will easily be able to sense the level of dryness of a batch of herbs by feel. A simple rule of thumb is that all parts should be easily 'snapped'. With most, but not all, herbs, any softness or bendiness indicates that the herb is not fully dry. If a batch is stored before the moisture content has been sufficiently reduced, it will deteriorate in storage. You need to be especially vigilant where there are different plant parts present. For example, when drying Calendula (*Calendula officinalis*) flowers, the petals may feel fully dry, while the green calyces can still feel pliable. If the Calendula flowers are stored with too high a moisture content in the calyces, these will act as a reservoir of moisture, causing rehydration of the petals, and could cause the whole batch to spoil. After all the work of growing, picking, and drying a batch of Calendula, you definitely want to avoid this. Some herbs are particularly good at pulling moisture out of the air and back into their cells. Dandelion leaf (*Taraxacum officinale*) is one of these. Even if the batch is completely crispy and brittle after drying, it can easily reabsorb enough environmental moisture to rehydrate and spoil in storage. To avoid this, you need to ensure very thorough drying and airtight storage.

Length of drying time

People often ask me how long it takes to dry each batch of herbs. This is one of those questions that is impossible to answer easily. It depends on the method of drying, the species, the plant part, and how it has been prepared. It also depends on the temperature used for drying, the degree of air movement, and the ambient humidity, as well as the moisture content of the herbs themselves. Herbs with a higher moisture content take longer to dry, hence the species of herb and the plant part will make a big difference to the speed of drying. Non-fleshy plant parts, such as simple flowers, will dry more quickly than will roots and fruits. Even different batches within the same species will vary in moisture content according to the prevailing weather conditions in the days leading up to harvest. A prolonged wet spell resulting in saturated soils will mean that harvested herbs have a much higher moisture content than those that have been harvested after a dry spell.

Another factor affecting drying times is the nature of the herb and how easily it gives up its moisture. Some herbs seem to hold on to their moisture more than others, and, in general herbs, that have been cut finely will give up their moisture (and their therapeutic constituents) faster than those that have been left whole. Passive drying will be slower than active drying in most climates, but in a hot, dry climate with good air movement in the drying area, there may be no difference.

I give some drying time guidelines in each of the sections below about different drying

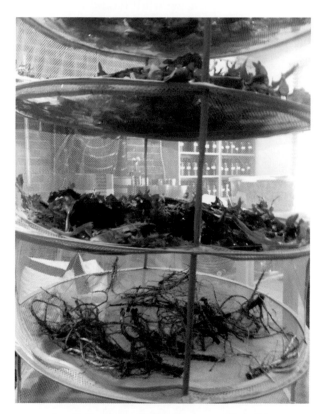

Dandelion leaves and roots on a collapsible cylindrical hanging herb-drying tower.

techniques, but I would like to emphasize that these can only ever be guidelines. There are inevitably quite large variations between different herbs and different years. A herbal practitioner living in a climate with high rainfall and humidity will have a completely different herb drying experience to one living in a hot dry climate. My best advice is to assess each batch individually to judge for yourself when it is thoroughly dry.

Drying methods

There are plenty of different options, and each of us must find a solution that is right for our situation, our budget, the space we have available, and the quantities of herbs that we wish to dry. There is no right or wrong way if we understand the principles of how to dry herbs effectively and preserve maximum therapeutic quality. Remember, drying is about so much more than just reducing water content.

The simplest way to dry herbs is to lay them out flat on trays, and leave them to dry in an airy, dark place. If you only want the leaves, for example in the case of Nettle (*Urtica dioica*), then it is best to remove the leaves from the stem before the herbs start to wilt. Hold each stem horizontally over the

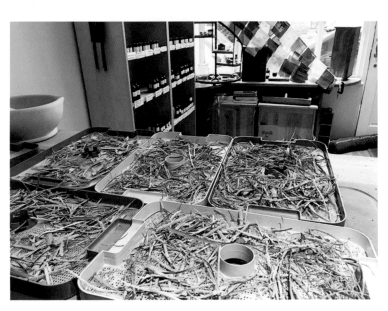

Cramp Bark laid out on trays

tray, and gently twist it around so that the leaves hang down in turn away from the stem. You can use scissors to snip each leaf off and let it fall onto the tray. Once all the leaves have been removed, you can gently spread them out, so that they form a single layer. Other herbs, such as Skullcap (*Scutellaria lateriflora*) and Hyssop (*Hyssopus officinalis*), are best dried in sections that include the stems. Evenly sized pieces of around 7.5–10 cm / 3–4 in are ideal. Roots should be cleaned and sliced into matchstick-shaped sections or slices of even thickness.

Make sure that the trays are off the floor and away from sources of contamination, such as cooking smells, pet hair, or household cleaning products. You can also cover a flat surface, such as a table, with a clean sheet and lay the herbs out on that.

Laying the herbs on suspended mesh screens or fabric will allow greater airflow from underneath and more efficient drying. You can buy drying racks consisting of mesh screens designed to keep the shape of knitwear after washing or collapsible cylindrical hanging herb drying 'towers', which come with several mesh compartments. The herb towers are hung from a hook in a beam or a ceiling joist. They can be quite heavy when filled with fresh herbs, so it is important to make sure they are properly secured in a place where weight-bearing is possible. When not in use, they can be stored flat – a great advantage for those of us where space is at a premium.

When I ran my practice from home, nearly every raised flat surface in the house was taken over by trays of herbs during the summer. As if that were not enough, one of the interior doorways periodically had a mesh herb tower hanging from the centre of its frame, so we had to squeeze past it if we wanted to enter that room. Luckily, I have a very supportive and understanding family.

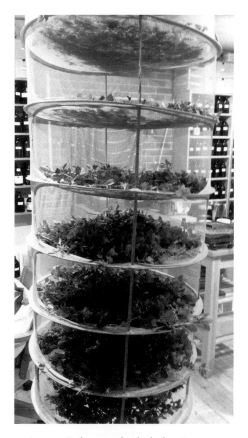

Lemon Balm on a herb drying tower.

Flat drying of leaves may take anywhere from 48 hours to over a week, depending on temperature, relative humidity, air flow, and the other factors discussed above. You should always avoid moving leafy crops while they are drying. Roots will take longer. Spread them out so that they are not in contact with each other, and leave them in an airy place to dry for between 10 days and two weeks. Once they have shrunk but are still pliable, you will need to finish off the drying process for a further few days in a warmer place. You can handle roots and turn them during the drying process, since there is much less risk of bruising.

A more picturesque option for herb drying is to dry them in bunches. Harvest whole plants near ground level and remove the lower discoloured or faded leaves, leaving a length of clear stalk for tying. Gather 5–6 stems together into a bundle and tie them tightly near the base with string, leaving

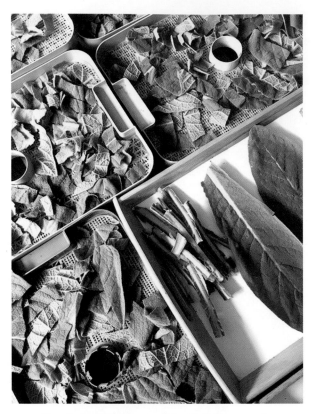

Flat drying of leaves such as Mullein may take anywhere from 48 hours to over a week, depending on temperature, relative humidity, air flow, and other factors.

the usable parts hanging upside down below. You can either hang individual bunches or you can suspend pairs of bunches over beams or 'washing lines' suspended across the ceiling. If you have clothes airing racks, you can peg smaller bunches to the cross-pieces. You can also dry large leaves, such as Mullein (*Verbascum thapsus*) or Comfrey (*Symphytum officinale*), individually on drying lines.

It is possible to buy beautiful cast-iron ceiling-suspended herb drying rings specially designed to create a country-kitchen look. Part of me has always wanted one, but although they look very pretty and rustic, sadly if sited in the kitchen, they do not result in particularly good-quality dried plant material. The drying process will be helped by the warmth of the kitchen, but the herbs are exposed to degradation by light, dust, and cooking aromas.

Herb stems shrink as they dry. Soak the string in water before tying the bunches, so it shrinks, as the herbs do. Do not be tempted to pack too many herbs tightly together, but aim to create light, open bundles that allow good airflow to the centre. The bunching technique relies on the herbs having structurally robust stems. Herbs with softer stems, such as Cleavers (*Galium aparine*), or herbs such as Dandelion (*Taraxacum officinale*) and Plantain (*Plantago lanceolata* and *Plantago major*), which do not form main stems, are best dried flat.

The time taken to dry herbs in suspended bunches is as variable as drying them flat, for the same reasons. Large bunches of herbs will dry more slowly than small ones. While the herbs on the outside of the bunch may be dry, the ones in the centre may remain damp for up to a couple of weeks. This is too long if you are aiming to produce high quality medicines. In wet years, even with small bunches, it may be impossible to get the moisture content low enough with passive drying alone. An airing cupboard – a hot-water cylinder

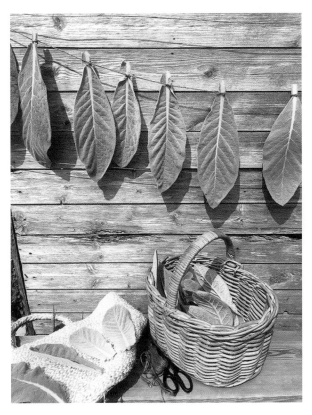

Large leaves such as Mullein can be dried individually on drying lines away from direct light.

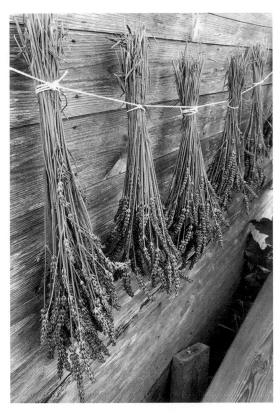

Preparing bunches of Lavender for drying. These will be dried away from direct light.

cupboard – is a perfect place to finish the drying process. Simply take the bundles down and place them on trays in the airing cupboard for 24 hours, to ensure that they are thoroughly dry before storage. Some people use the oven on a very low heat, with the door left open. This is not ideal, as it is difficult to ensure that the temperature does not rise too high.

If you do not have an airing cupboard, you may start to think about creating a drying cabinet with mesh or screen drawers. These can be filled with herbs and then a warm fan is directed through from one end in order to keep air movement and drying gradients constant. This is, in effect, a homemade dehydrator. The advantage of this is that you can tailor-make the drying cabinet according to the space you have available and your needs.

Another option is to buy one or several domestic food dehydrators. This is my personal choice. It is best to choose dehydrators with trays, which

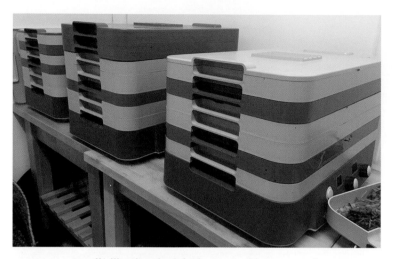

I really like L'Equip dehydrators and have several.

are stacked rather than slid into place. It is helpful if the stackable trays have as much depth as possible so that when the herbs are first placed on the trays they do not have to be squashed down as additional trays are stacked above them. Dehydrators that are fitted with timers, fans, and thermostats give a great deal of consistency and control over the drying process. I really like the L'Equip dehydrators and have been using them quite happily for many years. I have several, and these are, weather permitting, in nearly continuous use between May and September each year.

Having several small dehydrators allows you the option of drying batches of herbs in separate dehydrators rather than having one large dehydrator with trays of different herbs drying at varying rates. If you fill a dehydrator with trays containing different herbs and one tray is drying more slowly than the others, it will slow the drying of the whole batch by acting as a source of increased humidity within the dryer. There is also the potential for the scent from one herb to be absorbed by another. If I only have two trays of a herb to be dried I will dry them on their own in a dehydrator, even though the theoretical capacity of each dehydrator is to dry 6 trays at one time. If you are going to invest in one or more dehydrators, I recommend that you purchase additional spare trays. This will allow you to lay out herbs straight after harvest and leave them undisturbed until they can be placed into a free dehydrator.

The time it takes to dry different batches of herbs in a dehydrator varies. Since I always use L'Equip, I can only relate my experience with that brand. Other brands may dry more quickly or more slowly. Bear in mind that a dehydrator sited in a closed room will be less efficient than one sited in a room with ventilation. For more aromatic flower medicines, like Rose (*Rosa* spp.) petals or Chamomile (*Matricaria recutita*) flowers, 8 hours at under 33°C / 92°F may be sufficient, provided that there is good air movement and a low ambient humidity. Whole Calendula flowers need more time at a higher temperature in order to properly dry the fleshy green calyx. I have found that their drying time can vary between 12 and 36 hours in different years. The time taken to dry leafy crops in dehydrators does vary considerably, but I would suggest starting with 8 hours at 40°C / 104°F for leaves that have been removed from their stems. After 8 hours, move the trays around, bottom to top, then continue, for 2-hour periods, until the batch is perfectly dry. Do not be surprised in wetter years if the process takes up to double the original time. Cleavers (*Galium aparine*) dries more quickly than most leafy crops and may be completely dry within 9 hours at 40°C / 104°F.

Roots take longer to dry than aerial parts, and the timing of drying will also be affected by how they have been cut up. Washing roots is a necessity, but avoid soaking them for long periods, as it not only allows the medicinal constituents to leach out, but it greatly increases their moisture content before drying. It is a good idea to allow washed roots to dry passively on a tray at first in order to reduce their moisture content before starting the active drying process.

Barks are drier to start with, and I suggest starting aromatic barks like Cramp Bark off with 8–10 hours at 40°C / 104°F, increasing the drying time and temperature a little as necessary. Fruit takes a much longer time to dry, due to its high moisture content, and for this reason I hardly ever dry fruit. I do occasionally dry Pomegranate (*Punica granatum*) slices and find that at 42°C I am not surprised if I need to continue drying for 36 hours.

The times I suggest are only guidelines, and the time needed to dry each batch will vary according to the drying system and the prevailing temperature and humidity. Dehydrators that are loaded more sparsely will result in faster drying times than those that are packed with many trays. I find that 6 trays are maximum for efficient drying, but if I am drying a high-moisture-content plant part like Horse Chestnut (*Aesculus hippocastanum*) fruits, I will place only one tray in each dehydrator. When using multiple trays, it is important to change the trays around regularly, moving the bottom one to the top and

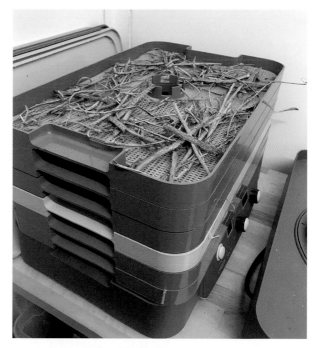

Cramp Bark ready for drying in a dehydrator.

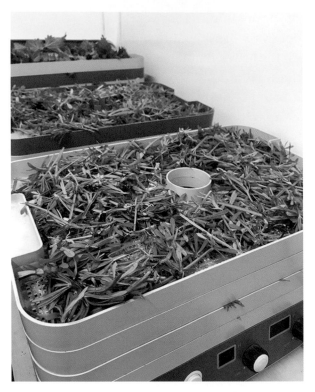

Cleavers drying. My dehydrators are in nearly continuous use between May and September each year.

swapping them all around, so that they dry as evenly as possible. The beauty of using moveable trays is that the herbs themselves are not handled, and therefore bruising of wilted and semi-dry plant material is avoided.

The moisture content of herbs varies hugely according to the weather conditions prior to harvest, and this, in turn, affects drying times. A couple of years ago there was a very wet spring. It rained so hard that I was worried I would not be able to harvest any Elder flowers (*Sambucus nigra*) at all. It looked as though all the Elder flowers on the trees would be battered and spoiled by high winds and storms before I could pick any. Finally, there was a dry day, which coincided with a day when I was not working in my clinic, and I was able to go out and harvest a couple of large baskets. I prepared the flowers for dehydration as usual and started the dryers off. I would normally have expected that Elder flowers harvested on a dry day would be very nearly dry after 12 hours in the dehydrator at 42°C / 108°F. I was shocked to find that after 14 hours of gentle drying they were still nowhere near dry – in fact, that particular batch took over 24 hours of active drying at a temperature of 42°C / 108°F. At the time, I did not want to increase the temperature, as I was worried about losing the volatile components of the Elder flowers, but in retrospect it may have been better to increase it a little, especially as the ambient humidity was so high. Drying our own herbs involves an ongoing learning process, and each year we discover more about how to get the best out of the drying system that we are working with.

If you have never dried Dandelion leaf (*Taraxacum officinale*), then I should warn you that it is a particularly tricky herb to dry. It can appear to be convincingly crispy and dry after perhaps 10 hours at 42°C / 108°F, but on closer inspection you will probably find that its fleshy midribs remain pliable. Do not be lulled into a false sense of security and decide to store them anyway at this stage. Dandelion leaves are experts at reabsorbing moisture from the environment and from their own moisture-laden midribs. Make sure that you carry on the drying process for a few more hours, until the midribs are brittle. On two unforgettable occasions, I stored batches of dried Dandelion leaves too early, and they spoiled. It is totally gutting to open a storage container and discover that all the hard work of gathering and drying a precious herb has been wasted. Nowadays I always take extra precautions with Dandelion leaf. I make sure that the midribs snap cleanly before I think of storing them, and I start by storing each batch in a small container with a minimal air gap, moving the crop to larger containers as more batches are ready to be stored. Also, I only ever store the Dandelion leaves warm from the dehydrator, so that they are as dry as possible at the moment of going into storage. Finally, I always check my storage container regularly for the first couple of weeks after first storing the leaves, to make sure there is no sign of moisture reabsorption. If I follow these steps carefully, I am rewarded with beautiful vibrant green Dandelion leaves that smell bitter and fresh for the whole year ahead.

As a self-sufficient herbalist, you need to rely on your senses to see whether herbs are thoroughly dry and to assess the quality of the herbs that you are processing. The most important thing is that the dried herb should retain the colour and fragrance of the fresh herb. When you open the lid of the herb storage container the fragrance and vibrancy should hit you. If it is your own crop, you will find that you are immediately transported back to the time and place of the harvest. This means two things: at a head level, on the one hand, we know that the medicinal constituents have been well preserved in that batch, since the aroma of the herb is true to its fresh version; on a heart level, on the other, we cannot help but to feel a strong connection with that batch of herb.

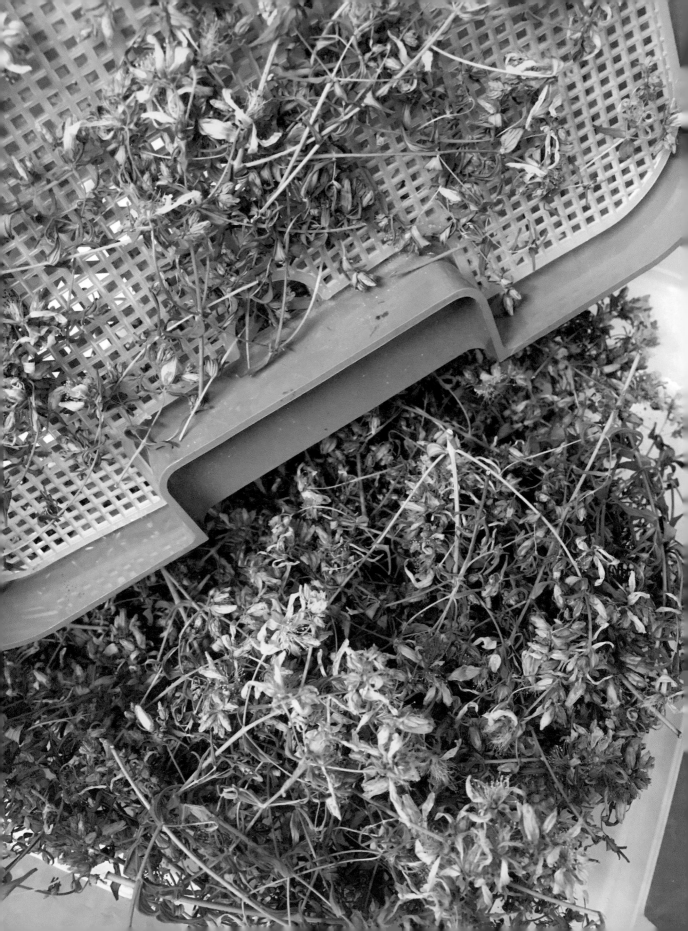

11

Storage

After all of the effort and attention to detail we put into harvesting and drying our herbs, we need to ensure that they are stored in a way that fully preserves their quality. The main principles are that they need to be kept totally dry, in the dark, and at a cool temperature, protected from dust, mould, and insect contamination.

The storage system that you choose will depend on your available space, the quantity of herbs that you wish to store, and your budget. The ideal is a dedicated herb store room that is kept at a constant temperature, is free from damp, and can be kept dark. Even indirect light will degrade the quality of your herbs, so make sure that if it has a window, you fit a good blackout blind and keep the overhead light off at all times. If you are using your stored herbs daily, you will need them to be organized and accessible.

On a small scale, individual herbs can be stored effectively in sealed foil sachets (as used by some herbal wholesalers) or large glass jars. If you want to store your herbs in recycled glass jars, store them in a cupboard or fit your shelves with blackout blinds. Another option is to cover each jar with a black sock that will keep out the light. As long as you label the lid clearly, you will be able to tell what is inside without taking off the sock.

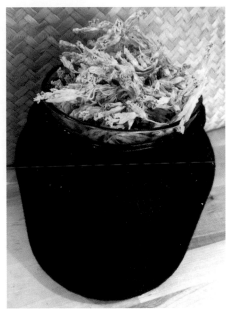

Dried Cowslip flowers being stored in a covered glass jar.

I have often read the recommendation that herbs should be stored in brown paper or cloth bags so that they can 'breathe'. This may seem a good storage solution if you live in a climate with a constant very low ambient humidity (or have a humidity-controlled room) but in temperate climates, herbs stored in brown paper or cloth bags will reabsorb moisture from the atmosphere and deteriorate in quality. In addition, breathable storage bags leave their contents vulnerable to infestation by insects and mould.

For a busy, full-time, self-sufficient herbal practice, these storage solutions are not practical in terms of scale, so you start to enter the realms of temperature- and humidity-controlled storage rooms lined with wooden drawers or, in my case, airtight food-grade plastic boxes that can be stacked on the shelves in my dark herb store. People do sometimes criticize me for using food-grade plastic boxes as my herb storage solution. I can understand that as an initial reaction. Quite rightly, we are all striving to minimize our use of plastics. It is my dream to have an environment-

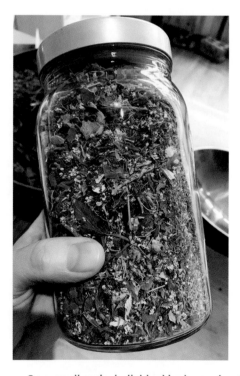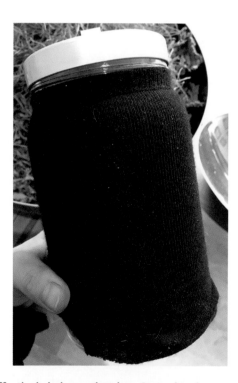

On a small scale, individual herbs can be stored effectively in large glass jars. Store clear jars in the dark or cover them with a black sock.

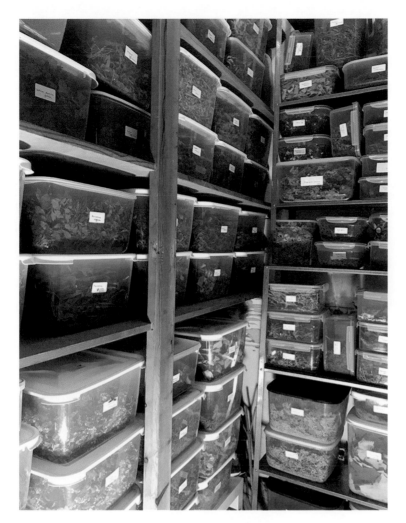

A view into my clinic herb store.

controlled herb store with floor-to-ceiling wooden drawers, each holding a particular dried herb. I have seen such rooms when doing clinical study in Tibet. They are incredibly beautiful and functional. Unfortunately, I am simply not in a position to have one of these at the moment. If you have the financial resources to create one, then absolutely do it, and please share photographs with me, so I can enjoy your herb store vicariously. Sometimes people ask me: if not wooden drawers, why not use glass? When I first started in practice, I used recycled glass pickle jars to store my bulk herbs, and I do always choose glass over plastic for liquids such as

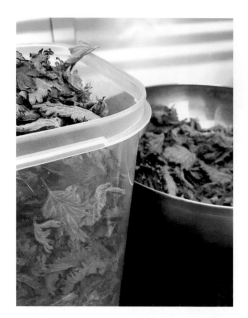

Dried Nettle leaves going into a storage box.

tinctures and oils. I have 'a thing' about jars and love to find uses for them, but my dreams of rows of jars filled with dried herbs on shelves evaporated when I realized that I needed to be able to store much larger volumes than could be accommodated in pickle jars. Food-grade plastic boxes were the practical solution for my circumstances. They are robust and safe, and I reuse them year after year, so I am not adding to the level of plastic waste that enters the environment. The boxes have been manufactured in order to avoid plastic compounds leaching into the contents, especially when those contents are totally dry. After all the love and care that has gone into growing, gathering, harvesting, and drying my herbs, the most important thing to me is that they are stored effectively and preserved safely to be available for my patients.

Whichever way you choose to store your herbs, each batch should be labelled clearly with the name of the herb and the date that it was gathered. You may end up with multiple batches of the same herb from the same year or from consecutive years. In my herb store, I start the autumn with five or six 15-litre boxes packed full of Skullcap (*Scutellaria lateriflora*), most of which will be used during the year ahead; with other herbs, such as Hawthorn (*Crataegus monogyna*) berry, I may have batches from two different years stored and labelled separately.

It is helpful if your storage system allows you to see at a glance where each herb is stored. In the early days, I had my jars of herbs stored in a cupboard with deep shelves and had to search through to find each one that I wanted. This is not really a problem if you are accessing the herbs only sporadically, but if you are using them daily, then you will need to find a more convenient system of storage. Arranging the herbs alphabetically helps, and shallow shelves allow a one-herb-per-piece-of-shelf-front arrangement.

Whichever system you decide upon to store your herbs, it is important to do your very best to preserve their medicinal qualities. This has to override aesthetics. Uncovered glass jars filled with herbs on the shelf of a dispensary or a shop may look very pretty, but they are losing their potency with every day that they are exposed to the light. All too often I see badly stored herbs

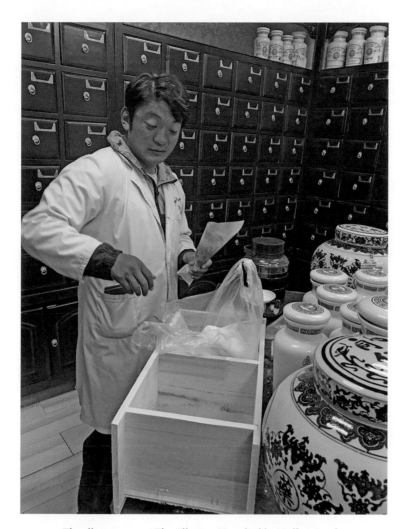

The dispensary at The Tibetan Hospital in Malho, Amdo.

losing potency. It seems such a terrible waste of healing potential. To create a well-maintained and effective herb store is not only the best way to look after your herbs, but it is also a wonderful place to hang out. Visitors to my clinic love looking into my herb store. They very often comment that they can really feel the vibrancy of the herbs and are reluctant to leave it.

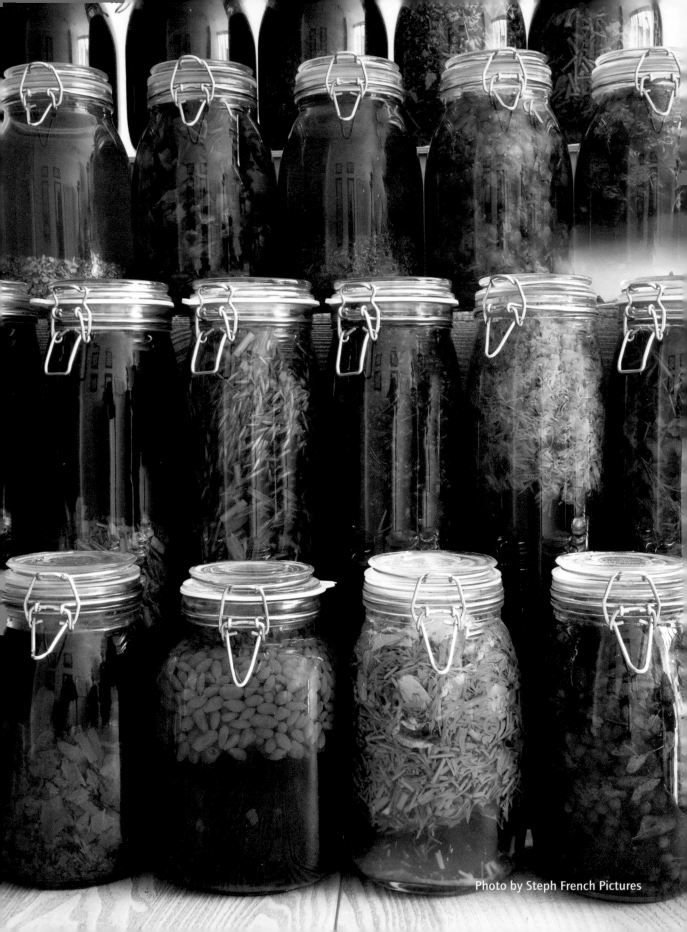

12

Processing

I was not going to write about processing when I originally planned this book. There are so many excellent resources out there telling people how to make tinctures, how to make capsules, and how to make infused oils and ointments. The information is freely available on the internet in numerous blogs and on herbal resource sites. I honestly felt that I had nothing more to add and wanted to concentrate my efforts on sharing information that is less easily available. However, over my years of posting on social media, a lot of people have asked me about my processing techniques. It is quite common for people to tell me that they would like to make their own products but feel daunted by the apparent complexity of herbal medicine making. They have concluded that it is easier for them to buy in ready-made products for their practice. Yet small-scale herbal processing is an integral part of running a self-sufficient practice. If we grow and gather our own herbs, we will want to use them for our patients and allow them to fulfil their healing potential. I hope that sharing my – perhaps rather unsophisticated – approach to processing will help to encourage more practitioners to start to explore the world of herb processing and find ways that work for them.

There are a great many different ways to process herbs. As long as the finished product is effective and safe and has a good shelf life, we can be sure that our method is a good one. If you are totally comfortable with the way that you process herbs, then you may prefer to skip over this chapter. If you are curious about traditional ways of preparing herbs and the way that these can be integrated into a self-sufficient practice, then I hope that what I share here may be food for thought, or at least a guide as to where to start.

Traditional herb processing is a matter of starting out with the methods that we have been shown by our teachers. As we start to process our own herbs, we may adapt the original instructions to suit our own situation and the way we work. Eventually, after many years, we may reach a point where we are comfortable and confident to do things totally differently.

The methods that we choose for processing our herbs depend on our scale of operation and what we intend to do with them. They also depends on our relationship with those herbs. If we are working on a small scale and making gifts or maintaining a home herbal dispensary, we can quite happily be more fluid and intuitive in the way that we do things. If, on the other hand, we intend to work on a relatively large scale and are aiming to supply other practitioners, herb processing needs to be done quite differently. In this latter case, we need to have in place prescribed, consistent, and fully traceable processes that provide exact information about how each herbal product has been made.

In-between these two scenarios, we have the self-sufficient herbal practitioner who is growing and gathering herbs to treat patients but not supplying other practitioners. This is the category that I fall into. In this scenario, we can process herbs our own way, because we are the only ones prescribing our products. Of course, we share the necessity of safety, effectiveness, and traceability, but beyond that we can vary the process a little if we want to. As long as we record how each batch has been made and use good labelling, we can choose to repeat the process for future batches of the same herbal product, or we can choose to adapt it in the light of experience or knowledge about the raw material that we have produced.

Take tincture making, for example. There seems to be a widespread belief that if we take the exact same amount of dried or fresh herb and we add the same amount of alcohol and water to it, at the same concentration, we will create a tincture that is exactly the same every time. This idea of consistency is somewhat illusory. Herbs are living and variable. The levels of their medicinal constituents vary according to where they have been grown, what variety has been cultivated, and the weather conditions that have prevailed each season. On top of that, the way in which they have been harvested, dried, and stored also has a very significant influence on the strength of the therapeutic constituents in each batch of a particular herb.

Not only are the herbs themselves variable, each patient taking those herbs also varies in constitution and nature. No matter how much we would like to make herb processing and herb prescribing an exact science, we should accept that, in the case of the self-sufficient herbal practice, we have the opportunity to adjust our methods of processing according to deeper knowledge and experience about our own herbs and how we prescribe them. We are using herbs that we will have observed over their growing season(s). These are herbs that we will have harvested ourselves, and these are herbs that we can touch and smell and connect with before we choose how to process them. It makes sense that we can allow that extra knowledge to influence the way that we process them. I have a good role model for this.

One of my main Western herbal tutors, Barbara Howe, made all of her own tinctures for her practice. She believed passionately that sourcing her own herbs was the 'proper' way to practise herbal medicine. It was at one of the annual student summer seminars that I learnt how she made tinctures., As it turned out, Barbara did not make tinctures according to a prescribed formula.

Tincture making

I remember to this day Barbara placing handfuls of fresh Comfrey (*Symphytum officinale*) leaf into a preserving jar. The Comfrey had been picked on the previous day, so that it was surface-dry and a little wilted. I remember her saying that if it had been raining on the day of the seminar and if the Comfrey had not been picked in advance, we would not have been able to make a tincture. She did not weigh the herb, she just judged the amount by eye, tearing the leaves into pieces and packing them into the jar. She poured an alcohol mixture in until it reached about three quarters of the way up the jar. At that point, she got out a pendulum and dowsed to see whether the tincture needed more alcohol or water. She announced that the herb was telling her that it needed a bit more alcohol. It was quite fascinating, especially as the whole process was carried out with the easy confidence of someone who had been doing it for many years and was quite sure that this was the best possible way to make tinctures. I remember being quite amazed and a little disconcerted. I had studied subjects like plant biochemistry and experimental analysis and design while at university and definitely was not ready to accept that tinctures could be made purely on the basis of intuition. Surely there had to be a proper recipe!

Despite the fluidity with which Barbara made her tinctures, she was very conscientious about recording how each batch was made. She kept a series of tincture-making books, and each batch was assigned a number and was labelled with the contents and the date it was made. The corresponding entry in the tincture book gave more details. The date, the herb and the part used, where it had come from, and the quantity of alcohol and water with the percentage used. This attention to detail felt comforting and went a long way to counterbalance my initial consternation over the intuitive way that the tinctures seemed to have been made. Also, there was no denying that Barbara got excellent therapeutic results with her tinctures in her practice. She had a large patient list and plenty of legendary cures under her belt. As students, we loved hearing about these. It seemed so exciting that one day we, too, would be able to help patients become well again through the use of herbs.

One summer, Barbara showed the students around her tincture room. I will never forget the sight of shelf after shelf filled with large jars of beautiful herbs macerating in the dark. All of the herbs in these tincture jars had been grown or gathered with her own hands. The scale seemed breath-taking. It was absolutely incredible to me that someone could have done all of this and that she was using these herbs to treat patients. I asked her about the amount of work that was involved, and she simply told me that it was her life's work.

I was hugely inspired by Barbara and wanted to emulate her way of working with home-grown and wild-harvested herbs. I realized that tincture making was going to be an integral part of that. She must have sensed the way I was thinking. She took me to one side at the end of that seminar and gave me a couple of litres of pure alcohol, saying: 'Start making tinctures Lucy! Don't wait until you are qualified. Create your dispensary! Apply for your alcohol license now!'

That was how my tincture-making began. I took the alcohol home and started making small batches of tincture with herbs that I had grown or gathered. In the beginning, I chose herbs that I knew quite well. Meadowsweet (*Filipendula ulmaria*) was one of the first, as I had been gathering and using the flowers for about 10 years already. I admit, though, that I did not really trust my dowsing abilities, so I had to find another way to work out alcohol and water percentages. I had a catalogue from a large herbal wholesaler who sold tinctures, and it showed weight-to-volume ratios as well as alcohol percentages. It seemed as good a place as any to start. I packed a jar with fresh

Meadowsweet flowers and poured the alcohol–water mixture in until it filled the jar. With some ceremony, I chose a hardback notebook and made the first entry, recording batch number 001, the date, and the words '*Filipendula ulmaria* flores, wild harvested in Cattistock'. I did not record the weight of the herb, but I did add details about the percentage and volume of the alcohol added underneath. I left plenty of space to record details about the date it was drained and pressed and to make notes about the final volume yield. I decided to use one page of the book for each batch, just as Barbara did.

I still remember the excitement of making that first tincture. I put it away in a dark cupboard and checked on it every day. As I saw the tincture beginning to change colour and the medicine being extracted, I began to see myself as one day being a herbalist practising self-sufficient herbalism. I have been making tinctures pretty much in that same way ever since.

I think perhaps this way of making tinctures combines the two main aspects of my herbalist personality traits. One part of me is very intuitive and likes to be guided by the herbs, the other part is much more prescriptive and pays close attention to material details. The first part is strongly influenced by my healer grandmother, who had taught me to dowse from an early age. The second part is influenced by my study of Agricultural and Forest Sciences at the University of Oxford. I am Piscean, and having opposing traits goes with the territory. You get used to it. The result of this contradictory constitutional manifestation is that the intuitive part of my nature likes to choose the amount of herb that is required for each batch, and the prescriptive part likes to ensure that the correct alcohol percentage is used. This works for me and my patients, but you may be more comfortable with another way. We are all different.

Let us start with the choice of alcohol percentages in tincture making. The percentage

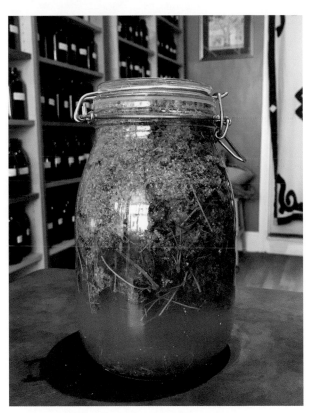

A jar of tincture made with wild-harvested Meadowsweet flowers.

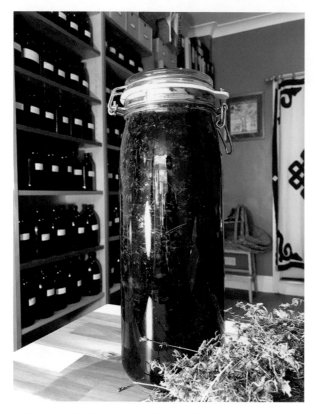

The very dark red of a well-made Hypericum tincture shows that there is a good extraction of medicinal constituents.

of alcohol used to make a tincture is very important. Each tincture is made with a mixture of alcohol and water. The alcohol extracts oil-soluble constituents and the water extracts water-soluble constituents, so both are important in allowing a herbal medicine to reach its therapeutic potential. As well as acting as a solvent, the alcohol preserves the tincture. If the alcohol is below a certain percentage, the tincture may not keep. Personally, I view 25% alcohol in the final product as being the minimum acceptable level for my needs, but I have seen different figures quoted. I prefer to be on the safe side. I remember a fellow student telling me that some bottles of tincture had once exploded on her shelf. She had made the batch with a lot of fresh high-moisture-content herb and had used a low-alcohol-proof vodka. Apart from the trauma of the exploding bottles, it had felt like such a waste of good herbs. She was determined never to make the same mistake again. Thanks to her telling me about it, I have never had a batch that has spoiled. I am very grateful to her.

Let me explain a little more about the principle of alcohol percentage in tincture making. First, herbs with more oil-soluble medicinal constituents require a higher alcohol percentage than do those with mostly water-soluble constituents. For example, tincture of dried Buchu (*Agathosma betulina* formerly *Barosma betulina*) is usually made with 60% alcohol, because it has quite a high proportion of oil-soluble constituents. Another herb that requires a relatively high alcohol content for good extraction is St John's Wort (*Hypericum perforatum*). If you make a tincture from carefully dried St John's Wort and use 60% alcohol, you will get a very dark-red tincture, which indicates an excellent extraction of the red constituent hypericin. If you use a lower alcohol percentage, the extraction will be much less, and the colour will be paler. Herbs with mostly water-soluble constituents, such as Pellitory-of-the-Wall

(*Parietaria diffusa*), require a lower percentage of alcohol for effective extraction. If you are using well-dried herb, the tincture can be made with 25% alcohol – just enough to ensure that the tincture will be preserved properly.

Second, fresh herb has a high proportion of water contained within it (usually around 75%), so adding 25% alcohol to a jar full of fresh herb would result in a final water content that is much too high – hence the exploding bottles on my friend's shelf. When making tinctures, we therefore need to adjust the alcohol percentage according to the water content of the herb. I add a higher proportion of alcohol if the herb is especially moist, a fresh root or fleshy leaves, for example, and a lower proportion if the herb has been dried thoroughly. When you look up how to make a tincture in a reference guide, it will generally refer to dried herb. Dried Buchu tincture is made with 60% alcohol in order to extract its oil-soluble constituents. If you are using fresh Buchu, you will need a higher alcohol percentage in order to compensate for the water content of the fresh herb. If you do make the tincture with 60% alcohol, it may be sufficiently alcoholic not to go off, but the resulting tincture will have a much lower concentration of oil-soluble active constituents and will therefore be less effective than one that has been extracted with a higher alcohol percentage.

Most people start out with using vodka or other spirits to make tinctures. This is a perfectly good plan, as long as the alcohol percentage is taken into account. Vodkas and other spirits are usually labelled in terms of their percentage 'proof'. In order to find out the alcohol percentage of a particular bottle of vodka, you need to divide the proof percentage by two. A vodka that is 60% proof is actually only 30% alcohol. If you are making a lot of tinctures using bottled and branded spirits, you will soon begin to wish that you could source higher-percentage

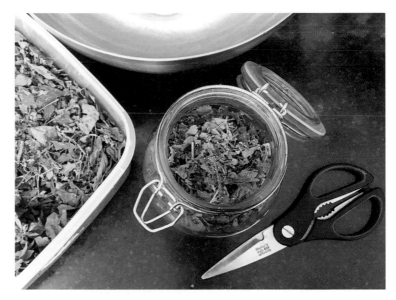

Preparing to make a tincture of Pellitory-of-the-Wall.

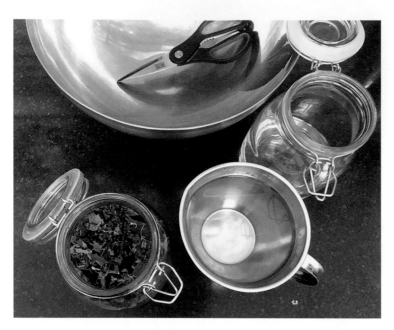

Herbs with mostly water-soluble constituents, such as Pellitory-of-the-Wall, require a lower percentage of alcohol for effective extraction.

alcohol and pay less tax on it. In the United Kingdom, we have a system where herbal practitioners and manufacturers can apply for a license to buy a certain amount of duty-free spirits each year. The applicant has to show that they will store the alcohol securely and account for every bit that has been used. Careful records need to be kept, and these can be checked by HM Customs and Excise. The record-keeping is not as onerous as it sounds, because if you are keeping a record of all the tinctures that you are making, you will already have a record of the amount of alcohol that has been used for each batch.

Once the license is approved, it is possible to purchase high-grade Neutral Spirit, which is 96% alcohol. As it is very rare that you would make a tincture using pure alcohol, the high-grade Neutral Spirit needs to be diluted before use. As it is not strictly 100% alcohol, you need to take into account when calculating the amount of water that needs to be added that it already contains 4% water. For example, if you want to end up with 40% alcohol, you will achieve this by using approximately 45% alcohol mixed with 55% water. I tend to use a graduated metric measuring jug and pour the high-grade Neutral Spirit into it to the required level and then top up to the 1-litre mark with filtered, purified water. I find this technique is accurate enough for my needs, especially since I err on the side of caution when choosing the alcohol percentages for my tinctures.

When it comes to choosing the volume of herb to tincture and the ratio of alcohol to add, I suppose you would call my way of making tinctures the 'folk' method because I usually do not weigh the amount of herb that has been used. Certain principles do apply, though. First, it is important that the herb material is properly submerged during the tincturing process. If there is herb material that is exposed to the air at the top of the jar, it will oxidize and spoil. Second, sufficient herb needs to be used in relation to the volume of liquid to make the finished tincture effective. If too little herb is used, the tincture will be very weak and may not produce the desired therapeutic results in practice. Third, the amount of herb used will be dictated by whether that herb is fresh or dry. When using fresh herb, I need to fill the tincture jar much more than when using the more 'concentrated' dried herb. Just as we are taught to use less dried herb than fresh when making a cup of herbal tea, the same applies to making herbal tinctures. Making a tincture using a whole jar of fresh herb makes perfect sense, but doing the same with a whole jar packed with dried herb may result in very little or no yield of tincture at the end of the process.

In practice, I choose the amount of herb for each batch of tincture on the basis of filling the jar to the level that feels right. I had been shown this technique by my tutor, Barbara, and it appeals to my intuitive side. For those who prefer a more solid starting point, a general guideline is that for fresh herbs we can use one part by weight of fresh herb to two parts by volume of solvent (known as the menstruum). For dried herbs, it is more appropriate to choose a 1:5 ratio. However, when making our own tinctures with a prescribed weight–volume ratio, we can run into problems. Sometimes, when using a powdered dried herb, you may find that the plant material has absorbed all of the liquid, leaving no yield of tincture at the end of the process. If that happens, you need to let go of your pre-prescribed ideas of what weight proportions should be used and just add more liquid until it looks right. We need to use common sense. Personally, I never powder herbs before tincturing them, I just cut them up by hand. Powdering for tincture making is contrary to the way that I was taught, and it just feels wrong to me. I know that many people do like to do this, though. If it works for you and you feel happy working in that way, then definitely carry on.

By feeling that we do not have to stick rigidly to a weight:volume ratio, we can

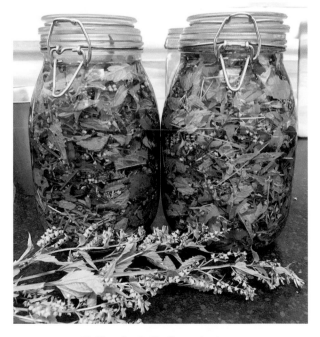
Making fresh Skullcap tincture.

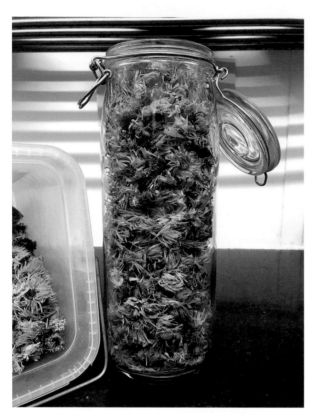

Making a batch of Calendula tincture.

take into account our own special knowledge and relationship with the herbs that we have grown or gathered. This is how I like to do it in my practice. For example, in a very good season we may find that the potency of a particular herb is really high. We can gauge this through a much more intense aroma and a very abundant crop, for example. We may decide to make extra tincture that year, because we can sense that it will be a very good batch. In other years, we may see that it has not been such a favourable growth season for that herb. It may not be quite as vibrant as usual, and its growth may be less abundant. It may smell and taste milder. In these circumstances, we may decide that we need to use a larger volume of herb compared to other 'average' years.

With dried herbs, we can be influenced by how well the drying process has gone and to some extent the age of the batch. If a herb was dried one year ago, we may decide to use more of it compared to a batch that has recently been harvested and dried. As self-sufficient herbalists, we have the knowledge to adjust the amount of the herb used, so it makes sense to do so. We can measure

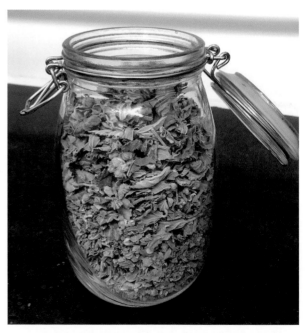

Making a batch of Marshmallow leaf tincture.

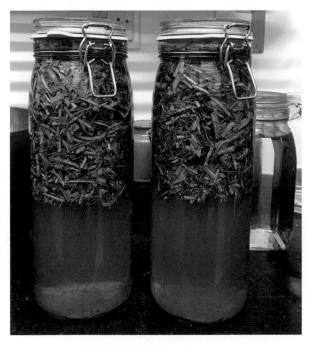

Making Cramp Bark tincture.

that amount using weight if we want to, or we can use volume if the herb has been cut up in the same way each time. I prefer to judge the amount by eye, basing it on how tightly the herb is packed into the jar and how far up the sides it reaches. I tend to cut herbs to a similar level of coarseness each time and use standard-sized tincturing jars, so this does provide a reasonable level of consistency and suits my purposes.

When tincturing fresh herbs, we need to consider a number of different factors. Some plants are higher in water content than others: for example, Wild Lettuce (*Lactuca virosa*) is moister than Rosemary (*Rosmarinus officinalis*). Then there is the weather prior to harvest. If the weather has been very wet in the days leading up to harvest, the moisture content of the harvested herbs will be much higher than of those that have been picked after a prolonged dry spell. I would always recommend harvesting on a dry day, but, as we have seen in the chapter on drying, the weather conditions even prior to harvest do have a significant influence on the moisture content of the herbs. Once we have harvested the herbs, we may decide to reduce their moisture content by wilting them. In this case, when deciding on the volume of herb for a batch of tincture, we need to take into account the length of time that the herb has been wilted prior to processing. If we need to wash the herbs – if they are roots for example – they will have an even higher water content, since they will absorb additional water during the washing process. Taking all

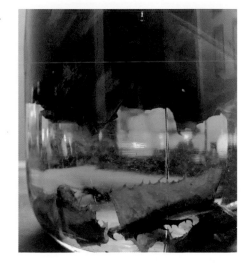

Wild Lettuce tincture.

of these different variables into account, we can see that not all batches of fresh herbs are equal.

Having made our tinctures, we need to record all of the details and then label the jar with a batch number, herb name, and date that matches the entry in our tincture-making record. It is then important to store the tincture in a cool, dark place. I use a cupboard in my clinic kitchen. You will often read instructions about shaking the tinctures daily, but I only do this from time to time, as I feel it is appropriate. Very frequent agitation exposes more of the plant

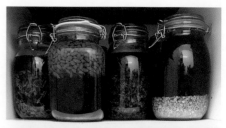

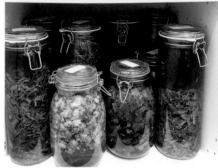

Once made, tinctures should be stored in a cool dark place. I use a cupboard in my clinic kitchen.

material to the top of the jar and may potentially increase the layer that becomes oxidized.

Once the tincture is ready, we can drain and press it. I use a conical stainless-steel colander lined with a muslin cloth. The colander happens to fit perfectly on top of a stainless-steel ice bucket, which has a capacity of around 5 litres / 1 gallon. Similar set-ups can be easily created with equipment widely available from kitchenware suppliers or large homeware retailers. The tincture and the herb are tipped out into the muslin-lined colander, and the liquid drains through into the ice bucket or whatever receptacle you have chosen. You can easily lift out the muslin and the herb and transfer it to your press after squeezing it by hand into the main lot of tincture. I use a small wine-making press purchased from a wine-making and home-brewing supplier.

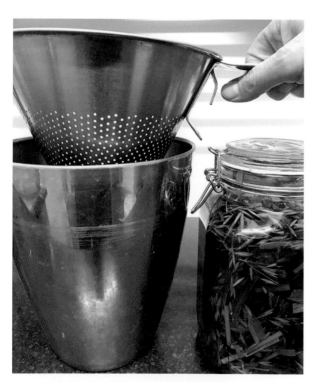

To drain tinctures, I use a conical stainless-steel colander that fits perfectly on top of a stainless-steel ice bucket.

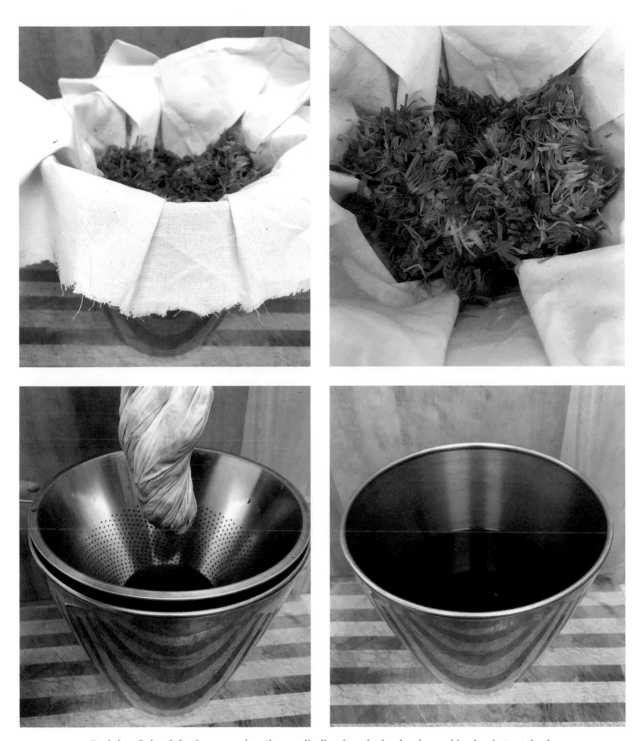

Draining Calendula tincture using the muslin-lined conical colander and ice bucket method.

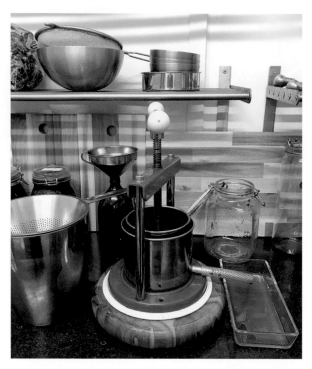

Pressing a tincture using a small wine-making press.

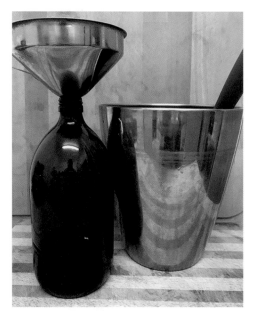

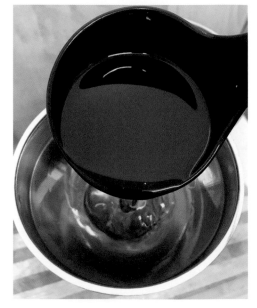

The tincture is ladled out of the ice bucket and put into bottles using a stainless-steel funnel.

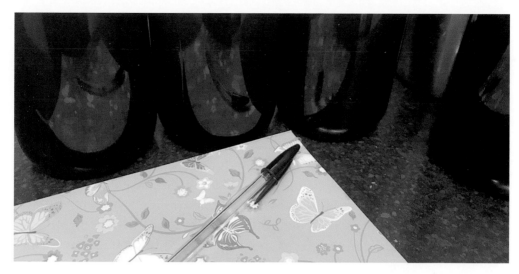

All the details are recorded in a series of tincture books.

You will find that some herbs do not seem to retain much of the liquid, and sometimes you find that wringing the cloth and the herb by hand is all that is needed to extract all that is going to come out. Other times you get a significant additional yield after pressing. Whatever I do, I am always conscious of the need to respect the herbs and not be wasteful. If I can press a batch and get enough medicine for another patient's daily dose, then that is a good aim.

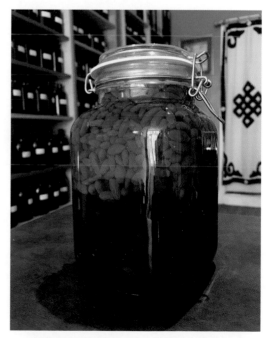

Once pressed, the spent herbs, or 'marc', are put to one side in their cloth. The herbs will later be added to the compost heap with respect and gratitude, and the cloths will be soaked and washed thoroughly. The tincture itself is ladled out of the ice bucket and put into bottles using a stainless-steel funnel. All that remains at that point is to label each bottle with the batch number, plant species, and the part used, such as root or leaf. All the other details are recorded in the record books. I store my tinctures in amber glass bottles on a shelf in my dispensary. If you are using clear glass bottles, you will need to store them in the dark.

Goji Berry tincture ready for draining and pressing, showing tincture storage shelves behind.

Making double-extracted tinctures

Before moving on to the making of other herbal products, I would like to describe the process of making double-extracted tinctures. It is something that I often get asked about. Simply put, it involves replacing the water fraction of a tincture with a cooled herbal tea or decoction. This technique is by far the best way to prepare medicinal mushroom extracts, because medicinal mushrooms traditionally require long, slow decoction in order to release their polyphenols. By making a double-extracted tincture, we are able to capture the valuable oil-soluble triterpenes as well as the water-soluble polyphenols in order to create a product that is highly effective, convenient, and long lasting. I love the fact that this technique enables us to extract the maximum possible medicinal potential from the mushrooms. I must admit that I am always a little sad when I see people taking medicinal mushrooms prepared as powders or capsules, because it feels like such a waste of the true healing potential of that precious natural medicine.

I use pretty much the same technique for all dried medicinal mushrooms. Here I use the making of a double-extracted tincture of Chaga (*Inonotus obliquus*) to illustrate the process. Chaga is a fungus that grows on mature birch trees in temperate zones, including the north of Scotland, Siberia, northern Scandinavia, and more northerly forests in the United States. I was very excited when I first got hold of some wild-harvested Chaga from the Highlands of Scotland. It had been gathered by a trusted professional forager, and I was delighted to buy some from someone who cared so deeply about ethical foraging and local sourcing. When I was in my twenties, I lived on Deeside, in the north of Scotland. I walked regularly in the Caledonian pine and birch forests among red deer and capercaillie, but sadly, in those days I did not know about Chaga. I may well have passed by trees with Chaga mushroom growth many times and have been totally oblivious to it. It is odd to think that there

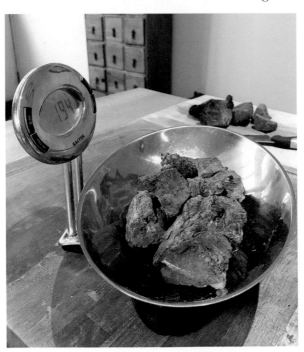

Weighing Chaga.

are so many medicines all around us, and unless we are familiar with how to use them, we are blind to them. Now that I have been using Chaga in my practice for many years, I know that I would always notice were I to see it, even if it was not appropriate to gather it. There is a beauty in noticing and appreciating a natural medicine for what it is. Every time that we do that, we are showing that the knowledge is preserved and is alive within us ready to be passed on.

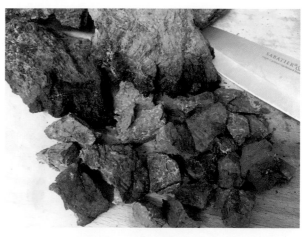

You first have to break the Chaga into small pieces. It is not as easy as it sounds.

The first time I held a chunk of Chaga in my hands, I was in awe of it. Even though it had not been gathered by my own hands, I knew how precious it was, how scarce in the overall scheme of things Chaga is, and how much this medicine should be respected and valued. It seemed to command respect, with its beautiful, rich, golden colour protected by a black, burnt-looking outer coating. Each chunk was woody in texture and hard as rock.

To make a double-extracted tincture of Chaga, you first have to break it into small pieces. It is not as easy as it sounds. At first, I tried sawing it using a mini hacksaw, but it seemed to be quite laborious and created a lot of sawdust. It was difficult to contain all of the pieces, and I was worried that too much would be wasted. I tried hitting it with a hammer, but pieces flew everywhere, and again there was a risk of wastage. Finally, I settled on pushing the point of a sharp knife into each large chuck, and once it was properly secure, twisting it slightly to cleave off a section. Perhaps, thanks to my study of geology, I felt that I could instinctively position the knife in such a way that the chunk would split. Maybe I was kidding myself, but it seemed to work. As the chunks got smaller, I realized that it was becoming increasingly risky to hold them steady, so I transferred the smaller pieces to my large pestle and mortar. That way I could break them down further and still keep all of my fingers. I still use this combination of

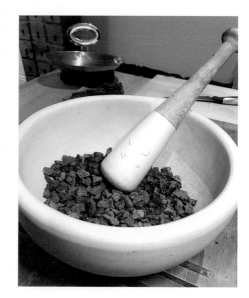

Once the chunks are small enough I break them down further using my pestle and mortar.

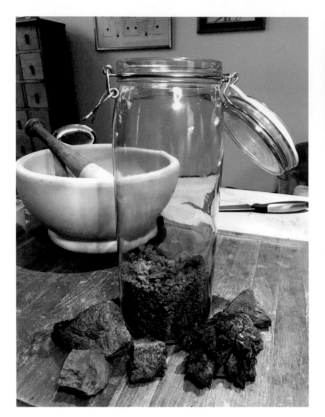 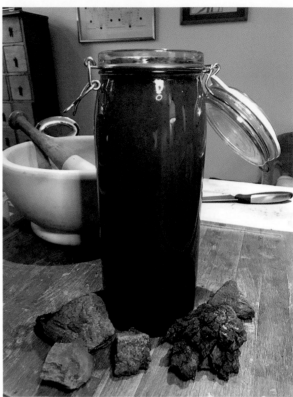

Place the chunks of Chaga into a Kilner jar ready to add the high strength alcohol. *Right*: Chaga tincture started off.

techniques to this day. Some people put the Chaga chunks into a clean pillow-case and hit it with a mallet. Whichever way you choose to break them down, you definitely need to make the chunks smaller before tincturing unless you have bought-in pre-cut material. I aim for pieces around 3–6 mm/⅛–¼ in in diameter. I think that powder would be too fine, but we may agree to differ on that point.

After you have reduced the size of the chunks, the first stage is to tincture the pieces in a high-strength alcohol. It is important to use a relatively high concentration of alcohol to start with, because later on in the process you are going to be adding more water to the mixture. You need to end up with a high enough concentration of alcohol that the final double extraction will be preserved properly. Since my Chaga is thoroughly dried, I choose 60% alcohol for this. If I were working with fresh mushrooms, such as Shiitake (*Lentinula edodes*), I would need to use a much higher strength to compensate for the water content in the mushrooms, and I would add less of the water extraction to the final double-extracted tincture.

If you use vodka to make your tinctures, you will need to find 120%-proof in order to make a 60% alcohol extract. A 40%-proof bottle will not be sufficiently strong to make a double extraction. It may well be that when the time comes for you to start making double extractions, you decide to look seriously at sourcing pure ethanol.

First, place the chunks of Chaga into a Kilner jar. I tend to work on the basis of adding approximately 650 g / 1.43 lb into a 1.5-litre / 2.5-pint jar and then adding 1.7 litres / 3 pints of 60% alcohol (remember: 60% alcohol is twice the strength of 60% proof). Label the tincture and place it in a cool, dark place for at least 4 weeks. After it has macerated, you can drain it in the usual way, but do not discard the hard-won pieces of Chaga in your draining cloth. Tip them out of the cloth into a large stainless-steel saucepan.

Measure the volume of the alcoholic extraction using measuring jugs and store it temporarily in a clean Kilner jar while you make the slow decoction. For every litre of alcoholic extraction you have made, you need to add twice that volume of water to the pieces of Chaga in the saucepan. You are going to

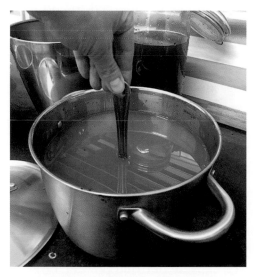

I measure the depth of the liquid in the pan by standing a knife in it and judging how far the depth must decrease before the volume will have reduced by 50%.

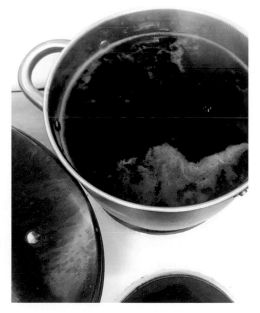

Decocting the Chaga.

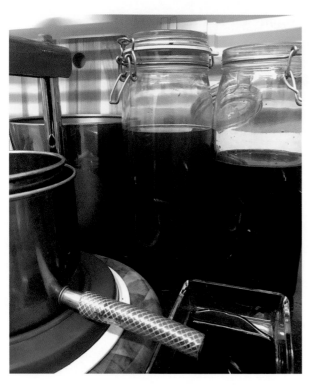

Once cooled the decoction is pressed. The jar on the left contains the tincture and the jar on the right contains the decoction.

decoct this slowly until the volume has been reduced by 50%. I measure the depth of the liquid in the pan by standing a knife into it and judging how far the depth must decrease before the volume will have been reduced by 50%. This is by far the best way of measuring the volume of boiling hot decoction part-way through the process. The decoction is simmered slowly for 3–4 hours. Once the volume is reduced by 50% and is therefore approximately the same volume as the tincture that you have set aside, you can strain it and cool it.

When the decoction is cool, you can measure its volume properly using measuring jugs. If your knife-measuring technique was good, you should have more or less the same volume as the alcoholic extraction. If you find you have slightly more of the decoction, put the 'extra bit' to one side and drink it as a tea yourself. Do not be tempted to add it to the final mix. It is not a good idea to add too much water to the final product.

Now you have an alcoholic extraction and a cooled aqueous extraction, which can be added together in a large mixing container before being bottled. You have made a double-extracted tincture that has sufficient alcohol content to preserve it properly. When making double-extracted mushroom tinctures, the idea is that you should end up with an alcohol content that is at least 25%. In my example, the final alcohol content would be 30%.

A well-made double extraction will keep for years and be richly potent and easily bioavailable. It is time-consuming to make but well worth the effort. Why would you assume that a human digestive tract can extract the goodness of a medicinal mushroom from a swallowed capsule of dried powder, or even powder added to a smoothie, when we know that traditionally it takes 3–4 hours of gentle decocting to extract the medicinal polyphenols in a bioavailable form? To make matters worse, medicinal mushrooms are often prescribed as part of a cancer-supportive strategy. In these circumstances, digestive capacity is often considerably reduced, because of stress, surgery, or the side-effects of allopathic treatments, and it is especially important that the medicinal compounds are as bioavailable as possible. In my practice, I make double extractions with various medicinal mushrooms as well as lichens such as Usnea. I thoroughly recommend the process. Once you see how effective these medicines are, you will be hooked.

As well as using decocted and reduced double-extraction techniques for medicinal mushrooms, you can make simpler double-extracted tinctures of herbs if you feel drawn to do this. For example, if making a tincture of Lemon Balm (*Melissa officinalis*) using high-strength alcohol (which would need diluting with water), you can replace the water part with an infusion of the herb.

If you are starting to make double-extracted tinctures, the main thing to bear in mind is that you must end up with a high-enough alcohol content in the double-extracted tincture that it is preserved effectively.

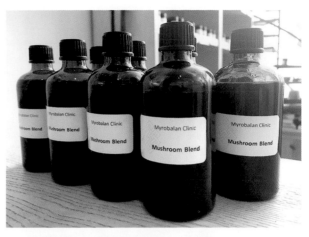

A blend of double-extracted medicinal mushrooms ready to go out to patients.

Capsule making

I think that the most important part of capsule making is making sure that we fill them with the best possible quality herbs. When we grow or gather our own herbs, it makes sense that we would want to use them to fill our own capsules.

Capsules can be made by blending herbs together in a formula or by encapsulating single herbs. In my practice, I have developed a range of standard capsule blends and single-herb capsules that support different systems of the body. I often prescribe these favourite blends alongside individually tailored tincture or tea prescriptions, which are totally unique to each patient. My standard capsule options include a kidney blend, a circulation blend, a gut-healing blend, a blood-building blend, and a nerve-calming blend, for example. These days I do not make up totally individualized capsule blends, because of the difficulty of grinding very small volumes of herbs without

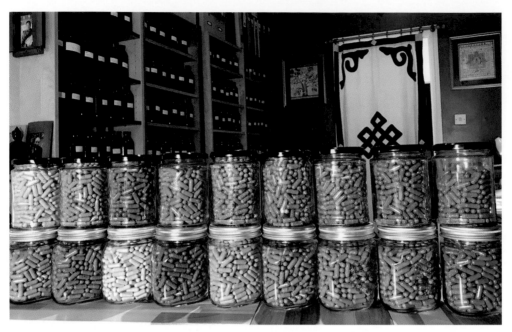

When we grow or gather our own herbs, it makes sense that we would want to use them to fill our own capsules.

waste. It is perfectly possible, though, to create tailor-made blends for pre-scribing, provided that you are sure that a particular blend suits the patient and that it will be required for a period of time. Capsules can be much more convenient for patients who travel frequently or for those who wish to avoid alcohol and cannot always make up a herbal tea. Once I supplied a Tibetan Lama with his own personal capsule blend so that it was convenient for him to take his medicine during a meditation retreat.

Capsule making requires that we have the means to break down the herbs into a fine powder. When I first started making my own capsules, I used a coffee grinder – or, more accurately, I should say, a series of coffee-grinders, because none of them lasted very long. After a while I realized that I needed to invest in something that was more robust. After some research, I bought a Vitamix 500, which came with both a 'wet' container and a 'dry' one. I have only ever used the 'dry' container. The Vitamix is a well-made and very powerful food processer. It grinds all sort of herbs and roots very well and is very good at tackling mixed batches of different-hardness plant material, such as you would get when grinding a capsule formula. It is not quite so happy when faced with very hard roots, but with repeated short bursts you can eventually get a reasonable grind. My machine is totally reserved for clinic use, so I do not use it for food preparation tasks where the 'wet' container would be needed. The Vitamix would be an excellent option if you generally do your herb preparation in your kitchen and are happy to have one machine that combines herb powdering and food preparation. Despite never having used the 'wet' container, I have found the Vitamix to be excellent value for money. My purchase was made over 12 years ago, and I hope I will not jinx it to announce here that my machine is still going strong. I have, however, recently upgraded to a C Goldenwall 4000g professional herb grinder because the volumes of herbs I am grinding have been increasing steadily. This is a very powerful machine that makes light work of even the toughest roots and seeds. I am impressed to see that it produces an excellent particle size even when faced with really tough roots, like Bloodroot

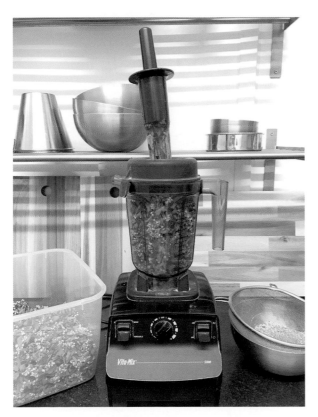

Powdering Hawthorn blossom in my Vitamix.

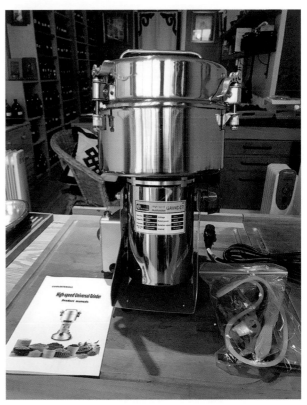

My C Goldenwall professional herb grinder.

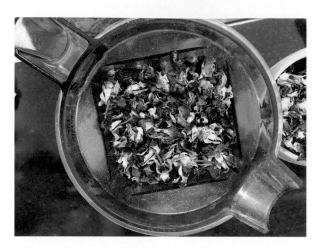

Powdering Rose petals for a capsule blend.

(*Sanguinaria canadensis*). The version I have can grind up to 4000 g / 8.8 lb of hard plant material in one batch, and I use it to grind capsule formulae that I am making in reasonably large quantities. The grinding blades need to be well covered by the herb in order for it to work efficiently, so you cannot grind small volumes in a high-capacity machine. If I need to grind small quantities of particular herbs or a small batch of a capsule formula, I stick to my Vitamix. C Goldenwall do have a range of different capacity machines, so if you are grinding small volumes and want a machine totally for use in your herbal work,

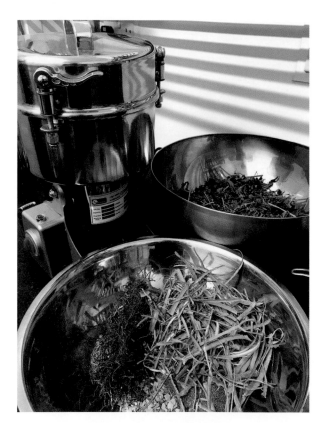

Powdering herbs for a calming capsule, blend 1.

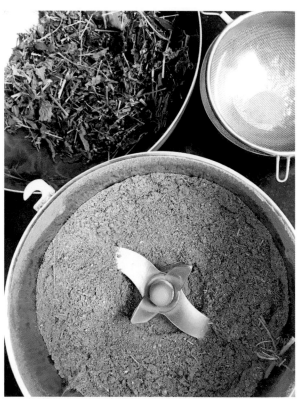

Powdering herbs for a calming capsule, blend 2.

I recommend that you consider one of their smaller machines. I am so impressed with the C Goldenwall machine that I am tempted to get a second smaller-capacity version myself.

Different herbs will break down to powder more or less efficiently. It is important to minimize a herb's exposure to heat, so I am careful to grind in short bursts, giving the machine a chance to cool down in between. I often grind whole formulae rather than individual herbs, especially when one herb in a formula is less easy to powder. Artichoke (*Cynara scolymus*) leaf, for example, has a tendency to become woolly rather than be powdered, but when mixed with other herbs it seems to be grind down much better. At the end of the grinding process, I sieve the herbs into a stainless-steel bowl. There is usually a small amount of coarser material left in the sieve, and this can be added respectfully to the compost. Once powdered, each formula

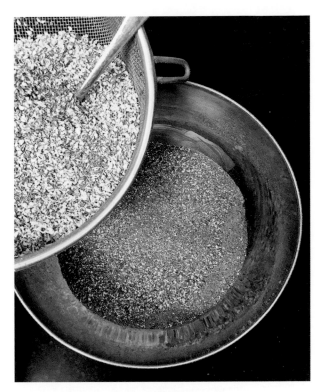

Sieving powdered Hawthorn blossom.

can be stored in glass jars in the dark until needed for capsule making. I grind and mix small batches as needed, since powdered herbs do not keep as well as whole herbs.

When you are ready to fill capsules with your powdered herbs, you will need to source empty capsule shells. Empty capsules are available from a wide range of herbal wholesalers and retailers. The price per capsule varies quite a great deal depending on the amount that you buy in one go. I tend to buy 15,000 at a time, which works well for my practice in terms of available storage space as well as getting a more favourable price per capsule. It makes perfect sense, though, to buy them in smaller quantities when first starting out.

Empty capsules are usually made of gelatin or vegetable cellulose; personally I always choose vegetable cellulose, so that the capsules are suitable for vegetarian and vegan patients. As you start researching capsule availability, you will see that there are different-sized capsules available. Size '00' is the largest, but I prefer size '0', which is slightly smaller. Some herbal practitioners worry

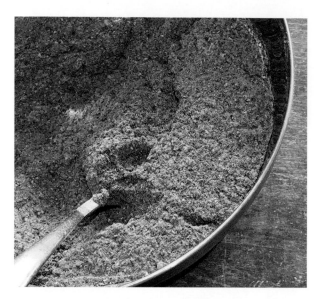

Powdered Rose petals.

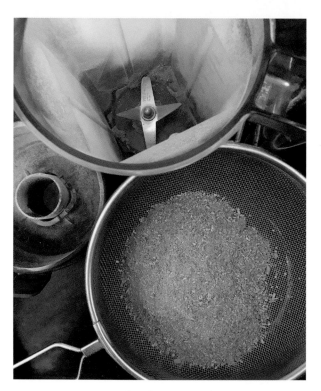

Powdered Cramp Bark.

that sizes smaller than size '00' would make it more difficult to deliver a therapeutically active dose. They have worked out the weight of the herb contained in a particular capsule size and conclude that with a size '0' capsule multiple capsules would be needed to deliver an effective dose. What I say to this is that the strength of herbs (and their weight per volume) probably varies quite widely. Herbs are living and variable products, and commercially sourced herbs may not have been treated optimally during harvest, drying, and processing. I know that my own dried herbs are the best possible quality, and I have found that size '0' capsules are most definitely therapeutically active. I should also report that many patients tell me specifically that they would not want to take larger capsules than the size that I prescribe.

Dosage can be varied by the number of capsules prescribed per day. Most often I prescribe patients one or two per day of each type required. In some circumstances, certain types of capsules are prescribed at higher rates: up to 9 a day for short periods of time. Like all aspects of herbal medicine, we adjust things according to the patient and their circumstances as well as our preferred way of working.

The easiest way to make capsules is by hand. I was shown how to do this by my amazing mentor, Edith Barlow, who used to make 3,000 capsules by hand every Monday morning. She told me that she would get up early and start at 7.30 am and would be finished by 11.30 am. She is still treating patients and making capsules at the age of

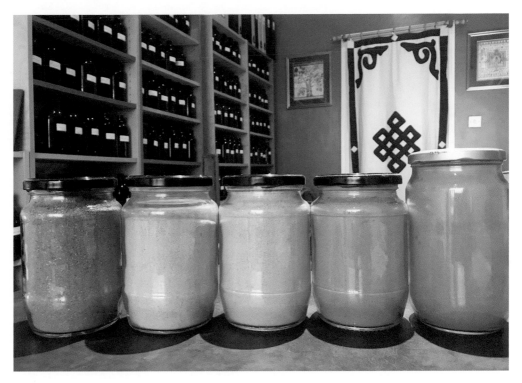

Once powdered, each formula can be stored in glass jars in the dark until needed for capsule making.

ninety, although I think that the quantities involved are a little more manageable these days.

I spent years making capsules in this way and learned to be very quick at it, to the extent that I was making and dispensing 700–800 capsules per day before I finally got a capsule-making machine. There is a story about how I got that machine, but first I want to explain the best way to make capsules by hand. I thoroughly recommend starting out in this way. You can start to get a feel for how you will integrate capsules into your practice, and by the time you are totally comfortable with how many you will be prescribing, you will be ready to invest in a decent-quality and efficient machine.

You need to have a clean surface and a series of small stainless-steel bowls, one for empty capsules, one for the herbal powder that is going into them, and another for the ones that you have made. With very clean hands (or wearing food-grade gloves) open each capsule and dab the larger end into the bowl of powder until it is totally filled. Place the smaller 'lid' on firmly

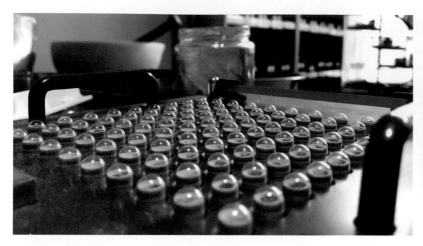

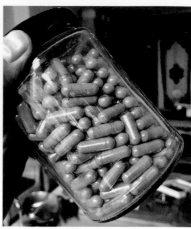

Making Turmeric capsules.   A jar of Turmeric capsules.

and push it down until it locks into place. Pop the finished capsule into the bowl, and start on the next one. It is much better to decant small quantities of empty capsules into a bowl than to reach into your main stock container with powdery hands as you work.

The next level up from making them by hand is a simple type of cap-

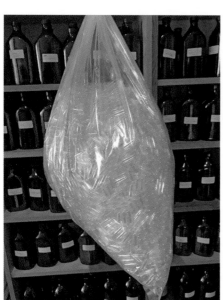

I buy in 15,000 empty capsules at a time.

sule filler that requires you to open each capsule and place the larger end into a holed tray template before filling them. I have two of these fillers but find them fiddly and inefficient. I soon realized that since you were already having to open each capsule by hand, it was much quicker to fill them immediately while holding them. I do still use one of them very occasionally to make oil-filled capsules in the very rare circumstances that I wish to treat patients in this way. Although it is inefficient, I only ever make very small quantities, and I do not want to get oils near my proper capsule filler.

The best capsule fillers are precision-engineered and allow you to remove the lids from 100 capsules and replace them in one go. The one I have is made by Adelphi Engineering in Haywards Heath, UK. I bought a Profiller 1100 capsule filler many years ago when I had been in practice for two or three years and was making

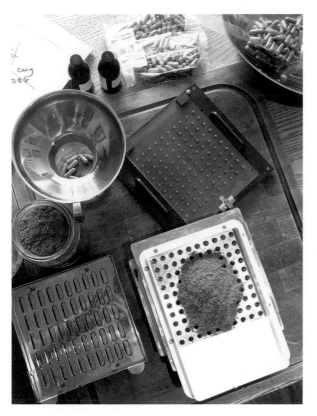

Making capsules for repeat prescriptions.

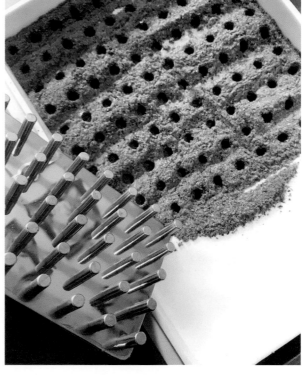

Tamping down the powder.

large quantities of capsules by hand. These fabulous machines are very easy to use once you get used to them. I can make capsules at a rate of around 100 in 2 minutes, provided that I have pre-blended my herbal powders. The machines are made to order, so when ordering, you have to specify the size of capsule that you require. Due to the relatively large investment involved, I would say that it is a sensible plan to have been working with capsules for a while in practice before purchasing. That way you will have settled on the size that works best for you and your patients and feel confident that the investment is worth it.

I said earlier that there was a story around how I got hold of my Profiller 1100 capsule filler, and here it is. When I first started in practice, I was working from a room in the beautiful and picturesque old barn conversion that we were living in. It had roses growing around the front door and a prolific Jasmine plant outside the window of my clinic and dispensary room. Between

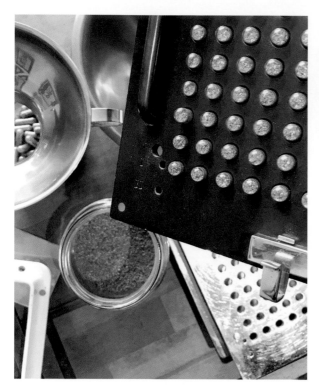

Finished capsules ready to be stored or dispensed.

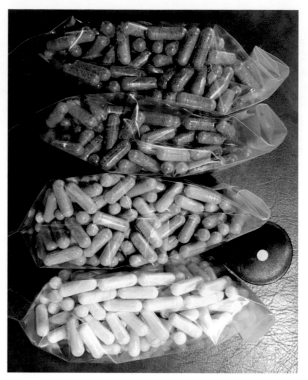

Capsules for a prescription.

patients I used to sit at the kitchen table in front of the Aga, making capsules. I had begun to dispense hundreds of capsules each day, so there was never a spare moment. Soon, making capsules by hand had started to take over my life, so I started to look seriously at alternatives. I bought a simple template filler from a herbalist who was retiring, but soon realized that I was much quicker at making them by hand. I did a bit of research and found that the best option for my needs was the precision-engineered type as made by Adelphi Engineering. At the time, they did not list prices on their website, responding instead to individual requests for quotations. I had sent off for a quotation, not knowing at all what to expect, and had recently received the reply that informed me that the machine, with accessories, would be around £1,300. I was still quite new in practice and was paying off debts accumulated during my clinical training, so was weighing up whether this was the right time to invest in the equipment or whether I could manage as I was for another year or two. I was mulling all of this over in my mind when my next patient arrived and immediately asked me what I was doing there at the kitchen table.

I explained that I had been making my capsules by hand for a few years, but had just reached the point where I was seriously considering upscaling, because making them by hand was taking over my life. She seemed very interested and asked me about the different alternatives, and I explained about the recent quotation for the Profiller 1100 and said that I was not sure whether I should go for it at this stage. Out of the blue, she suddenly announced that she would like to buy one for me! I was hugely embarrassed by this offer, because I was worried that she might have thought that I was hinting at that outcome by mentioning the price of the machine I was considering. I remember turning the colour of a beetroot, and I am not one to blush easily. I argued that although it was extremely kind of her to offer, it really was not necessary. I was so sorry that I had mentioned the details, and I hoped that she did not think I was hinting that she should buy it. She said that of course she did not think that for a minute, she just really wanted to buy it for me. She felt that the herbal treatment that I had given her had been instrumental in her recovery from what had seemed like a hopeless situation. In her mind, I had saved her life. She told me that it would give her the greatest pleasure to repay me in some bigger way than my normal fees, and she would not listen to my remonstrations. She took out her cheque book, wrote me a cheque for the amount, tore it out, and handed it to me with a flourish. She said, take it, I really want you to have it. So, after a bit of an awkward hesitation, I did, thanking her profusely. I am still embarrassed about it in a way, because up until that point she had paid the going rate for her treatment, and I felt that there had already been a fair exchange between us. She was very insistent, though, and my overriding feeling is one of enormous gratitude to her. I never charged her for consultations or medicines again, and I think about her every time I use that machine – almost a daily occurrence. Her spontaneous generosity quite literally changed my life and made it possible for me to treat the increasing numbers of people that were finding their way to my door.

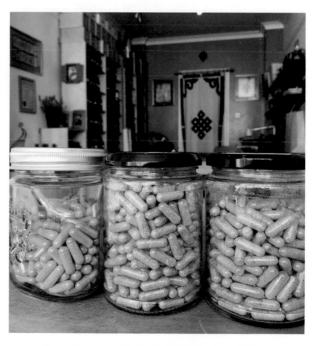

Capsules stored in jars ready for prescribing.

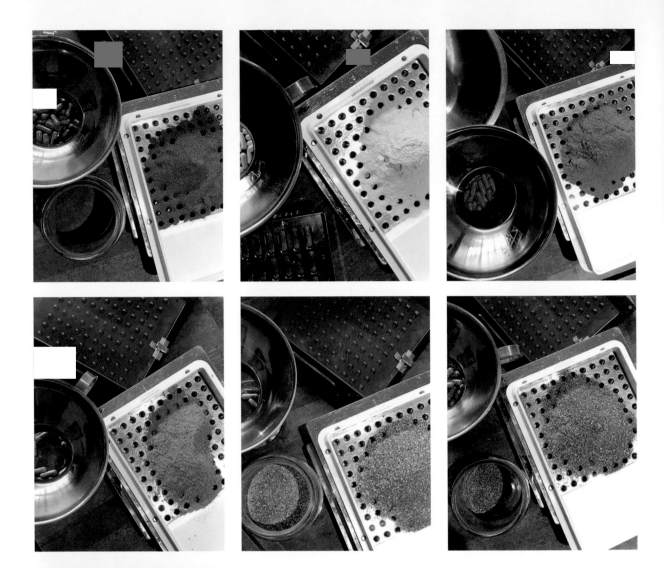

Top row: Anaemia blend; Ashwagandha; Cats Claw

Middle row: Circulatory support; Hawthorn; Hawthorn and Motherwort

Bottom: Meadowsweet and Celery Seed

Fourteen different capsule blends being encapsulated.

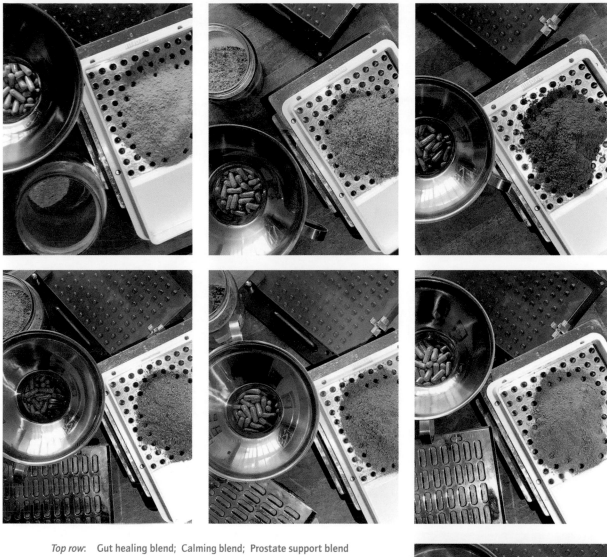

Top row: Gut healing blend; Calming blend; Prostate support blend

Middle row: Rose and Hawthorn blend; Seaweed blend; Sendru Dangné Tsawa

Bottom: Turmeric

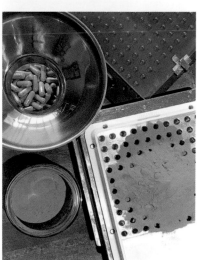

Infused-oil making

It is a wonderful thing to be able to make infused herbal oils as topical treatments. The oils can be used as massage oils or topical rubs, or they can be set into ointments for convenience. You can also use them to make creams or body butters by emulsifying the infused oil with a water-based infusion or decoction.

I usually choose mild and light olive oil as the basis for these infused oils. The mild olive oil is not too scented, so it does not mask the scent of the herbs that are infused into it. If you choose cold-pressed olive oils, they tend to have a stronger smell, but they are richer in naturally occurring Vitamin E, which helps to extend their shelf life. You can always add some Vitamin E into the finished product, though, if you like.

Although I mostly choose olive oil for my infused oils, I use other oils for particular herbal products, as needed. Sesame seed oil is excellent as an external treatment for 'wind' conditions in Tibetan medicine, almond oil is lovely as a face oil when infused with Rose petals, Green tea and Hibiscus, and Safflower oil makes a very good basis for a bruise ointment due to its own inherent medicinal properties.

There are so many different possibilities for making infused oils depending on the properties and actions that you require. You can use either fresh herbs or dried herbs. It is worth noting here, though, that you should not

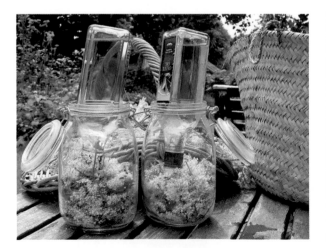 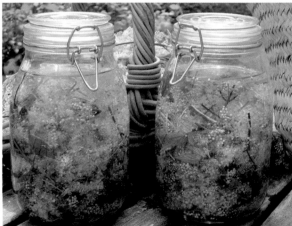

Making infused Meadowsweet oil.

take oils made from fresh herbs internally. This is due to the small risk of anaerobic bacteria such as *Clostridium botulinum* growing in the infusion. This cannot happen if dried herbs are used.

My favourite infused oils are made with fresh St John's Wort (*Hypericum perforatum*) flowers, or Comfrey (*Symphytum officinale*), Lavender (*Lavandula angustifolia*), Agrimony (*Agrimonia eupatoria*) and Calendula (*Calendula officinalis*) flowers. I also make a lot of Nettle (*Urtica dioica*) seed and Rosemary (*Rosmarinus officinalis*) infused oil each year, as well as others like Chickweed (*Stellaria media*), Arnica (*Arnica montana*), Yarrow (*Achillea millefolium*), Pine (*Pinus sylvestris*) shoots, Dandelion (*Taraxacum officinalis*) flowers and Meadowsweet (*Filipendula ulmaria*) flowers. We all have our own favourites, but whatever we choose, the process is pretty much the same.

If using fresh herbs, it is important to pick them on a perfectly dry day. If you are working with a fleshy high-moisture-content herb such as Comfrey (*Symphytum officinale*), it is advisable to wilt the herb for about 12 hours before infusing in order to reduce the moisture content. Herbs like Rosemary (*Rosmarinus officinalis*) or Pine (*Pinus sylvestris*) shoots do not have such a high moisture content and can be used straight away if their surface is dry. When using fresh herbs, the water eventually collects in a murky layer at the bottom of the infusing container. You can

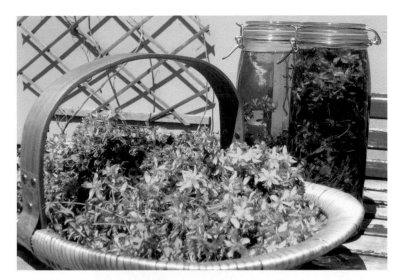

St John's Wort oil just started off.

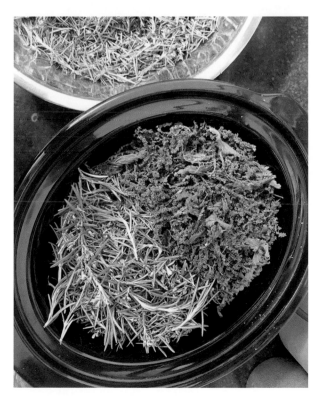

Making Nettle seed and Rosemary infused oil in a slow cooker.

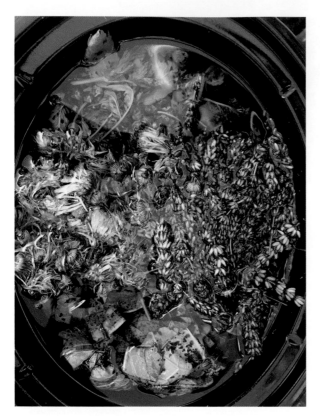

Making a batch of Comfrey blend infused oil.

carefully decant the oil and leave the moisture to be discarded. If using dried herbs, you can simply use the whole infused batch, without worrying about any moisture.

There are various different techniques for making infused oils. The simplest and most beautiful to observe is passive solar infusion. You pack the chosen herb or herbs into a glass preserving jar and fill it to the top with the oil of your choice, ensuring that all of the herb material is submerged below the surface of the oil. You may need to devise a way of weighing the herbs down. I find that if I fill the jar with oil to the very top, this is not necessary. Once filled, the jar is placed on a sunny window sill for a few weeks. It is magical to watch the beautiful red colour developing in an infusing St John's Wort (*Hypericum perforatum*) oil.

If you do not have a sunny windowsill or have already filled your available space, then you might consider methods that use gentle heat. It is not a good idea to heat the oil directly, as you could damage the herbal properties and affect the keeping quality of the oil. A double boiler or bain marie is an excellent piece of equipment for the self-sufficient herbalist. I have a porringer, which is a double boiler designed for making porridge. It consists of a base pan that is used to simmer boiling water and a second pan, which fits snugly inside it. A porringer allows you to gently warm the oil without applying direct heat. The oil pan should be packed with herbs, but, as with the passive infusion method, all the herbs should be submerged below the oil. You warm it for around two hours before straining, cooling, and bottling. It will be necessary to keep topping up the water in the base pan, as only a shallow layer is possible, and this tends to boil dry quite quickly. I always set a timer to remind me to check it every 15 minutes or so. I have learnt from bitter experience how easy it is to lose track and let it boil dry.

Another option is to use a slow cooker on the 'warm' setting. Be aware that not all slow cookers have a 'warm' setting. I like the slow-cooker option because there is no risk of it boiling dry, and it requires less intensive tending. It can still over-heat the oil, though, if it is left on continuously. I avoid this by pulsing the slow cooker on and off on the 'warm' setting over a period of a few days. I generally allow it to have an hour on 'warm' daily, which because of the insulated nature of the slow cooker means that it stays warm for several hours each day. This is much easier for me to manage between seeing patients than the porringer option.

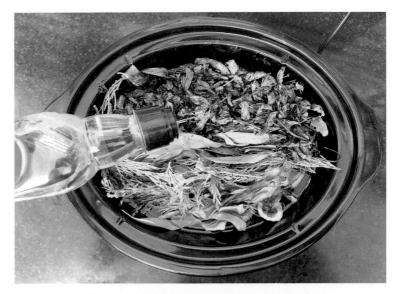

Making a batch of decongestant blend infused oil.

If you only have a 'low' setting on your slow cooker, this will be too harsh unless you create a makeshift double boiler. This is done by adding water to the slow cooker pan and sitting a bowl of herbs and oil in it. You will need to have a close-fitting lid on the bowl of herbs so that drips of condensed water do not collect on the slow cooker lid and fall into the oil. Alternatively, you can leave the whole thing without a lid and keep topping up the water as needed.

Once the oil is ready you will need to strain out the herbs and decant the oil. I use a conical colander lined with filter paper, which sits over an ice bucket, so that the oil can drip through. The whole filter paper and spent herbs can then be removed and added to the compost. In the early days, I used a muslin cloth, but it was quite a lot of extra work to get the oily cloths clean afterwards. I still use muslin cloths for tincture straining, though.

Once the oil has been drained, it can be filtered for a second time by using another coffee filter paper in a funnel as you decant it into bottles. The infused oil is ladled into

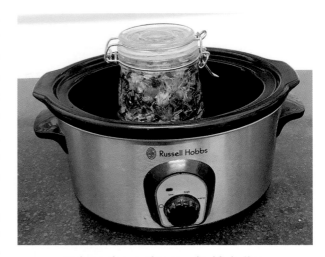

Using a slow cooker as a double boiler.

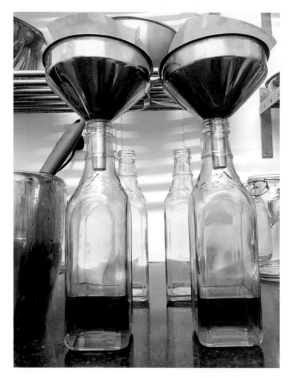 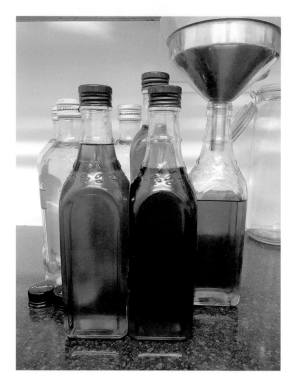

Filtering infused oil as it goes into the storage bottles.

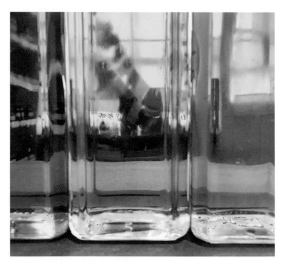

Filtering twice results in a very clear oil and is
worth the time and effort.

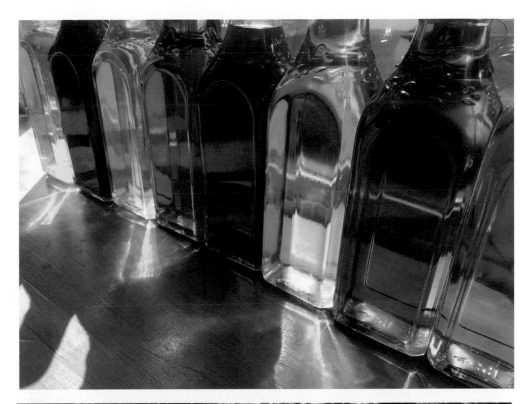

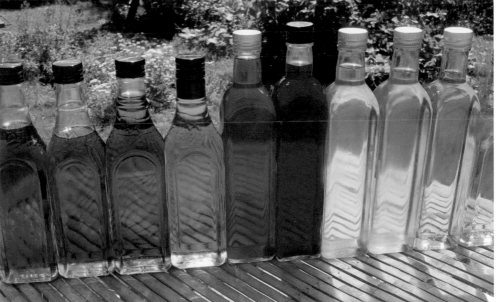

Infused oils are beautiful to look at but should be stored away from direct light.

the funnel, from which it can drip slowly into the bottle. I use glass olive oil bottles. These days it can be hard to find olive oil in glass bottles, but if you do you will be able to use the bottle to store the oil once it has been infused. For this reason, I think it is well worth paying a little bit more for the olive oil if you find it in a glass bottle. Over the years, I have built up quite a collection of glass oil bottles, which are washed and re-used again and again.

Filtering a batch of oil often takes a couple of days or more. I have a dedicated herbal processing kitchen in my clinic, so it is not a problem for me to leave herbal oils filtering for this length of time. What you will find is that the oil tends to stop dripping through the filter paper once a certain amount of oil has collected in the funnel. Occasional lifting of the filter paper in the funnel releases the surface tension and allows the built-up oil to run through into the bottle. I lift the filter papers hourly if I can, or at least every time I walk through the kitchen during a clinic day. The extra effort is worth it as the double-filtering process results in a very clear oil. Take care to leave the watery cloudy fraction behind, though. Once the oil is in the bottles, these are labelled and then stored in a cool, dark place until needed.

Making ointments

In my practice, I use my store of infused oils to create small batches of various ointments, as needed. I find it more efficient in terms of storage space to store the bulk of the infused oils in bottles and make batches of 20–30 jars of ointments, as needed. As the bulk of my ointments are prescribed, the rate at which they are used varies according to the patients whom I am seeing at any one time. I can never predict which ointments will sell out fastest. I do not want a lot of jars and labels tied up unnecessarily, so it is more efficient in terms of working capital requirement to make batches as needed. You may feel that it makes more sense to make the whole batch of oil into ointment in one go. If you do keep some as infused oil, you have the leeway to make the ointments when it suits you. The infused oils have captured the medicinal properties of the herbs while they were in season, so there is no urgency to process it further until it is needed.

Making ointments involves warming the oil with a setting agent until it melts. I use beeswax, which I add at a ratio of 1 g per 7 ml of infused oil. Different oils may require different ratios, and the amount of setting agent you use will be influenced by how hard or soft you wish the finished product to be. The oil and wax are heated in the double boiler so they are not exposed to direct heat. Once the wax is melted I pour the oil from the pan into a jug and then, carefully, into jars. It is important not to move the jars once the ointment has started

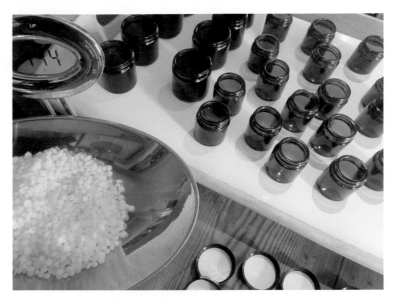

Weighing the granules of beeswax.

to set. Undisturbed jars set with a nice flat surface, especially if you slow the cooling process by covering them with a piece of kitchen paper. Once the jars of ointment are set, they can be picked up to put the lids on and apply labels without spoiling their appearance.

I make a wide range of ointments using my home-grown or wild-harvested herbs. Ointments are convenient and popular. Patients often buy multiple small jars, so they can have one in their handbag and another at home in the bathroom, for example. Smaller travel sizes are a good option too. My products include a topical treatment for haemorrhoids and varicose veins, ointments for arthritic fingers, aching muscles, bruises, congested sinuses, general healing, and scars. I also make a Fennel (*Foeniculum vulgare*) ointment – using bought-in Fennel seeds – for women suffering with vaginal dryness. As a self-sufficient herbalist, you

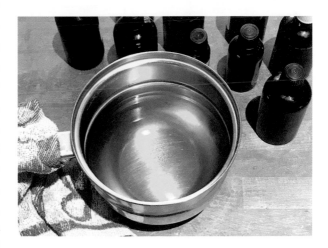

Preparing to pour the oil once the beeswax has melted.

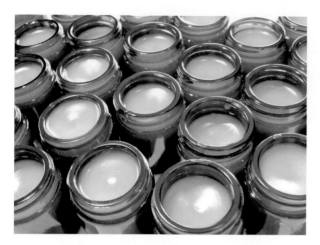

Undisturbed jars set with a nice flat surface.

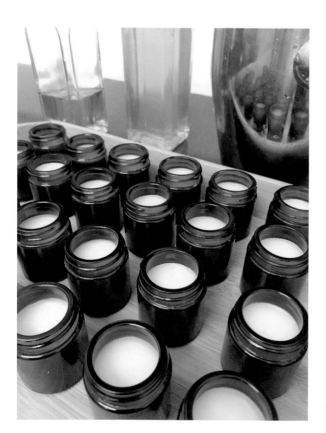

Jars of ointment setting in the clinic kitchen.

will soon know or discover which infused oils and topical products fit best into your own work.

In summary, then, tinctures, capsules, and ointments are the most often used processing techniques in my practice. I use simple and straightforward processes, which have resulted in tried, tested, and effective herbal medicines for many years. I hope that this little tour gives you the confidence to process more of your own herbs. I do worry that so many herbal students whom I meet seem to be daunted by the apparent complexity of making herbal products 'correctly'. I cannot help but wonder whether the way students are taught about herbal processing these days is overly influenced by a desire for herbal medicine to be fully embraced by the allopathic community. We know that herbal medicine uses whole living plants, which are inherently different from therapeutic, artificial substances made under laboratory conditions. We also know that herbal medicine works on the basis of supporting the patient and allowing their body to move back into a more balanced and 'at-ease' state. It is quite different from the way that allopathic medication works. I am not arguing that allopathic medication is wrong or totally undesirable. Not at all. All practitioners have gone into a healing modality with a genuine desire to help patients feel well and get more out of life. We are most fortunate to live in a world where we have a choice of approaches that we can turn to when we need help. I am just saying that our approach is different, and therefore the way that we prepare and prescribe our

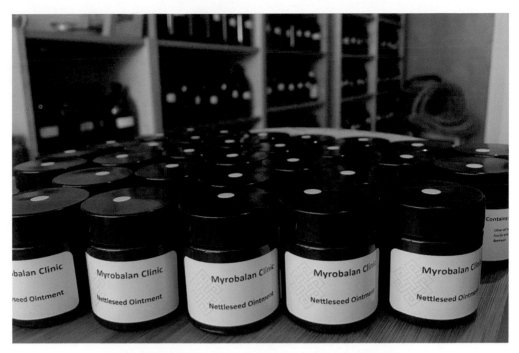

Finished ointment ready to go out to patients who need it.

medicines will, inevitably, be different. Of course, all medicinal products, whether herbal or otherwise, must be safe and therapeutically effective, but our benchmarks are not the same as those used for allopathic medicine. We must ensure that our processing techniques are grounded in good practice, but just as we use our detailed understanding and knowledge of the actions of herbs to adjust the way we formulate prescriptions, I think that there should also be scope for more fluidity and intuition when processing herbs for our own practice. This is the difference between working with herbs purely as 'bundles of chemicals' and working with herbs as living beings that have a purpose and an energy to offer us beyond the physical make-up of their cells.

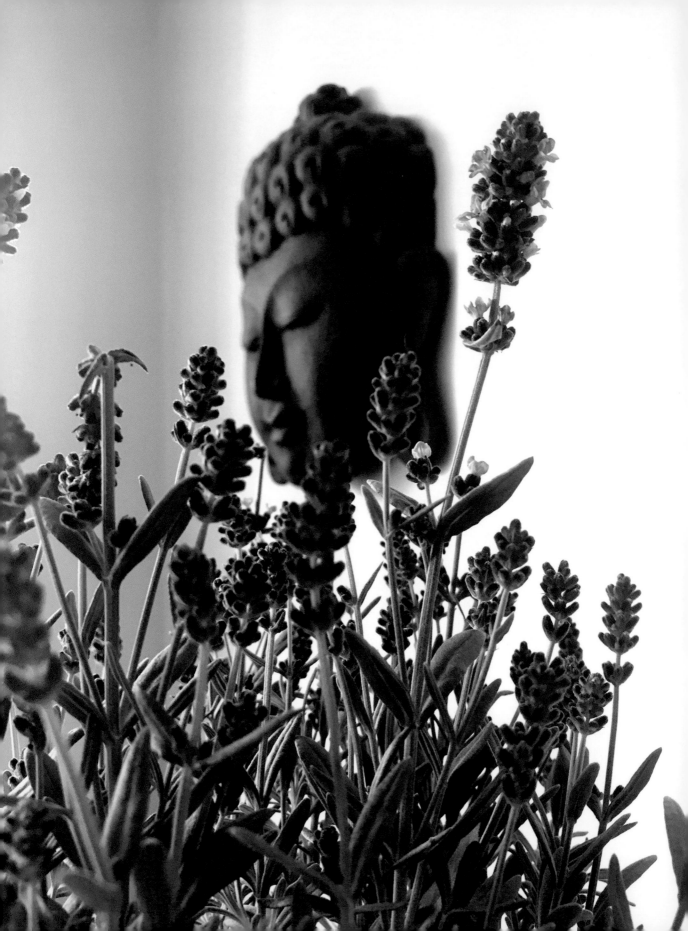

As well as sharing practical information about how to grow, gather and process our own herbs for medicine, I have explained that there are very many reasons why this way of working is one well worth exploring. It not only allows us to create high quality and vibrant herbal medicines, but also through the environmental benefits that it brings, it helps us to play our part in reducing harmful impacts on this precious planet. Working more closely with the herbs that we use for medicine benefits our patients, the herbs, and our relationship with them. It nourishes and grounds us, helping us to feel more connected to the land where we live and it allows us a greater capacity to help others without depleting ourselves.

These reasons for practicing self-sufficient herbalism are compelling in themselves but there is another far wider reason why I hope that many more of us will work in this way. I believe that an understanding of how to grow, gather, and process our own herbal medicines is vital if herbal medicine itself is to survive and thrive. Those of us who love herbs and respect their medicinal properties are custodians of an ancient and precious tradition. We are links in a chain of teaching and knowledge that stretches back through countless generations. Our lineage represents far more than just an understanding of how herbs work and how they should be prescribed. To be complete and resilient, it must include practical knowledge of herbal sourcing and of the preparation of safe, effective natural medicines. If we are unable to source particular herbs, or if obtaining them literally costs us the earth, then we will be unable to continue using them. Equally, if the quality of herbs available to us becomes significantly diminished we will not feel comfortable using them.

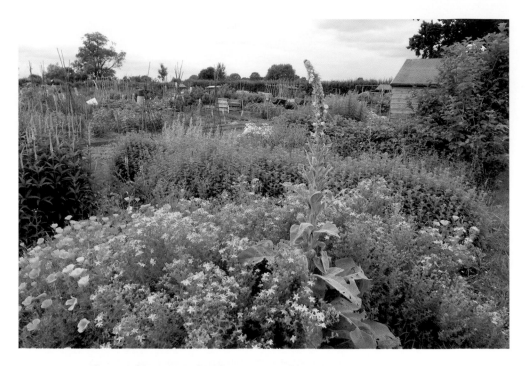

Above: Mid-summer abundance at my allotment.
Below: Baskets of freshly harvested, vibrant herbs ready to be made into medicine.

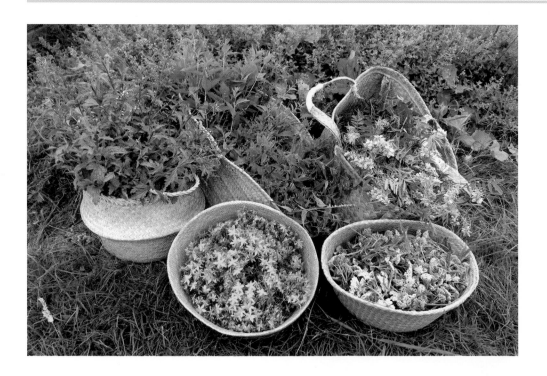

The more that we rely on the vagaries of the market economy to source our herbs and herbal medicines, the more vulnerable we will be to a potential erosion of our beautiful and sophisticated tradition.

When I first graduated in Western herbal medicine, I assumed that most herbal practitioners grew or gathered their own herbs. It has taken me many years to understand how far from the mark this idea is. As the number of people who are comfortable with, and understand, the process from seed to medicine dwindles, so does the resilience of our herbal lineage. I accept that not every one of us will feel able to grow and gather their own herbal medicines, but I strongly believe that if we are treading this herbal path, it is important to at least learn and understand all of the processes involved and to hold that knowledge for future generations. Self-sufficient herbalism is far more than simply a quaint idea: it could actually be the means by which our herbal tradition is able to thrive and continue to play a valuable role in modern sustainable health care.

I sincerely hope that you, as a fellow herbal lineage holder, will take the thoughts that I have shared within these pages as a starting point and will build on them for yourself with your own experiences. I invite you to join me on this path, to find your own way along it, and to pass on what you have learnt.

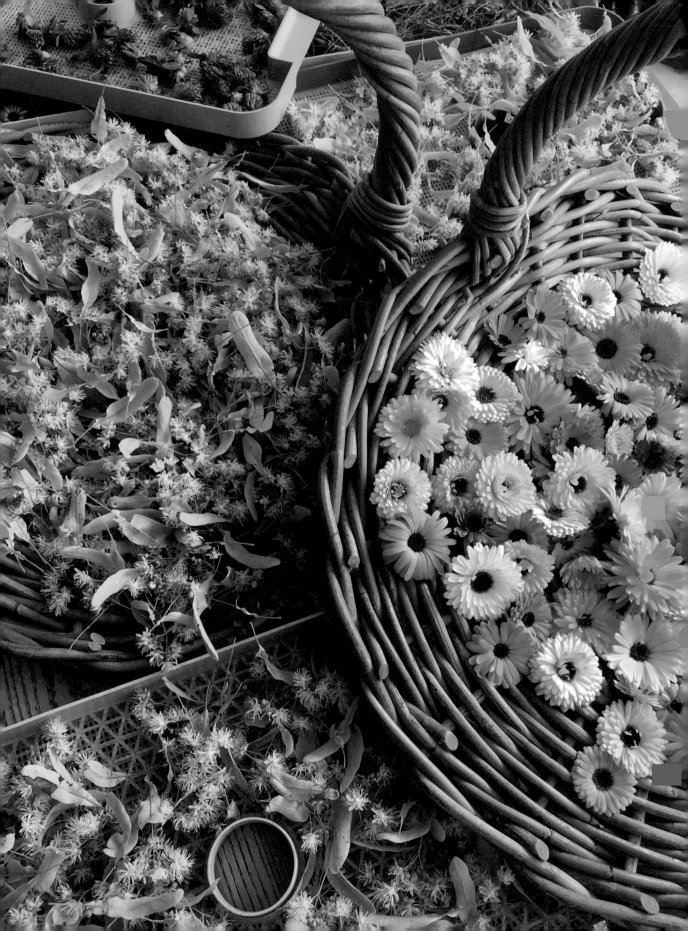

THE HERBAL HARVESTING YEAR

In this part of the book, I describe specific techniques that I have found helpful when harvesting and processing 108 of the herbs that I grow or gather for my own practice. I had to limit this section to around 100 herbs for practical reasons but chose 108 due to that number's significance in Tibetan Buddhism. I hope that what I describe, both here and in the preceding chapters, will help you to extrapolate the information to other herbs that I have not covered in detail.

I include instructions for drying each herb using a dehydrator, such as temperature ranges and guidelines on timing, as well as notes on passive drying. For those herbs that I tincture, I have included notes on how I do this usually: whether I use fresh or dried herb and the alcohol percentage that I generally choose. Please be aware that this is just my way of doing things, and there are many other ways that people choose to tincture their herbs. I am not suggesting that my way is the right or only way: I am simply sharing what works in my practice in case that is helpful to you.

I discuss each species in the approximate order that you would be harvesting them during the growing season in the United Kingdom. This means that regardless of whether you have chosen to cultivate a plant or whether you are planning to wildcraft it, you should be able to find helpful information on harvesting techniques in this part.

We can never be rigid about the timing of each harvest, so it is impossible to specify the months when plants are ready to be harvested. As with everything else in the natural world, the timing of the seasons varies quite significantly. There are early springs and late springs. There are 'Indian summers' or early autumns with unexpected frosts. In some years spring and summer seem to be compressed, with many species becoming ready to harvest within a very short space of time or even simultaneously. Although those years are glorious in their sheer abundance, I find them challenging, because so much needs to be gathered and processed within a very short window of time. In other, more spread-out years, harvesting feels calmer and more rhythmic, the timing of one harvest flowing smoothly to that of another at a steady pace.

The harvesting techniques discussed here are intended to serve as a guide rather than an instruction on the 'only right way' to do it. Not all species are covered, but if you find my techniques useful, you can easily apply them to other plants with a similar growth habit. In the end, we all find our own way of gathering and working with wild plants. We live in different areas, and we all have a different repertoire of plant species that we like to collect. I can only share those methods that have worked for me in my area.

This section is not intended to include information on medicinal properties of herbs: there is an abundance of excellent sources you can refer to for this information. However, I do grow some herbs that are no longer commonly used as medicines, and in these cases I have included a very brief description of their medicinal properties, so that those who are not familiar with them have a starting point for further consideration and research.

I do include harvesting and drying information for some species that are restricted in terms of how they can be prescribed in herbal medicine due to concerns over toxicity. Regulations as to which plants are affected, what level of dosage is acceptable, and in what form vary widely between different countries and are constantly being revised. Please check the current situation in your own country before prescribing herbs that contain known toxic constituents, such as pyrrolizidine alkaloids or arbutin. My reasons for including information about these species is simply to preserve the traditional knowledge of how to grow and harvest them.

Calendar for 108 herbs

Teasel (*Dipsacus fullonum*) ❖ roots

Hardy biennial herb ✦ **full sun to partial shade** ✦ **any moist soil** ✦ **spacing: 0.3–1 m ⁄ 1–3 ft**

Growing Teasel is easily grown and can be invasive. Collect seeds, and scatter them in a corner of your garden or wild harvest, with permission.

Harvesting The roots are harvested after the first year of growth. At this stage, the plants form a rosette of leaves that lies close to the ground, and they have a strong, vibrant root system with a thick supportive tap root. You can also harvest Teasel roots in the autumn, but I prefer to harvest when there is less pressure on my processing facilities. Dig up the young plants, and shake off the excess soil. Separate the roots from the foliage with a pair of secateurs, cutting the root system away from below the point where it becomes a stem. Wash and scrub them thoroughly, but do not leave them to soak.

Passive drying Cut the clean roots into matchstick-shaped sections, and lay them out to air-dry.

Active drying Start with 12–14 hours at 43°C ⁄ 110°F before swapping the trays around and continuing for periods of 1–2 hours, as necessary.

Tincturing I use dried root and 25% alcohol.

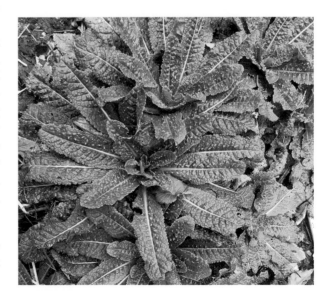

Dandelion (*Taraxacum officinale*) ❖ roots

Hardy perennial herb ◆ full sun to partial shade ◆ any moist soil ◆ spacing: 15–30 cm / 6–12 in

Growing It is easiest to harvest Dandelion root from cultivated ground. Weeding well-grown plants from your herb garden is a great way to combine harvesting with weeding. You can establish your own colony by transplanting small seedlings, using root cuttings or seeds.

Harvesting Unearth plants, and trim the foliage away from the roots. Once the roots are thoroughly washed, cut them into matchstick-shaped sections of even thickness and air-dry for 24 hours on a tray lined with absorbent paper.

Passive drying Lay the roots out on a dry tray, and leave in a warm, airy place, away from direct light. Turn the roots regularly.

Active drying Lay the roots out onto dehydrator trays. Air-dried roots should dry in around 16–24 hours at 43°C / 110°F. Store in an airtight container as soon as they are thoroughly dry.

Tincturing I use dried root and 45% alcohol.

Coltsfoot (*Tussilago farfara*) ❖ flowers

Hardy perennial herb ◆ full sun to partial shade ◆ any soil, especially disturbed areas ◆ spacing: 15–30 cm / 6–12 in

Growing Establish from roots in late autumn or early spring. One of its country names is 'Son before Father' because the flowers appear before the foliage. Later in the season the leaves appear.

Harvesting Coltsfoot contains pyrrolizidine alkaloids, which are considered to be a health risk. As a result of this, in many countries its medicinal use has been restricted or banned. The flowers and the flower stalks are gathered when they first appear in early spring. The plant is easily uprooted, so if you are gathering flowers, support the base of the plant with one hand while you pick the flower stem. The leaves are gathered later in the spring, when they first appear and are still young and fresh.

Passive drying Lay the flowers out on trays in a single layer, and allow to dry in a warm, airy place, out of direct light.

Active drying Dry at 42°C / 108°F for 12 hours, with further time periods, as necessary. The leaves are also dried at 42°C / 108°F for 12 hours or so.

Tincturing I use dried flowers (or leaves) and 45% alcohol.

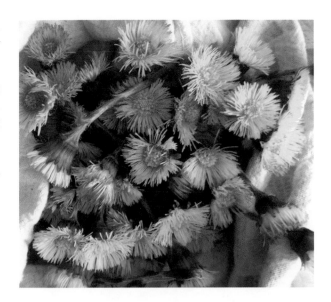

Cramp Bark or Guelder Rose (*Viburnum opulus*) ❖ bark

Hardy perennial shrub • full sun to partial shade • any soil • spacing for coppice: 1–1.25 m / 3–4 ft

Growing Wild harvest or grow your own, and manage by coppicing on a 4–year rotation. Cramp Bark plants are easily obtainable from hedging suppliers; they can also be grown from seed or cuttings.

Harvesting Harvest in early spring, just before the buds burst. If you have four large, established plants, you can harvest one each year. When coppicing plants, you should always angle your cut outwards, to allow rainwater to be channelled away from the centre of the coppiced plant. If you are wild harvesting Cramp Bark, the technique you use will depend on the nature of the plants that are available to you. If they are small, open-grown trees, it is best to prune a few small-diameter branches, making sure that you remove them using a sharp pruning saw. If you are harvesting Cramp Bark from bushes managed as a hedge, try to select stems that are as straight as possible in order to have a reasonable length for bark stripping. Aim for branches that have a diameter of less than 3.75 cm / 1.5 in at the point where you prune them. The bark on these younger sections of stem is thinner and more vibrant. Also, by cutting smaller branches, you are causing less damage to the tree and creating smaller wounds, which heal more easily. Support each branch as you cut through it in order to avoid it tearing the bark at the point of attachment as it falls. In choosing which branches to cut, be mindful of maintaining a balanced and healthy crown in the tree. The branches of open-grown trees usually fork and divide multiple times and therefore tend to have rather short internode

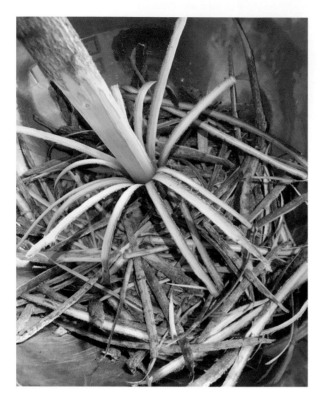

the bark from one internode at a time, twisting it as you go, so that in a series of strokes you end up with a peeled internode section and a star shape of peeled bark strips attached to the stem around the basal node. Remove these by hand, and let them fall into your collecting bowl. Long stems will need to be cut into a more manageable size with the saw or turned the other way up when you have stripped the bark from the lower half. This stripping method is quick and easy, and you soon fall into a relaxed rhythm, perhaps made even more relaxed by the heady scent of the valerenic acid in the freshly peeled bark.

Passive drying   Lay the bark strips out on trays to dry in a warm, airy place.

Active drying   Air-dry the bark for a day, and then dehydrate at 42°C / 108°F for about 12 hours. The bark pieces should be brittle and still smell strongly of valerenic acid. Pack into your storage containers while they are still warm.

Tincturing   I use dried bark and 45% alcohol.

sections where bark stripping is possible. This slows the process down considerably and is one of the reasons why I prefer to grow my own coppiced (and straight) stems these days. Strip the bark as soon as possible after harvest. I use a small-bladed sharp knife and a large stainless-steel bowl. Support each stem or branch upright in the bowl with one hand while you remove the bark with the other. Make a nick in the bark below the first node and run the knife down to the end of the branch in a single, fluid motion so as to remove the bark and the green inner bark. Keep the angle of the knife very shallow: if it is angled too deep, it will not run easily, as it will be trying to cut into wood. Experiment with slightly different angles. You will find a 'sweet spot' where the knife just runs down the stem and the bark peels away like butter. This is the correct angle. Always push the knife downwards or away from yourself for safety reasons. Strip

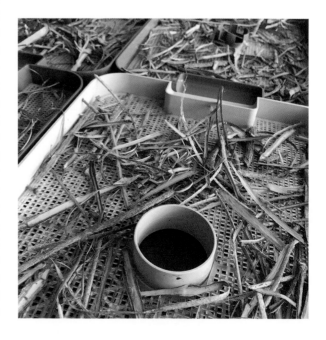

Wild Cherry (*Prunus avium*) ❖ bark

Hardy deciduous tree ◆ full sun ◆ fertile, well-drained soil ◆ spacing for coppice: 1.8 m / 6 ft

Growing Wild Cherry can be grown from seed or can be propagated by relocating root suckers. If you wish to establish Wild Cherry for bark in your herb garden, manage it by coppicing on a 4–5-year rotation, using a technique as described for Cramp Bark.

Harvesting Cut the stems in the early spring, just before the buds burst. Strip the bark straight away, and dry using the technique described for Cramp Bark.

Tincturing I use dried bark and 45% alcohol.

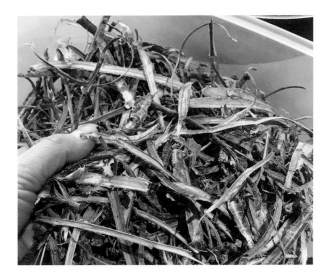

White Willow (*Salix alba*) ❖ bark

Hardy deciduous tree ◆ full sun to partial shade ◆ moist soil ◆ spacing for coppice: 1.8 m / 6 ft

Growing Willow is very easy to grow from cuttings. Place sections of young Willow branch into moist soil, and within 4 weeks it should have rooted and will be producing foliage. After two years, you can coppice your young trees. Continue to coppice them on a two-year rotation.

Harvesting Cut the stems in the early spring, just before the buds burst. Strip the bark straight away, and dry according to the instructions given for Cramp Bark.

Tincturing I use dried bark and 45% alcohol.

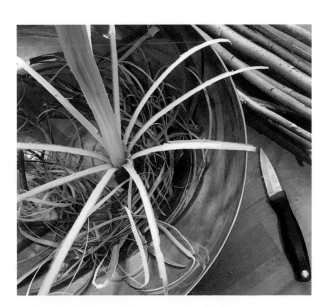

Witch Hazel (*Hamamelis mollis* or *Hamamelis virginiana*) ❖ bark

Hardy perennial shrub ◆ partial shade to full sun ◆ moist, fertile soil ◆ spacing for coppice: 1.8–2.5 m / 6–8 ft

Growing Propagation of Witch Hazel can be tricky, so it is recommended that you buy in a young plant. It prefers a sunny spot, with moist soil in summer. Mulch the plants generously.

Harvesting Take a harvest after the flowering is over. This can be done by pruning or coppicing. Suckers that come up around the base of the plant should be removed. Strip the bark straight away, and dry according to the instructions given for Cramp Bark.

Tincturing I use dried bark and 45% alcohol.

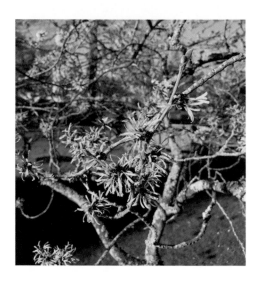

Birch (*Betula pendula* and *Betula pubescens*) ❖ bark

Hardy deciduous tree ◆ full sun ◆ moist, moderately fertile soil ◆ spacing for coppice: 1.8–2.5 m / 6–8 ft

Growing Plant bare-rooted whips in autumn and ensure that they are well watered and weed-free in the first year. If you have a wet site, choose Downy Birch (*Betula pubescens*). Manage by coppicing on a 4–5-year rotation.

Harvesting Coppice the chosen plant or plants in early spring, before the buds burst. Strip the bark straight away, and dry according to the instructions given for Cramp Bark.

Tincturing I use fresh bark and 50% alcohol.

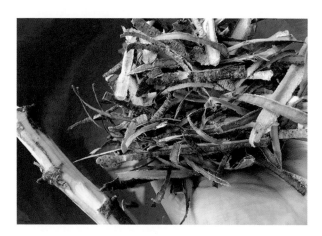

Pilewort (*Ranunculus ficaria*) ❖ whole plant

Hardy perennial herb ◆ partial shade ◆ any soil ◆ spacing: 7.5–10 cm / 3–4 in

Growing   Pilewort or Lesser Celandine is often present as a weed in gardens and is a common wild flower. If you wish to cultivate it, gather a few tubers from a suitable source and plant them. They will establish readily. Pilewort emerges in early spring and then dies down, seeming to disappear during the summer. Do not worry, it will definitely be back.

Harvesting   The whole plant, including tubers, leaves, and flowers, is harvested. Since you will be uprooting the plants, you need to obtain permission from the landowner. Carefully dig around each chosen plant to uproot it, including the tubers. Shake off as much soil as possible, place the plants into a bucket or tub, and bring them back to your processing place for washing. Tease the soil away from the tubers and rinse the whole plant very thoroughly. Even if you are very careful, some of the tubers will become detached from the plants. Try to salvage

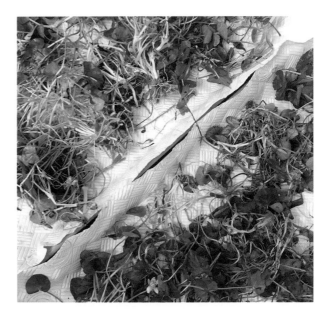

these detached tubers from the bottom of your washing vessel, otherwise there is a risk of wasting precious medicine. Do not soak the plants in the washing water. Once they are clean, lay them out in a single layer on a tray covered with absorbent kitchen towel to air-dry for a couple of days. Turn them repeatedly, being careful not to handle the leaves. Once all parts are surface-dry, gently move them to your drying system.

Passive drying   Leave on the trays in an airy, warm place, out of direct light.

Active drying   The time that they take to dehydrate varies greatly, depending on the amount of water that has been absorbed during the washing process. Start with 12 hours at 42°C / 108°F, and then continue for 2-hour stints, as needed.

Tincturing   I use dried plants and 45% alcohol.

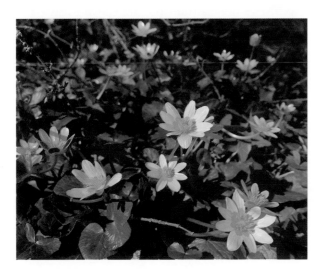

Cowslip (*Primula veris*) ❖ flowers

Hardy perennial herb ✦ **full sun to partial shade** ✦ **moist but well-drained soil** ✦ **spacing: 15 cm / 6 in**

Growing Cowslips are scarce in the wild and should not be wild harvested. It is easy to establish a population of your own Cowslips from seed. Increase plants by allowing self-seeding and transplanting, or collect and sow fresh seed in autumn, as it requires a cold period before germination. I started with three plants about 15 years ago and now have a large colony that has developed entirely from self-sown plants.

Harvesting It can be hard to steel yourself to pick the flowers in early spring, when they look so beautiful. Once your colony is large enough, you can harvest more lightly, if you prefer. Either snip the flowers from the stems and then tidy up the plants by removing the cut stems afterwards, or you can cut the flowers with their stalks and then remove these once you get to your processing area.

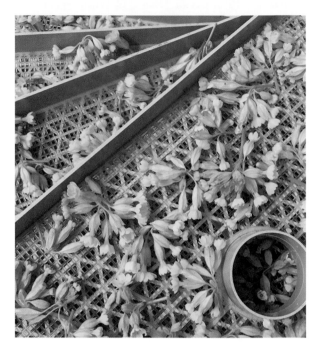

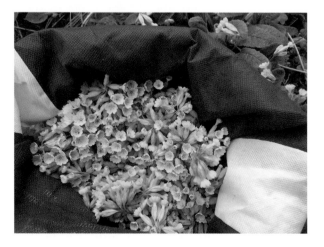

Passive drying Cowslip flowers deteriorate rapidly, so they should be laid out on trays in a single layer and left undisturbed in a warm, airy place as soon as possible.

Active drying Place into the dehydrator immediately. Start them at 38°C / 100°F for 10 hours, and then continue the drying time for short periods, as needed. In order to assess whether the flowers are properly dry, test the calyces with your fingers. If there is any sign of moisture, you will need to continue the drying process.

Tincturing I use dried flowers and 45% alcohol.

Daisy (*Bellis perennis*) ❖ flowers

Hardy perennial herb ✦ full sun to partial shade ✦ moist but well-drained soil ✦ spacing: 7.5 cm / 3 in

Growing Daisies are easiest to harvest from lawns or mown grass.

Harvesting Daisies are time-consuming to pick, but it is much easier if you find a patch where they are very abundant. Be careful not to uproot the plants when picking: support the rosette of leaves with one hand while you pluck the stalk with the other. Use a shallow basket, so that the Daisies you have harvested are not piled too deeply before you are able to spread them out at your processing place.

Drying I generally do not dry Daisies. I air-dry them for a few hours and then infuse them fresh in oil. If you do wish to dry them, follow the basic instructions as given for Cowslip.

Tincturing I use fresh flowers and 60% alcohol.

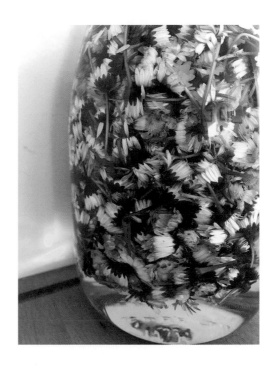

Lily-of-the-Valley (*Convallaria majalis*) ❖ flowers, leaves, roots

Hardy perennial herb ✦ partial shade ✦ deep, fertile, well-drained, moist soil ✦ spacing: 15 cm / 6 in

Growing Divide the rhizomes in autumn, and plant in a well-prepared site, with plenty of organic matter.

Harvesting Leaves and flowers are harvested in early spring, while the plants are in full flower, before the lowest flowers on each scape are beginning to fade. Some people use roots too, and these are harvested in the autumn. Generally, the flowers are considered to be the most medicinally active part. Lily-of-the Valley is potentially toxic, so should be taken only under supervision of a medical herbalist. The flowers turn brownish yellow on drying, and the sweet fragrance almost disappears. The dried material takes on a bitter, narcotic odour.

Passive drying Hang small bunches upside down in a warm, airy place, out of direct light.

Active drying Dry leaves whole, and leave the flowers on the scapes. Start the drying at 38°C / 100°F for 12 hours. Continue for small periods of time, as needed. You may need to separate out moister stalks for drying longer on their own.

Tincturing   I use dried flowers and leaves tinctured in 45% alcohol.

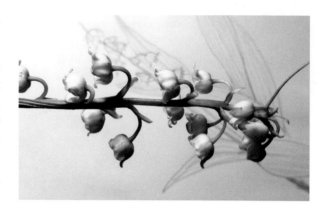

Pasque Flower (*Pulsatilla vulgaris*) ❖ flowers and leaves

Hardy perennial herb ◆ full sun ◆ well-drained chalky soil ◆ spacing: 20 cm / 8 in

Growing Sow fresh seed in spring and early summer or transplant self-sown seedlings. After flowering, rhizomes of established plants can be divided and replanted.

Harvesting Once the flowers are in full bloom, snip off mature leaves and flowers using a pair of scissors or secateurs. Leave the plant with enough young leaves to recover after harvest. Place your harvest carefully into a shallow basket.

Passive drying I was taught that Pasque Flower is a medicinal herb that should always be dried before use, in order to moderate the caustic compounds that are present. Lay the leaves and flowers on trays immediately after harvest, and leave to dry in a warm, airy place, out of direct light.

Active drying Lay your harvest out on dehydrator trays immediately after harvest. Start the drying process at a temperature of 42°C / 108°F and continue for 12 hours before moving the trays around and continuing for further short periods, as needed.

Tincturing I use dried herb and 45% alcohol.

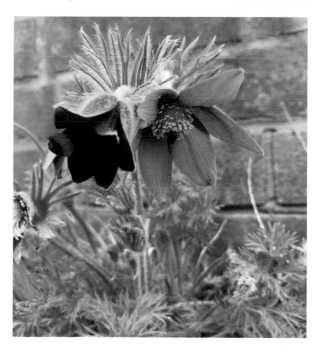

Dandelion (*Taraxacum officinale*) ❖ flowers

Hardy perennial herb • full sun to partial shade • any moist soil • spacing: 15–30 cm / 6–12 in

Growing Easily grown from seed, but you will probably be able to gather all that you need through weeding or wild harvesting.

Harvesting The best time to harvest Dandelion flowers is before any of them have gone to seed. There is a glorious moment in the early spring when the Dandelion flowers all burst open, and the meadows, verges, and green lanes are decorated with bright yellow, cheerful flowers. Pick them one by one, and snip the stems close to the flower head. You will find that the flowers are very popular with little black bugs. Lay the flowers in a flat basket, and when you have harvested what you need, cover the basket with a white sheet and place it in the shade for an hour or so. The bugs are attracted to the light and should fly up to congregate on the underside of the sheet. Lift it carefully and shake the bugs off, away from your basket. Repeat if necessary. You may find that harvesting flowers on a cloudy day reduces the number of bugs that find their way into your harvest. I spend a lot of time repatriating bugs at this time of the year.

Passive drying Dandelion flowers can take a surprising amount of time to dry, as they are very prone to reabsorbing moisture from the atmosphere and their fleshy calyces hold on to water. If possible, use some active heat for this process.

Active drying Mature Dandelion flowers tend to turn to seed heads in the dehydrator, so it can be a tricky process. However, if your harvest is of newly opened flowers and you dry them gently and steadily, you can end up with a reasonable proportion of yellow flower heads rather than fluff. Start at 38°C / 100°F for 12 hours and adjust timing and temperature, as needed.

Tincturing I use fresh flowers and 60% alcohol. I also make a separate preparation of fresh seed heads, also using 60% alcohol.

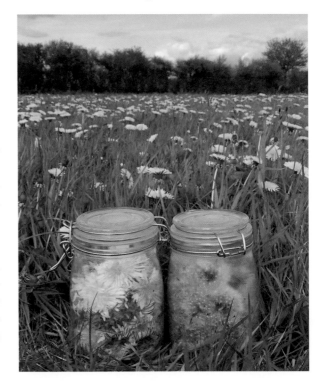

Oak (*Quercus robur* and *Quercus petraea*) ❖ bark

Hardy deciduous tree ✦ full sun ✦ fertile, well-drained soil ✦ spacing for coppicing: 3.5 m / 12 ft

Growing Oak can be grown from acorns; manage it by coppicing on a 7–10-year rotation, using a technique similar to the one described for Cramp Bark.

Harvesting If you have your own coppice, cut the stems in the spring as the buds are first bursting. If you are wild harvesting, search for small freshly wind-fallen branches after a spring storm, or carefully harvest small-diameter branches from a suitable – and willing – tree. Strip the bark straight away and dry according to the instructions given for Cramp Bark.

Tincturing I use dried bark and 25% alcohol.

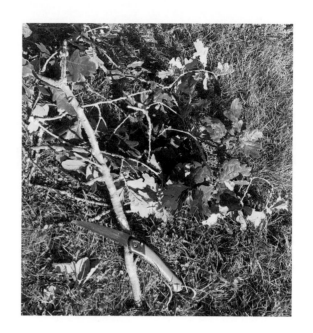

Chickweed (*Stellaria media*) ❖ aerial parts

Hardy annual herb ✦ full sun to partial shade ✦ moist, free-draining, fertile soil ✦ spacing: 15 cm / 6 in

Growing Chickweed grows naturally as a 'weed' on cultivated ground, but if you wish to grow it, gather ripe seeds and scatter them *in situ*.

Harvesting Chickweed can be harvested both in spring and in autumn. It is easily removed from cultivated ground, and I often combine my harvest with weeding. I harvest the Chickweed before starting more general weeding, while my hands are still soil-free and clean. Pull the plants out, carefully snipping off the roots before putting them into your basket so that you avoid contaminating your harvest with soil. If you are careful about this, you will not need to wash your plants, and the harvest will be of a much higher quality as a result. If the plants are affected by soil splash or your harvest was contaminated by soil, rinse them gently, taking care to minimize bruising. Lay the plants out on a tray lined with absorbent paper, and air-dry for 24 hours before starting the active drying process.

Passive drying Lay out the plants onto dry

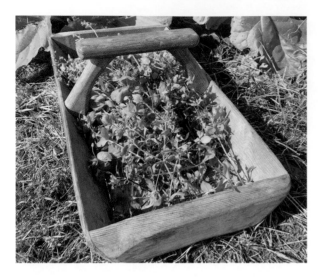

trays, and leave them in a warm, airy place in the dark.

Active drying   Lay the plants onto dehydrator trays, and dry at 42°C / 108°F for around 10 hours before swapping the trays around and continuing for 2-hour periods, for as long as necessary. Chickweed is a moist herb, and its moisture content is much affected by weather conditions in the days leading up to harvest. It gives up its moisture quite readily, but actual drying times will vary according to the season and the time of the harvest. Make sure it is thoroughly brittle and dry before storing.

Tincturing   I use dry herb and 45% alcohol.

Greater Celandine (*Chelidonium majus*)   ❖   aerial parts

Perennial herb ◆ well-drained soil ◆ full sun to partial shade ◆ spacing: 30–40 cm / 12–16 in

Growing   Greater Celandine self-seeds very readily. Gather seeds and scatter in your chosen location, or transplant seedlings.

Harvesting   This is a plant that is harvested for its yellow sap and should therefore be processed fresh. I make both a tincture and also an infused oil from the fresh plant. Greater Celandine sap will not only stain your skin but will also irrevocably stain your clothes, so do not wear a favourite outfit or use your favourite basket when harvesting this plant. Cut whole plants, including flowers. Return to your processing area immediately, and cut the fresh plant material into small pieces before tincturing or infusing in oil. I do not dry this herb.

Tincturing   I tincture fresh and use 60% alcohol.

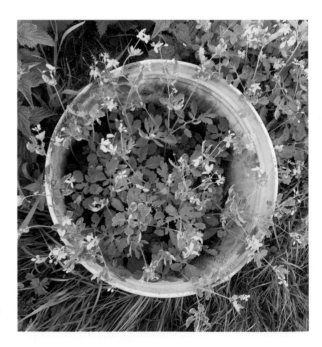

Cleavers (*Galium aparine*) ❖ aerial parts

Hardy annual herb ✦ full sun to partial shade ✦ moist, fertile soil ✦ spacing: 7.5–12.5 cm / 3–5 in, with support

Growing It should not be necessary to grow Cleavers, but if you do need to, gather ripe seed and sow it in a very moist trench, with support. Most people will be able to wild harvest from hedgerows and field edges.

Harvesting Cleavers is harvested at two main times of the year. In early spring the young, tender shoots make a wonderful and delicate medicine. They are snipped from their growing spots, usually under the shelter of a hedge, taking care not to uproot them and avoiding other plant material, such as Ivy shoots or other

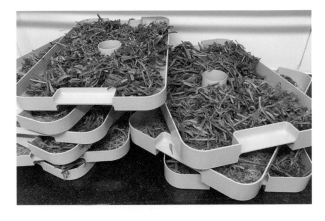

emerging herbaceous plants. Later in the spring and early summer, Cleavers reaches its height of vibrancy for medicine, developing long, green, leafy stems with beautiful, delicate white flowers at the ends. This is the time to take your main harvest. Fully grown Cleavers can be well over 1.75 m / 6 ft long, and I find it easiest to pull handfuls of plant out of the hedge, together with the roots. Hedgerow Cleavers thrives where it can root into the wet soil of a ditch and therefore comes away easily in one piece. I gather all the plants into a large bundle, with the stems all orientated the same way. At this point I usually drape the stems through a forked hazel stick and walk along the road with them, in the style of a fairy-tale character leaving home with her worldly belongings wrapped in a cloth on a stick. It is a sight that has been known to cause much amusement to the few passing vehicles and horse-riders on the quiet country lanes where I gather this herb. By keeping all the stems aligned in the same direction, it is easier to efficiently trim the roots and discoloured stem bases from the plants once you return to

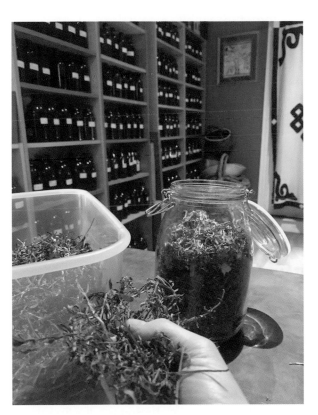

your processing area. It also means that usable stems will not be contaminated with mud or soil. Remove any leaves of other hedgerow species, such as Hawthorn, that have become caught in the sticky stems. These are very straightforward to remove, as you are preparing the harvest for drying. If you leave your Cleavers harvest too late, it becomes brown and dried out, with abundant sticky seeds not suitable for use as medicine. The seeds can be roasted and used as a coffee substitute.

Passive drying Cut the stems into lengths of approximately 10 cm / 4 in and arrange them evenly on trays. Alternatively, drape stems over

a drying rack or hang over a taut rope. Leave in a warm, airy place, out of direct light.

Active drying Cut the stems into lengths of approximately 5–10 cm / 2–4 in and arrange them evenly on your dryer trays. Start with 12 hours at 42°C / 108°F, and then reverse the order of the trays, moving the bottom tray to the top and continuing for additional 2-hour periods, for as long as necessary. Once it is thoroughly brittle and dry, pack the herb away into storage straight from the dryer while it is still warm.

Tincturing I use dry herb and 45% alcohol.

Nettle (*Urtica dioica*) ❖ leaves

Hardy perennial herb • full sun to full shade • moist, rich soil • spacing: 15–30 cm / 6–12 in

Growing Most people will prefer to wild harvest from wild places, waste ground, or field edges. The advantage of cultivating the crop is that it can be kept weed-free, making harvesting quick and efficient. I have cultivated Nettle in the past by planting root cuttings. Alternatively, transplant seedlings, or gather ripe seed and scatter in your chosen location.

Harvesting Nettles are often found growing among Cleavers. Their harvest periods coincide, as do their locations. I harvest large quantities of Nettle leaf each year, so I spread my gathering period over the spring and early summer. I try to concentrate my Nettle harvest in the earliest part of the season, while the stems are still soft and the leaves are young and vibrant, but it is not possible to harvest all that I need at this time of the year. You should not harvest Nettle leaves for medicine once the plants have

flowered, since the uric acid levels in the leaves become much higher at this time. Some people like to harvest Nettles without gloves, but I wear thin cotton gloves that reduce the amount of stinging but do not completely stop it. Use secateurs or scissors to cut the stems down to a point that is 15 cm / 6 in from the base, or, alternatively, to just above the point where the condition of the leaves deteriorates. Later on in the season, Nettle leaves develop quite a lot of damage due to insect predation, and some leaves are folded over as part of the cocoon construction for moths or butterflies. At this time, you need to select your stems carefully to avoid both damaged leaves and cocoon-containing leaves. By late spring and early summer the stalks are quite fibrous and will not dry at the same rate as the leaves, so at this time I prefer to keep my harvest to leaves only. I tend to snip off individual leaves from the stems, allowing them to fall directly into my basket. If harvesting to more of a deadline – before a threatened spell of wet weather, for example – it can be better to snip off good-quality stems and then remove the leaves when you get back to your processing area. You can return the stalks to the gathering area in due course, or compost them, if a return trip is not possible. Once the Nettles flower, it is time to turn your attention to the gathering of other species while the Nettles work on producing seeds.

Passive drying   Make small bunches of leafy stalks and hang them upside down in a warm, airy place, away from direct light. Alternatively, you can remove the leaves and spread them onto trays to dry.

Active drying   Spread the leaves on dehydrator trays evenly. Start the drying at 42°C / 108°F for 12 hours, then swap the trays, and continue for additional 2-hour periods, for as long as necessary.

Tincturing   I use dried leaves and 45% alcohol.

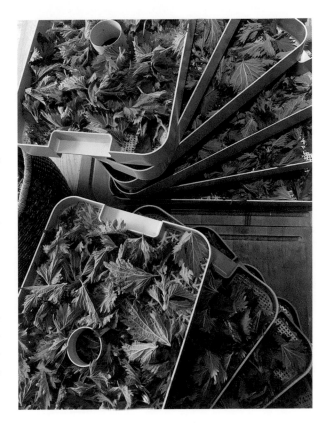

Birch (*Betula pendula*)   ❖   leaves

Perennial tree ◆ full sun ◆ deep, moist soil ◆ spacing for coppicing: 2.5–3.5 m / 8–12 ft

Growing   Wild harvest or grow as a coppice crop in your herb garden. In late summer you can gather ripe seed and sow it immediately. Keep the seed bed moist until the seedlings are established. Alternatively, you can take softwood cuttings in early summer or buy in young bare-rooted plants and plant in autumn.

Harvesting   Birch leaves are gathered when they are newly emerged, fresh, and green. It can be a challenge to find Birch trees with low-enough branches to harvest the leaves, but the dedicated forager will already have located suitable trees during the winter or in previous seasons. The trees are very distinctive with their striking, pale bark, so it is an easy task to locate suitable trees within your foraging territory. If you are growing your own coppiced Birches, you should be able to reach the leaves by gently bending over the young stems. Carefully prune

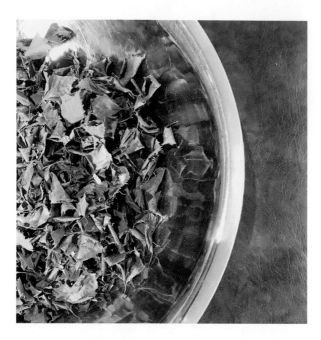

Active drying   Spread the leaves out on dehydrator trays, and start the drying process at 42°C / 108°F for 8 hours, and increase the drying time in stints of 1 hour, for as long as needed. Once the leaves are dry and are brittle enough to snap cleanly, put them away into storage while they are still warm.

Tapping   Many people also tap Birch trees for their sap in early spring. When I was studying Western herbal medicine, my tutor, Barbara Howe, told us that she had once tapped a large Birch tree in her garden and had collected a good quantity of sap. When she returned to the tree to remove the sap container and to plug the hole she had made in the bark, she had a very strong sense that the tree was not at all happy about it. She tipped all the liquid that she had collected back into the ground by the roots of the tree and apologized to it. I have never been able to bring myself to try it, although I completely accept that careful and responsible tapping is not harmful to trees.

off some of the very small lower branches, and remove the leaves back at your processing place. You can use them fresh to make an infused oil, or you can dry the leaves for your dispensary.

Passive drying   Spread the leaves out on trays, and leave to dry in a warm, airy place, out of direct light.

Tincturing   I use dried leaves and 45% alcohol.

Wood Avens (*Geum urbanum*)   ❖   aerial parts

Hardy perennial herb ✦ partial to full shade ✦ moist, fertile soil ✦ spacing: 30–50 cm / 12–20 in

Growing   Sow seeds in spring or pot up self-sown seedlings and replant where you want them to grow. I usually gather all that I need from the wild.

Harvesting   Wood Avens is one of those plants that produces plenty of lush foliage early in the summer, but this becomes sparse once the plant flowers and starts to seed. I like to take my har-

vest early on, when the volume of plant material is at a maximum and the leaves are in good condition. Loosely gather together a handful of leaf stems and cut them together. Be careful not to bunch them tightly together, as it could cause bruising.

Passive drying   Create small, loose bunches and hang them upside down in a warm, airy place to dry. Alternatively, spread leaves thinly on trays to dry in a warm, airy place.

Active drying Spread the leaves evenly on dehydrator trays. Start the drying at 42°C / 108°F for 12 hours, and then swap the trays, and continue for additional 2-hour periods, until the leaves are brittle.

Tincturing I use dried herb and 45% alcohol.

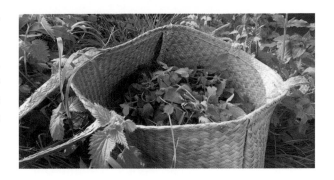

Shepherd's Purse (*Capsella bursa-pastoris*) ❖ aerial parts

Hardy annual or biennial herb ✦ **full sun to partial shade** ✦ **any well-drained soil** ✦ **spacing: 15 cm / 6 in**

Growing Most people will be able to fulfil their need for this medicine by wild harvesting. It can be grown readily from seed, though. Gather ripe seeds and sow them outdoors immediately in a large pot. Keep the soil watered, and they will germinate and can be transplanted in the spring.

Harvesting Shepherd's Purse is prone to being affected by blackfly later in the season, so it is a good idea to catch it early, while the aerial parts are vibrant and clean. In the early part of the season it produces abundant leafy material, ideal for harvesting; you can also harvest it later in the season, though by then it concentrates its energy into producing the characteristic and easily identified seed heads. These late-season leaves are much smaller and look rather different, so get confident about identifying this plant at different growth stages in order to maximize your harvest. It is a weed on arable land and can easily be found on field edges and in gateways. When picking, be very careful not to uproot the plant; it is best to use secateurs or sharp scissors. If you do not have scissors with you, support the

basal rosette with one hand while picking with the other. This is one of the few plants that must be tinctured while fresh, so you need to gather sufficient for your tincture needs for the entire year ahead. I do not dry this herb.

Tincturing I use fresh herb and 60% alcohol.

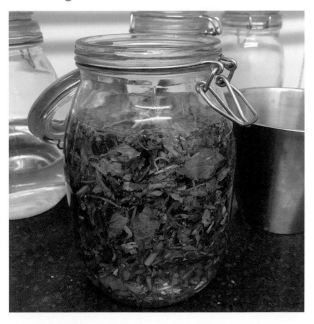

Hawthorn (*Crataegus monogyna*) ❖ blossom

Hardy perennial shrub or small tree • full sun to partial shade • any well-drained soil • spacing: 30 cm / 12 in for hedging, and up to 10 m / 30 ft for trees

Growing Hawthorn grows abundantly in hedges, woodland edges, and waste ground. It can be grown as a hedge or shelter belt for the herb garden. Buy in bare-rooted hedging stock, or gather seeds in autumn and plant immediately into pots. Transplant once established.

Harvesting It is definitely worth researching suitable foraging locations for Hawthorn before the blossom comes out. Hawthorn is generally very abundant, but many plants are not suitable for foraging blossom (or berries later in the year) because they are trimmed as hedging. Closely trimmed hedges are usually altogether devoid of blossom. Hedges are designed to be barriers, and Hawthorn is very thorny, so sticking your arms in to reach blossom is not a pleasant option. The ideal trees are abundantly covered in blossom and have branches low enough for easy picking. If you want to gather Hawthorn, I recommend that you walk your area and identify suitable trees in advance. Once the blossom is out, support the main branch with one hand, and with the other grasp bunches of blossom and pluck them from the tree. Aim to avoid including too many woody twig pieces, although inevitably some of these will find their way into your basket and will need to be removed from the blossom later. You will inevitably pick some young leaves alongside the blossom. That is absolutely fine. Choose branches that are most laden with flowers, and pick them with whichever leaves happen to be included within them. The approximate ratio between blossom and leaves will probably end up as being 60:40 or so, but even if it is 50:50, your harvest will still be perfectly good. Leaves are medicinal too. Fill your baskets, but aim to spread the blossoms out in a single layer within an hour of picking.

Passive drying Spread the flowers and leaves out onto trays, and leave them in a warm, airy place to dry away from direct light. Make sure that leaves are brittle before storing them.

Active drying Spread the flowers onto dehydrator trays, and start the drying at a temperature of 42°C / 108°F for 12 hours before rearranging the trays and continuing for hourly stints, for as long as needed. Pack the dried Hawthorn away while it is still warm. It should be vibrant and fragrant, smelling the same as the day it was picked.

Tincturing I use dried blossom and 45% alcohol.

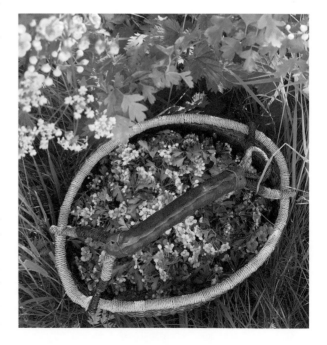

Elder (*Sambucus nigra*) ❖ flowers

Hardy perennial shrub • full sun to shade • moderately fertile, moist, well-drained soil • spacing: 1.8–4 m / 6–13 ft

Growing It is usually possible to gather all that you need of this abundant wild medicinal, but it can be grown in the garden if gathering is difficult in your location. Grow from seed, or buy in young plants.

Harvesting Elderflowers are another medicinal herb for which you need to identify your gathering shrubs in advance. Not all Elder shrubs are suitable for gathering from. If they are growing in the close company of other woodland shrubs, they will be tall and will carry their flowers high up out of reach, unless you use a ladder. Some people do use ladders to

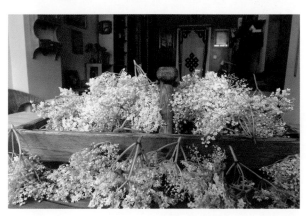

harvest, but I prefer the fluidity of walking along a hedgerow picking the best flowers from the lower branches. I am very happy to leave the higher flowers for wildlife. Choose only the best and most vibrant flowers. The moisture content in Elder is very dependent on the weather conditions a few days prior to harvest. If you are harvesting on a dry day that follows a spell of very wet weather, you will be picking Elderflowers with a very high moisture content. In some years this cannot be helped, but if the weather stays good, pick after a spell of dry weather if you can. It is preferable to pick Elderflowers when they are releasing abundant pollen. I find it best to harvest them by cupping each flower in my left hand and running the stalk through my fingers, until the flower is cupped in my palm and the stalk can be snipped from below my fingers. This keeps the flowers whole and minimizes the length of extra fleshy stalk, which I cut. I continue snipping off flowers, forming a little fragrant stack of 3–4 flower saucers in my left hand, before I bend down to put them gently into my basket. Sometimes it is easier just to cut them over an open basket, so that they fall into it. Elderflowers are quite easily bruised, so be careful and do not press them down to get more in. Lay the flowers out in a single layer within an hour of picking.

Passive drying   Spread the flowers on trays, and dry in a warm, airy place, out of direct light. Make sure that the flower stalks are thoroughly dried before storing. Store the flower heads whole.

Active drying   Spread the flowers evenly on dehydrator trays, trimming off any particularly fleshy stalks. Start the drying process at 42°C / 108°F for 12 hours and then swap the trays around. Continue at a lower temperature, 38°C / 100°F, for additional 2-hour periods, for as long as necessary. Make sure that the stalks are brittle and snap cleanly before packing the flowers away.

Tincturing   I use dried flowers and 45% alcohol.

Pellitory-of-the-Wall (*Parietaria diffusa*)   ❖   aerial parts

Hardy perennial herb • full sun to partial shade • prefers dry soil but will tolerate moist conditions • spacing: 30 cm / 12 in

Growing   This plant is dioecious, so you will need both male and female plants if you plan to increase your population by seed. I have established my own population of Pellitory-of-the-Wall in my garden, as the most abundant populations locally are along the side of busy roads and therefore are not suitable to be gathered. Transplant small seedlings or gather seed, and sow it outdoors in a seed bed in autumn. Transplant into its final growing location once the young plants are established.

Harvesting   This is a herb that, earlier in the season, produces abundant lush foliage, which becomes sparser on flowering. I prefer to take my main harvest of this herb before it starts to flower. I also sometimes take a late harvest once the flowers have turned to seed. I avoid harvesting during the actual flowering stage due to the very abundant pollen that forms at this time. While there is nothing medicinally wrong with the pollen, provided that you are not pollen-sensitive, it does make the herb rather 'dusty'

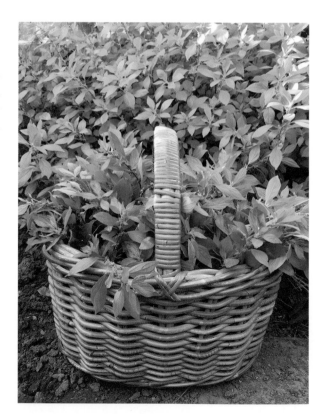

for using as infusions. Cut stalks individually, or, if you have a large population, gently gather together groups of stalks and cut them together.

Passive drying   Hang in small bunches to dry upside down, away from direct light. If possible, finish the drying process in a warm place, such as an airing cupboard, for 24 hours.

Active drying   Cut the stems into 80–100-mm / 2–2.5-in sections, and lay them out on dehydrator trays. Start the drying process with 12 hours at 42°C / 108°F. Swap the trays around and continue for periods of 2 hours, for as long as needed. This is a herb that is very prone to reabsorbing moisture from the atmosphere after it has been dried. Once it feels dry and stems snap cleanly, I recommend continuing the drying process for an additional 2 hours and then immediately storing in an airtight container while still warm from the dryer. I wonder whether the herb's affinity with the water systems of the body is in some way related to he

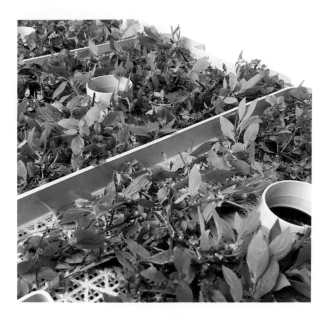

herb's ability to reabsorb water so readily from the atmosphere. I have noticed the same tendency in Dandelion leaf.

Tincturing   I use dried herb and 25% alcohol.

Dandelion (*Taraxacum officinale*) ❖ leaves

Hardy perennial herb • full sun to partial shade • any moist soil • spacing: 15–30 cm / 6–12 in

Growing   Easily grown from seed, but you will probably be able to gather all that you need through weeding or wild harvesting.

Harvesting   Open-grown Dandelion in grazed pasture land grows in rosettes with the leaves lying flat on the ground. In these situations, you will find that the majority of plants bear many small leaves rather than a few large ones. For a self-sufficient herbalist, few larger leaves are more efficient to gather than a multitude

of very small ones, but if you have the time to gather small ones, they will be perfectly good medicine. I find it much better to find a place where Dandelions are growing among taller vegetation. This could be an unmanaged piece of land, an unmown field edge, or a woodland clearing. In these situations, you can find large Dandelion leaves up to 1 ft / 30 cm in length, which makes filling your basket much easier. It is also a good idea to search for well-grown Dandelion plants at your local allotments or community garden. I have a couple of favourite spots to find large Dandelion leaves, one being my own allotment, where I let them grow large before harvesting them, and another being on a local shady bank. If you are harvesting from a cultivated area, you will probably find that the Dandelion leaves are affected by soil splash, in which case you will need to wash the leaves before processing them. Wash them gently, swirling them around with your hand. Avoid using salad spinners, as this can cause bruising. Allow the leaves to drain passively in a colander, rearranging them frequently with great care. Spread them gently onto a tray lined with absorbent kitchen towel to air-dry.

Passive drying Lay the leaves out on a dry tray, and leave in an airy place, away from direct

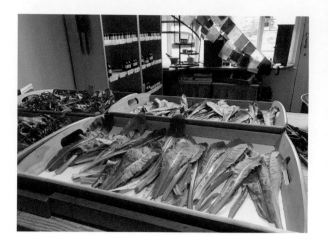

light. If you need to turn them, only pick them up very gently by the very base of the leaf. If possible, finish the drying process in a warm place, such as an airing cupboard. Please see the comments on storage in the active drying section below.

Active drying Air-dry the leaves overnight or for a whole day, before commencing active drying. Start the dehydrator at 42°C / 108°F for 12 hours and then swap the trays around. Continue at the same temperature for additional 2-hour periods, for as long as necessary. If atmospheric humidity is very high, increase the temperature to 43°C / 110°F. Make sure that the midribs are completely brittle and snap cleanly before packing the leaves away. Dandelion leaves are very prone to reabsorbing moisture from the environment. I tend to continue drying for an additional 2 hours once the leaves reach a point that for any other herb I would have said was perfectly dry. Always pack the leaves away while they are still warm from the drying process. If your dryer has a timer and it has been off for a few hours before you get to it, set it for at least one more hour, so that you can ensure that any slight moisture reabsorption is redressed. Use a

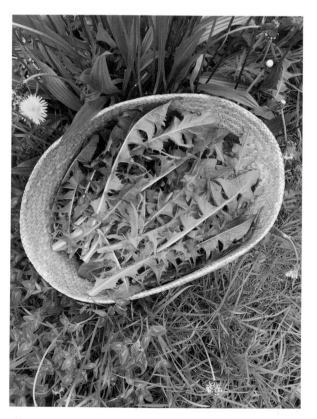

small storage container at first, so that there is a minimal reserve of 'damp' air available for reabsorption of moisture. As your harvest progresses through the season, increase the size of your storage container, as needed. I usually store each new batch separately in a temporary container for a fortnight and check on it several times to ensure that the leaves are remaining properly dry. Once I am satisfied that the leaves are stable and well dried, I will add them to my main batch, releasing the temporary container for another harvest.

Tincturing   I use dried leaves and 45% alcohol.

Motherwort (*Leonurus cardiaca*) ❖ aerial parts

Perennial herb ◆ full sun to partial shade ◆ moderately fertile, well-drained soil ◆ spacing: 30–45 cm / 12–18 in

Growing   Motherwort is a very vigorous self-seeder, so once you have an established colony, you will never be without new replacement plants, provided you allow one or two to seed.

Harvesting   I prefer to make my harvest when this herb is just about to flower. Not only is it at peak potency during this time, but also this harvest timing is a good way of avoiding self-seeding and the resulting hours and hours of weeding later in the year. Like the other labiates, once the plant is flowering, the stems get tough and woody, and the foliage becomes much sparser. If you have plenty of Motherwort, it is a good idea to take an early harvest of the leafy soft-stemmed growth and then take a later harvest just prior to flowering.

Passive drying   Hang small bunches upside down to dry in a warm, airy place, away from direct light. Once the leaves are dry, carefully remove them from the stems and store them. Return the stems to the compost heap.

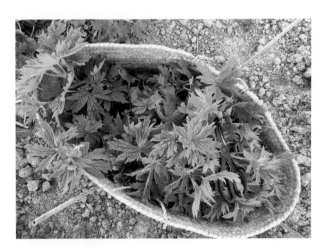

Active drying   The softer, early-season stems can be dried by cutting them into 7.5-cm / 3-in sections and starting them off for 12 hours at 42°C / 108°F. If you are harvesting later-season stems, carefully snip off the leaves and the flowers and put the stems into the compost or dry them separately.

Tincturing   I use dried herb and 45% alcohol.

Mullein (*Verbascum thapsus*) ❖ leaves and flowers

Hardy biennial herb • full sun to partial shade • any well-drained soil • spacing: 0.6–1.75 m / 2–4 ft

Growing   Mullein can be grown from seed or by transplanting self-sown seedlings.

Harvesting   Some herbals recommend harvesting second-year leaves, but if you want to harvest Mullein leaves, you have to get to them before the Mullein Moth caterpillar (*Cucullia verbasci*) does. The caterpillar of this species is a voracious feeder on Mullein and Figwort leaves, leaving only the midribs and main veins. They are creamy in colour, with black and yellow spots, reaching a length of 5 cm / 2 in when fully grown. I generally harvest leaves from second-year plants before the flower spikes start to form, leaving plenty of leaves so that the plants can recover before flowering. Aim to harvest

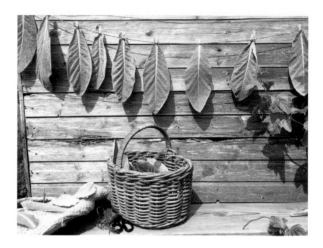

the leaves when they are dry to the touch. This can be tricky, as they are furry and tend to hang on to their moisture in the early part of the day longer than other plants. Check for caterpillars before cutting and place the leaves in your basket in a single layer if they are still a little moist. The flowers are harvested later on in the season, once they are out. You can either cut the flower spikes and remove the fully open flowers back at your processing area, or you can carefully remove individual fully open flowers without damaging the spike, so that you can harvest more flowers as they mature. The fresh flowers are infused in oil.

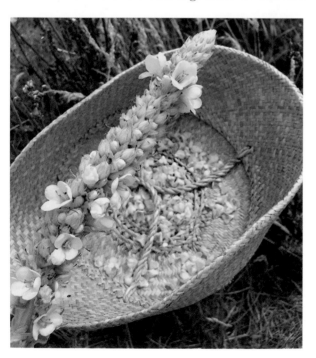

Passive drying   Thread and hang individual leaves on a line in a warm, airy place, out of direct light, in the manner of Tobacco drying. Alternatively, cut leaves into lateral strips approximately 5 cm / 2 in wide and lay them out on trays. Individual flowers can be dried on trays, but I tend to use the flowers fresh for infused oils. Mullein easily absorbs atmospheric moisture, so, if possible, place your dried harvest into an airing cupboard for 24 hours to finish the drying process before storage.

Active drying Once they are surface-dry, cut the leaves into lateral strips approximately 5 cm / 2 in wide and spread them onto dehydrator trays. Dry them for around 12 hours at 43°C / 110°F swapping the trays around and continuing for smaller periods of time. Once thoroughly dry, store while they are warm. Flowers can be dried at 38°C / 100°F for 10 hours before reassessing. Once dry, finish for 1 hour at 42°C / 108°F before storing immediately in a small container.

Tincturing I use dried leaf and 45% alcohol. I do not tincture the flowers. I tend to make an infused oil from fresh flowers, but sometimes I top this up with additional dried flowers, so that the preparation is 50:50 fresh and dried flowers. This can be helpful when taking small harvests from the same plants over a few weeks.

Small Flowered Willowherb (*Epilobium parviflorum*) ❖ aerial parts

Hardy annual herb ◆ full sun to partial shade ◆ well-drained, moderately fertile soil ◆ spacing: 10–15 cm / 4–6 in

Growing I usually encourage a small population to grow among my cultivated crops as a 'weed', rather than specifically cultivating it. It is easy to grow from seed: gather ripe seed heads, and scatter immediately in your chosen area. Once established, it self-seeds freely.

Harvesting This plant produces seed heads that explode on drying, releasing fluffy seeds, so it is preferable to harvest it before the flowers start to turn to seed. At any one time in early summer you will find plants that are going to seed and some that are just starting to flower. Choose the ones that are just starting to flower. If you are pulling the plants out by the roots as part of your weeding operations, be careful to snip off the roots before placing the aerial parts into your basket in order to avoid contaminating the aerial parts with soil.

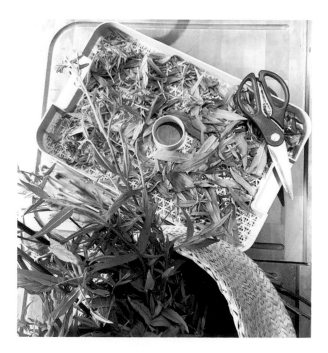

Passive drying Hang small bunches upside down in a warm, airy place to dry.

Active drying Once back in your processing area, cut the softer stems so that you have pieces that are approximately 10–13 cm / 4–5 in long. Remove the leaves from larger, tougher stems, and either dry the stems separately, or return them to the earth. Lay them out on dehydrator trays immediately. You can air-dry them for about 12 hours before starting the active drying process, provided that you leave them on the trays that you intend to use in the dehydrator. Start with 10 hours at 42°C / 108°F, and then continue drying in additional stints of 2 hours, as needed. Once completely dry, as indicated by the stems snapping cleanly, store them in an airtight container.

Tincturing I use dried herb and 45% alcohol.

Feverfew (*Tanacetum parthenium*) ❖ aerial parts

Hardy perennial herb ⬩ full sun ⬩ well-drained, fertile soil ⬩ spacing: 30 cm / 12 in

Growing Sow seeds in spring or autumn. Mix them with a little dry sand before sowing, in order to get better spacing. They can also be propagated in summer from non-flowering stem cuttings, and in the autumn large plants can be divided.

Harvesting Feverfew should be harvested while it is in full flower. The timing of this will vary according to how well established your plants are. Cut the aerial parts, leaving the coarsest stems and any faded or damaged leaves at the base of the plants.

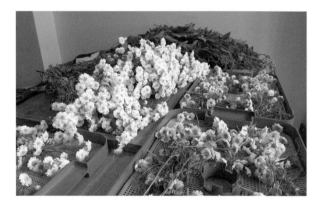

Passive drying Make bunches of stems or hang individual plants upside down to dry in a warm, airy place, away from direct light.

Active drying If you have quite long stems in your harvest, cut them so that you have pieces approximately 15 cm / 6 in long. Feverfew is rather aromatic, so take care not to dry at too high a temperature. If the ambient humidity is low, use a lower temperature, perhaps 38°C / 100°F, but if the ambient humidity is quite high, then it will be preferable to increase the temperature to 42°C / 108°F for 6 hours before reducing it. Once the herb is thoroughly dry, store it in an airtight container immediately.

Tincturing I use dried herb and 45% alcohol.

Gotu Kola (*Centella asiatica*) ❖ leaves

Tender perennial herb ◆ **full sun to partial shade** ◆ **rich, moist soil** ◆ **spacing: 20–30 cm / 8–12 in**

Growing Gotu Kola will not tolerate temperatures below 10°C / 50°F, so if you are in a temperate climate, you will need to give your plants protection during the winter. It naturally spreads prolifically, provided it has plenty of water available to it. Propagation can be carried out at any time during the growing season by dividing and rooting the runners.

Harvesting Cut the individual leaves in late spring or early summer, depending on the growth of your own crops.

Passive drying Spread the leaves onto trays, and leave to dry in a warm, airy place, away from direct sunlight.

Active drying Spread the leaves onto dehydrator trays, and start the drying process at a temperature of 42°C / 108°F for 12 hours. Rearrange the trays, and continue drying for periods of 2 hours, for as long as needed. Store immediately while still warm.

Tincturing I use dried herb and 45% alcohol.

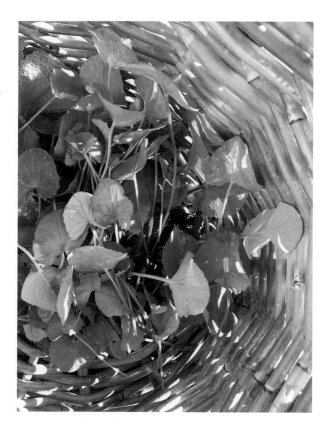

Mid-summer

Plantain (*Plantago lanceolata* and *Plantago major*) ❖ leaves

Hardy perennial herb • full sun • well-drained, moderately fertile soil • spacing: 15–23 cm / 6–9 in

Growing   Most people will be able to wild harvest Plantain leaves, but if you do not have access to a clean source, then consider growing your own, either in a wildflower 'lawn' or in a cultivated bed. Commercial sources of Plantain leaves are almost invariably *Plantago lanceolata,* since these are easier to harvest from field-scale cultivation. Gather ripe seed heads and scatter in your chosen place, or transplant self-sown seedlings. Growing Plantain in a grassland environment rather than in cultivated soil will result in cleaner leaves.

Harvesting   If harvesting by hand, it is perfectly acceptable to harvest both types and either mix them together, or use them separately. Whichever species you are collecting, pick the leaves individually, including the stalks. Plantain leaves are extremely prone to bruising, so it is preferable to avoid the need to wash them; however, if the leaves are affected by soil splash, washing them will be necessary. I usually harvest both species, and mix them together, since I use them interchangeably, but in recent years I have found that I am gathering a higher proportion of *Plantago lanceolata* because of the better availability of good-quality clean leaves in my area.

Passive drying   If you have washed the leaves, air-dry them on a tray lined with absorbent kitchen towel for 24 hours. Be very careful about how you handle the leaves. It is ideal to harvest clean leaves and spread them onto trays immediately.

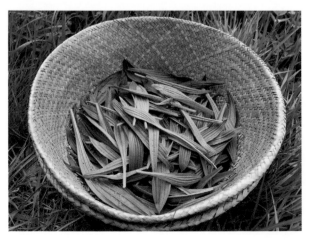

Active drying Spread surface-dry leaves onto dehydrator trays immediately. Do not touch them or move the leaves on the trays until they are completely dry. Start them at 42°C / 108°F for 12 hours and then swap the trays around. Continue at the same temperature for additional 2-hour periods, for as long as necessary. The first time you touch the leaves after laying them out should be to test whether they are brittle and thoroughly dried.

Tincturing   I use dried leaves and 45% alcohol.

Lime (several species and hybrids, including *Tilia x europaea*, *Tilia platyphyllos,* and *Tilia cordata*)   ❖   flowers

Hardy deciduous tree • full sun • moderately fertile, well-drained soil • open-grown trees are best

Growing   Widely grown in parks and gardens, so foraging should be possible, but plant a tree if you have room. Lime trees reach enormous heights (up to 40 m / 130 ft) at maturity. The inner bark can also be used medicinally, so it may be worth establishing a couple of coppice plants to provide bark harvests. Limes managed by coppicing will not produce flowers.

Harvesting   Foraging for Lime flowers first requires you to identify a tree or trees with branches low enough from which to pick flowers. The second challenge with gathering Lime flowers is to monitor the progress of the flowers and to catch them when they are just at the right stage to harvest. Lime flowers are ready at any time between late May and early July, depending on the season and your location. Within the same area, trees in less sheltered or less sunny microclimates can flower up to two weeks later than the earliest ones. Lime flowers develop bracts first, with a little flower bud hanging down. The bracts make it look as though the trees are in flower, but actually, on closer inspection, they are not. When the buds burst, they transform into fluffy balls of fra-

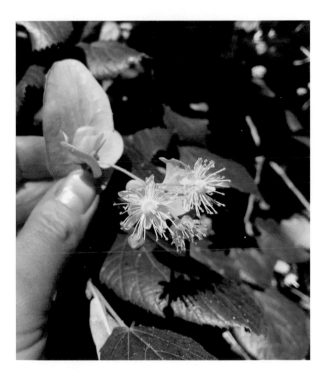

grance, and you can smell the Lime trees from quite some distance. This peak of flowering lasts only a very short time, so you have to make the most of it. I always hope that the weather is kind: a prolonged spell of wet weather can mean that

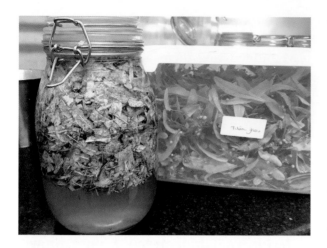

you can drop the flowers, as you pick with two hands. With one hand, support each branch and pick all the flowers with their bracts that are hanging down below it. You will see the flowers more clearly if you look beneath the branches. It is a wonderful experience to be there among the Lime flowers and the leafy branches, listening to the buzzing of the bees and drinking in the heady fragrance. You will find that your basket will contain a mixture of flowers yet to burst, flowers that are open, and a few that have started to form seeds. That is fine. It is the large, very mature seeds that should be avoided.

the Lime flower harvest is missed completely. Once the flowers go over, they transform into hard, round seeds hanging below the bracts, which by now are looking a little more tattered and brown about the edges. It is not advisable to harvest a large proportion of flowers that have gone to seed, since these are reputed to be quite narcotic and not particularly good medicine. Assuming that you have identified a suitable tree and you have a dry day when the flowers are ready, you can venture out with your basket to harvest some. Choose a wide basket into which

Passive drying   Lay the Lime flowers and bracts out on trays, and leave in a warm, airy place, out of direct light.

Active drying   Lay the Lime flowers and bracts out on dehydrator trays. They are quite naturally 'dryish', so you can start with 8 hours at 36–38°C / 95–100°F. Change the trays around, and continue for 1-hourly stints, for as long as needed. Store immediately.

Tincturing   I use dried flowers and 25% alcohol.

Agrimony (*Agrimonia eupatoria*)   ❖   aerial parts

Hardy perennial herb ◆ full sun to partial shade ◆ any soil ◆ spacing: 30–60 cm / 12–24 in

Growing   Easily grown from seed. Plant seeds in spring or transplant self-sown seedlings from the garden to increase your colony.

Harvesting   If you are harvesting for teas, take a cut before the flowers burst open, as at this stage the plants are leafier and the stems softer.

Later in the season the stems become woodier and the leaves are sparser, as the plant puts all of its energy into forming flower spikes. Harvest by cutting the entire stems down to the last green vibrant leaf or to about 15 cm / 6 in from the ground. Lay the stems in your basket in the same direction, since it makes it easier to avoid damage when removing the leaves from the stems back at your processing area.

Passive drying Hang whole plants or stems in bunches upside down to dry in a warm, airy place, out of direct light. Alternatively, remove leaves and flower spikes from the stems and lay them out on trays. You may need to cut larger flower spikes into shorter sections, as they tend to be fleshy and will dry more slowly than the leaves.

Active drying In order to prepare for drying, remove the leaves from the stems, or, if it is early in the season and the stems are very pliable, you can cut them and dry them at the same time as the leaves. I like to start by passive drying overnight on trays and then 12 hours in a dehydrator at 42°C / 108°F. Continue drying in 1-hour stints, for as long as needed. Be careful not to over-dry as you wish to preserve the aromatic lemony quality of this herb. To be in the clinic while Agrimony is

drying is quite literally a blissful experience. Store immediately in an airtight container while the herb is still warm.

Tincturing I use dried herb and 45% alcohol.

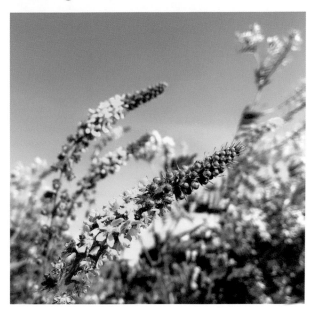

Meadowsweet (*Filipendula ulmaria*) ❖ flowers

Hardy perennial herb • full sun to partial shade • moist, rich soil • spacing: 30 cm / 12 in

Growing Easily grown from seed. Gather ripe seed in the autumn, or buy it in. Sow *in situ* in autumn or spring. This is a good herb to grow in a damp part of the herb garden.

Harvesting Commercial sources of Meadowsweet consist of aerial parts, which includes flowers, leaves, and stems. I prefer to harvest and use just the flowers. Choose flowers that are fresh and vibrant, rather than those that are starting to go to seed. It is acceptable to include some younger, immature flower heads too, but I

prefer the bulk of my harvest to be of open flowers. Cut the stems below the main flower heads, so that you maximize the number of flowers and minimize the amount of stalk that you harvest. Later in the season Meadowsweet can be rather prone to developing powdery mildew; avoid flowers that are affected. If you harvest on a cloudy day, you will reduce the number of bugs that are gathered with the flowers.

Passive drying Spread the flowers evenly onto trays, removing any particularly large, thick

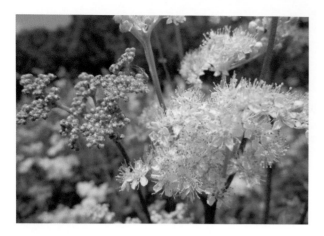

stalks. Spread the trays in your processing area, away from direct light, with the windows open for several hours. Any remaining bugs should be attracted to the light from the windows and find their way out, or congregate on the glass, where you can gently collect them on a piece of paper and let them out. Leave the trays in an airy place, away from direct light, until the stalks are brittle when snapped.

Active drying Spread the flowers evenly onto dehydrator trays, removing any particularly large, thick stalks. Allow the bugs to escape, as described above. During this stage it is a good idea to place a sheet or a solid tray under the dehydrator trays, as Meadowsweet flowers drop copious amounts of yellow pollen and little florets, which fall through the gaps in the trays. Once you are ready to move the trays to the dehydrator, you need to remove the solid trays or sheets that you were using to collect the fallen blossoms and pollen. When drying, I leave an empty dehydrator tray at the base of each tray stack, to catch most of this and reduce the amount that will find its way into the filter. Start the drying process at 42°C / 108°F for 12 hours. Swap the trays around, and continue for additional 2-hour periods until the flowers are thoroughly dry. Store immediately.

Tincturing I use dried flowers and 45% alcohol.

Skullcap (*Scutellaria lateriflora*) ❖ aerial parts

Hardy perennial herb • sun to partial shade • moist, fertile soil • spacing: 15–30 cm / 6–12 in

Growing Grow from seed, or divide and replant roots in early spring. I grow a lot of Skullcap, and I usually take a couple of harvests from the same patch during each season. If you are harvesting intensely, give the plants a top-dressing of compost or well-rotted manure in the autumn.

Harvesting Start as the plants begin to come into flower, and continue until the flowers turn to seed. Since I grow it in a dedicated patch

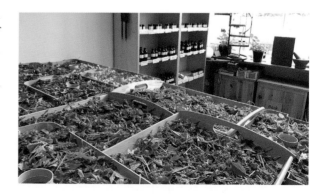

that is kept free of other species, I can harvest it by gathering together loose handfuls of the growing herb and cutting them together, rather than cutting individual stems. When harvesting Skullcap – whether you are using the bunching method or cutting individual stems – be very careful not to pull upwards on the plants. Skullcap is quite shallow-rooted, and during dry conditions it can easily be pulled out of the soil. Do not cut the stems too close to the ground, as this can introduce soil into the basket and also may deplete the plants and prevent them from re-growing for a second cut later in the season. If you do notice any unwanted weed species in your basket, pick them out as soon as you see them. Skullcap is one of those species that I always tincture from fresh plant. I have to make enough tincture at this point to supply my clinic's needs for the entire year. In my practice, I aim to make around 15–20 litres of tincture, depending on how much tincture I still have remaining from the previous year. Any additional Skullcap that is harvested can then be dried, for use in infusions. People have asked me whether using dried Skullcap for infusions is effective, as I tincture fresh herb. I have been prescribing my own dried Skullcap in infusions and capsules for many years, and it is most definitely effective. I am sure that tincture made from dried herb would also be effective, I just prefer to make tincture from fresh plant. I do not think I can give a perfectly logical explanation for this: it is based on how I was taught, and my own feelings when I contemplate this herb and how to prepare it.

Passive drying Form small bunches of perfect, undamaged leaves and flowers. Dry upside down in an airy place, away from direct sunlight. Ensure that the stems are properly brittle before packing the harvest away into your herb store.

Active drying Cut the stalks into sections that

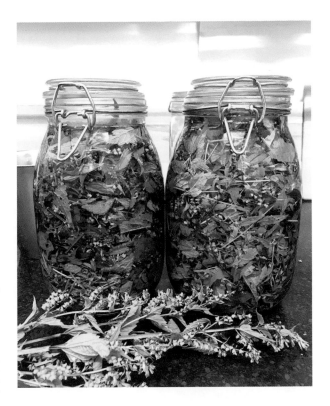

are 7.5–10 cm / 3–4 in in length, and spread them onto dehydrator trays. Remove any discoloured or insect-damaged leaves that may have found their way into your basket at the time of harvest. Start the drying process at 42°C / 108°F, and allow 12 hours before changing the trays around and continuing for additional 2-hour periods. The drying time will be very dependent on the weather conditions prior to harvest and the resulting moisture content of the plants. Ensure that the stems are properly brittle before packing the harvest away into your herb store. The plant material should be bright green. Over the year in storage it may darken slightly, but it will still be green and still retain the scent of fresh Skullcap.

Tincturing I use fresh herb, wilted for 12 hours, and 50–60% alcohol, depending on the moisture content.

Wormwood (*Artemisia absinthum*)   ❖   aerial parts

Hardy perennial herb   ◆   full sun   ◆   well-drained, sheltered site   ◆   spacing: 60 cm ∕ 2 ft

Growing   Plant seeds in spring under shelter, and harden off when established. You can also propagate Wormwood using softwood cuttings from the early summer growth, or divide large, established plants in spring or autumn. It does not do well in exposed sites or on persistently cold, wet soils.

Harvesting   Wormwood is very easily bruised, so great care must be taken when harvesting it.

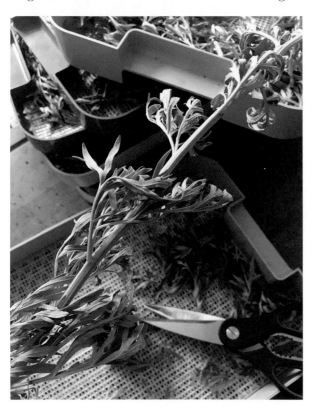

I prefer to harvest whole stems shortly before flowering. Transport the stems back to your processing area without crushing them.

Passive drying   To tie the stems together tightly in bunches will cause bruising. Create small, open bunches to hang upside down, or carefully remove the leaves from the stems and dry on trays.

Active drying   Use a pair of scissors to snip the leaves from the stem. It may seem quicker to run your hands down the stems, pulling off the leaves in your fist, but if you do this, you will be affecting the long-term quality of your crop due to bruising. Hold each stem horizontally over a tray with your left hand (if you are right-handed), and twist it slowly around while snipping off the leaves that hang down with your right hand. If you are left-handed then reverse the instructions. Spread the leaves thinly onto dehydrator trays. Start with 12 hours at 42°C / 108°F, continuing for 1–2-hour periods if more drying is needed. The dry leaves will be softly brittle. Store immediately while warm. If you really want to include the stems, then you should cut them into 2.5-cm / 1-in sections and dry them separately, as they will take much longer than the leaves. If you do not want to use them, then add them respectfully to the compost.

Tincturing   I use dried herb and 45% alcohol.

Marshmallow (*Althaea officinalis*)   ❖   leaves

Perennial herb   ◆   full sun   ◆   moist, rich soil   ◆   spacing: 90 cm / 36 in

Growing   Divide roots and replant in spring or autumn. This is a good candidate for growing in a moist part of the herb garden.

Harvesting   The traditional time for gathering Marshmallow leaves is when they are in flower; however, I quite often harvest the leaves a little before this point. This herb is a very important crop for me. I use a great deal of it in infusions for patients with digestive sensitivities who cannot tolerate tinctures. Marshmallow is rather prone to developing rust in wet years, so keep a close eye on your crop, and at the very first sign of rust, immediately harvest all the remaining healthy leaves. Do not include any leaves affected by rust in your harvest: they will not

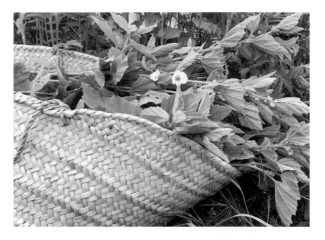

keep well. Cut the stems at the lowest healthy leaf.

Passive drying   Make small bunches and hang them upside down to dry in an airy place, away from direct light. Check your harvest frequently for the development of rust, removing affected leaves and stems immediately.

Active drying   Once back at your processing place, remove the leaves, checking each one carefully for any blemishes or fungal infection. Lay them out immediately on dehydrator trays in a single layer. Start the drying process for 12 hours at 42°C / 108°F. You may need to increase drying times when the ambient humidity is high. Once thoroughly dry, the leaves should snap cleanly. Be especially vigilant about the leaf stalks. They should be brittle and not have the slightest hint of flexibility. Once you are satisfied that they are thoroughly dry, store them while they are still warm from the dryer.

Tincturing   I use dried leaves and 25% alcohol.

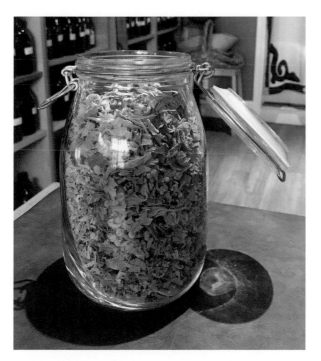

White Horehound (*Marrubium vulgare*)   ❖   tops

Hardy perennial herb ◆ full sun ◆ well-drained neutral to alkaline soil ◆ spacing: 30 cm / 12 in

Growing White Horehound prefers a sheltered site and dryish soil. It can be sown straight into prepared ground in spring, or cuttings can be taken in early summer. Large plants can be divided in autumn.

Harvesting Cut flowering tops as they come into flower. Preferably choose softer stems on plants that have not yet gone to seed, but if you miss this phase, the more mature stems are still fine.

Passive drying Hang small bunches upside down in a warm, airy place, out of direct light.

Active drying Cut the stems into sections approximately 7.5–10 cm / 3–4 in in length. Spread them onto dehydrator trays, and start the drying process at 35°C / 96°F for 12 hours, continuing in small time stints, as needed. If ambient humidity is high, you may need to increase the drying temperature to 42°C / 108°F. Properly dried stems should be brittle but still

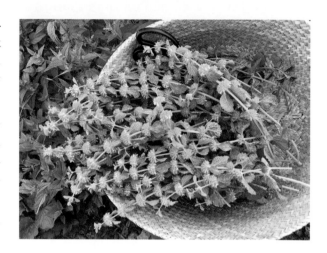

smell faintly aromatic and have a bitter taste. Moisture tends to be retained around the flower and seed heads. Be vigilant when you first place your harvest into storage. Check regularly over the first few days to make sure that it has not reabsorbed moisture.

Tincturing I use dried herb and 45% alcohol.

Wild Oat (*Avena sativa*)   ❖   aerial parts

Hardy annual or perennial grass ◆ full sun ◆ moisture-retentive soil ◆ spacing: 15–20 cm / 6–8 in

Growing If you live in an area where organic arable farming is practised, you should be able to forage Wild Oat. Alternatively, you can grow your own crop from seed. Plant the seeds in a well-prepared seed bed in spring at a depth of 12 mm / 0.5 in.

Harvesting Wild Oat is harvested when the seeds are at the milky stage. This means that if you squeeze a seed, it will be filled with a milky liquid. Wild Oat has not been bred, like cultivated cereals, to have consistent, uniform ripening, so the point at which you can say they

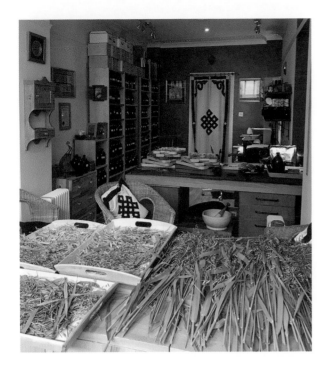

are at the right stage to harvest is not definitive. You will need to look at the seeds from a selection of plants in the population, and choose a time when most of them are at the milky stage. Some will not yet be at that stage, and others will be past it. That is fine, as long as the majority are at the milky stage. Commercially available Wild Oat is divided into 'milky oats' and 'oat straw'. I prefer to harvest the stems while the seeds are at the milky stage, so that my crop contains seed heads and straw. Well-grown Wild Oats are around 2–2.5 m / 7–8 ft tall and are often lodged (have fallen over) by the time they are mature. Avoid stems that are contaminated by soil. If the crop has lodged, harvest stems from the top of each swathe rather than from underneath. Cut the stems to a length that you can deal with. In practice, I find that cutting them about 1.25 m / 4 ft from the top is adequate. Keep the stems the same way up, and tie them loosely in a bundle, or balance the bases in a large basket so that you can carry them by sup-

porting the stems with one hand and holding the basket with the other. You are aiming to maximize seed heads in your harvest, but the amount of straw and leaves will probably make up around 50% or so. Once back at your gathering place, remove any leaves affected by rust as well as any stems affected by eye spot fungus.

Passive drying Create bundles of healthy stems, and hang them upside down to dry in a warm, airy place, out of direct light. Place a tray or a sheet underneath to catch seeds as they fall.

Active drying Cut the healthy leaves, stems, and seed heads into evenly sized lengths, approximately 10–13 cm / 4–5 in long. Spread them evenly on your dehydrator trays. You can fill the trays, making layers several stems thick, since Wild Oat is quite tough and resilient to bruising. It should dry well in 12 hours or so at a temperature of 42°C / 108°F. Store immediately once you are satisfied that it is thoroughly dry. Especially check the thickest stems for pliability. They should be tough and brittle. If you are harvesting just the milky oat seeds, you may prefer to tincture fresh.

Tincturing I use dried herb and 45% alcohol. If you are tincturing fresh seeds, use 60% alcohol.

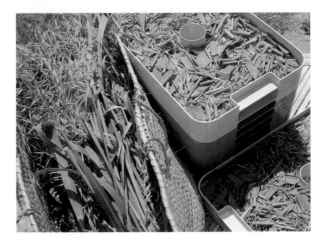

Lemon Balm (*Melissa officinalis*)   ❖   aerial parts

Hardy perennial herb ◆ **full sun to semi-shade** ◆ **moist, rich soil** ◆ **spacing: 60 cm / 24 in**

Growing Divide in spring or autumn, or transplant self-sown seedlings. Keep your Lemon Balm patch weed-free. After flowering, cut the dead stalks down and remove them, if you want to reduce self-seeding.

Harvesting Lemon Balm starts the season as a mass of soft-stemmed leafy herb; it becomes harder and more 'stalky' once it starts to flower. If your Lemon Balm is destined for teas, it is a good idea to harvest early, before flowering. Loosely grasp a handful of stems, and cut them with the other hand. You can only use this 'bulk

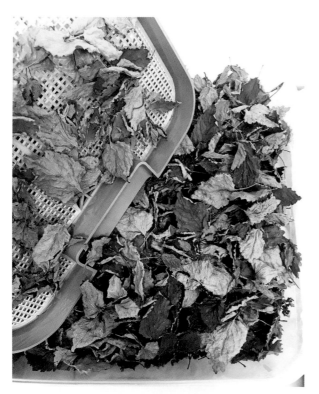

harvesting' technique if your patch of Lemon Balm is nicely weed-free and you have removed the dead stalks left from the previous year's growth. Add each little bundle of stems and leaves to your basket the same way up. This makes it much easier when you are processing them.

Passive drying Make small bunches of stems, and hang them upside down to dry in an airy place, away from direct light. Alternatively, cut the stems into sections approximately 7.5 cm / 3 in long, and lay them on trays.

Active drying Once back at your processing place, cut the stems into sections approximately 7.5 cm / 3 in long, and lay them on dehydrator trays. Start by drying at a temperature of 38°C / 100°F for about 10 hours, then rearrange the trays, and continue for short periods, for as long as needed. Take care not to over-dry them, or you will reduce the aromatic constituents. Later in the season the stalks become quite twiggy and do not dry easily. You can either cut the flowering stems very near their tips to avoid woody growth or you can cut longer stems and then remove the leaves from the stems before drying, adding the stems to the compost. Use the same drying principles and monitor your harvest to avoid over-drying. A well-dried harvest will smell very intensely lemony and still be green.

Tincturing I use dried herb and 45% alcohol. If your drying system does not allow you to produce intensely fragrant dried herb, then choose fresh herb and use 60% alcohol.

Peppermint (*Mentha piperita*) ❖ aerial parts

Hardy perennial herb ⬦ full sun to partial shade ⬦ moist, rich soil ⬦ spacing: 50–60 cm / 20–24 in

Growing Divide root runners during the growing season to establish new plants, or root some cuttings in water and plant when roots appear. Establish well in pots before planting out.

Harvesting Peppermint can get quite woody stems towards the end of the season, so the length of stem you cut will depend on the stage of the season and the desired end product. I like to take a good harvest of younger stems early in the season if they are intended for infusions. This way I avoid the inclusion of hard, woody stalks. Later in the season I choose to cut the flowering stems near their tips, to avoid woody growth.

Passive drying Make small bunches, and hang upside down to dry in a warm, airy place, away from direct light.

Active drying Once at your processing area, snip away soft, leafy growth from hard woody stalks, which should be respectfully discarded. Cut the softer stems into sections that are

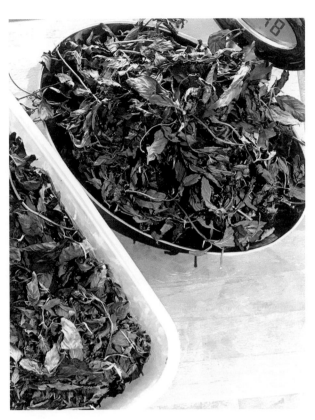

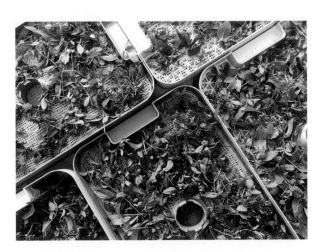

7.5–10 cm / 3–4 in in length. Start the drying process straight away at 38°C / 100°F, and allow 12 hours before changing the trays around and continuing for additional 2-hour periods. Make sure that the stalks are thoroughly dry and brittle before placing the crop into storage, but also be careful to avoid over-drying. The end product should be green and smell very intensely of Peppermint. You will find that this scent is much, much more intense than that of commercially sourced dried Peppermint or shop-bought Peppermint tea.

Tincturing I use dried herb and 45% alcohol.

Spearmint (*Mentha spicata*)   ❖   aerial parts

Hardy perennial herb • full sun to partial shade • moist, rich soil • spacing: 50–60 cm / 20–24 in

Growing   Divide root runners during the growing season to establish new plants, or put some cuttings in water and plant when roots appear. Establish well in pots before planting out.

Harvesting   Like the other labiates, Spearmint develops quite tough stems towards the end of the season. I take my main harvest of younger stems early in the season if they are intended for infusions. Later in the season I cut the flowering stems near their tips, avoiding woody growth.

Passive drying   Make small bunches, and hang upside down to dry in a warm, airy place, away from direct light.

Active drying   Like Peppermint, this is a plant the leaves of which are best removed from hard, woody stalks. Cut softer stems into 7.5–10-cm / 3–4-in sections and start the drying process straight away at 38°C / 100°F Allow 12 hours before changing the trays around and continuing for additional 2-hour periods. Make sure that the stalks are thoroughly dry and brittle

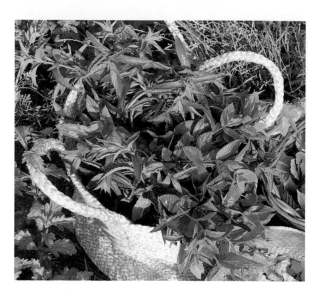

before placing the crop into storage. The herb should be green and smell very intensely of Spearmint. Do not over-dry it, as you will lose the aromatic constituents.

Tincturing   I use dried herb and 45% alcohol.

Catmint (*Nepeta cataria* and *Nepeta mussinii*)   ❖   aerial parts

Hardy perennial herb • full sun to partial shade • moist, rich soil • spacing: 50–60 cm / 20–24 in

Growing   Sow seeds in spring, take soft-wood cuttings, or divide mature plants.

Harvesting   I harvest Catmint in two phases. I take a good harvest early in the season, while the stalks are soft and the leaves are abundant. Provided your crop is weed-free, you can gather together handfuls of stems, and cut them in one go. I usually take an early cut from about half of my Catmint patch, leaving the rest to form flowers. Once the crop is in full flower, I harvest the flowering stems individually, cutting them below the end of the flowering section of the stem. This will also include some foliage. The two harvests are mixed together once dried.

Passive drying   Create small bunches to hang and dry upside down, or, if your harvest is of flower spikes, spread them onto a tray, and dry in an airy, warm place.

Active drying   Cut the stems and flower spikes into 7.5–10-cm / 3–4-in sections, discarding any large, woody stems. Spread onto dehydrator trays, and start the drying process straight away, at 38°C / 100°F. Allow 12 hours before changing the trays around and continuing for additional 2-hour periods. Make sure that the stalks are thoroughly dry and brittle before plac-

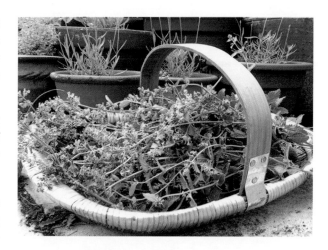

ing the crop into storage. It should be light green and smell intensely of the characteristic slightly musky aroma of Catmint.

Tincturing   I use dried herb and 45% alcohol.

Wild Lettuce (*Lactuca virosa*)   ❖   leaves and flower spikes

Hardy biennial herb ✦ full sun to partial shade ✦ moist, rich, free-draining soil ✦ spacing: 30–60 cm / 12–24 in

Growing   Sow the seeds on the surface of moist compost in spring: they need light to germinate. Transplant to the growing site once the seedlings have at least three sets of leaves. In the first year, the leaves form a rosette that grows close to the ground; in the second year, the plant grows a very tall stem, bearing spikes of little yellow flowers, which turn into wind-borne fluffy seeds that spread far and wide. Once you have enough Wild Lettuce in your garden, you will probably want to limit the number of flowering spikes that go to seed in any one year. When I first grew Wild Lettuce, I found it quite difficult to source seed. After the second year, I let them all seed, hoping

to maintain my population. My Wild Lettuce plants seeded so prolifically that, years later, I still find seedlings popping up in all sorts of places surrounding my allotment. It is lucky that Wild Lettuce is a native plant that is entirely appropriate to the area.

Harvesting   You can harvest from either first-year or second-year plants. Tradition would have it that plants on the point of flowering are the most potent, but I have used first-year plants on many occasions and have made excellent medicine from them. Wild Lettuce exudes copious amounts of white milky sap when cut. The sap is the part that we want to preserve for its sedative

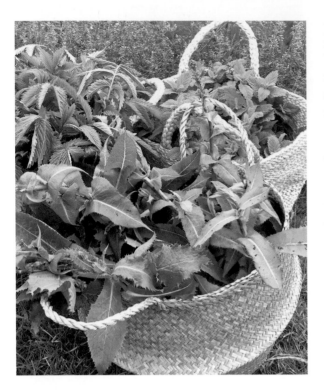

properties, and for this reason it is important to make tinctures from fresh plant, if at all possible. Choose a very dry day, and be prepared to make your tincture immediately. Cut the leaves at the point where they join the stem. If you are including flowers, cut the spikes where they join the main stem. The stem is very high in water content, so I avoid including it in my harvest. When you get back to your processing area, cut the leaves into small pieces, and make your fresh tincture straight away.

Tincturing   I use fresh herb and 60–70% alcohol, depending on the moisture content of the harvest.

St John's Wort (*Hypericum perforatum*)   ❖   flowers

Hardy perennial herb ◆ full sun to partial shade ◆ moist soil types ◆ spacing: 30–45 cm / 12–18 in

Growing   Sow seed in spring, or divide large plants in autumn.

Harvesting   This herb is traditionally harvested at Midsummer. When I harvest St John's Wort, I like to cut only the very tips of the stems, where there are fully open flowers or flowers that are about to burst open. Some people take the entire aerial parts of St John's Wort, but I prefer to harvest just the flowering tops. I have a large patch of St John's Wort and harvest the flowers by gathering the flowering stalks loosely together and cutting them just below the lowest flowering area. This is usually about

10–15 cm / 4–6 in from the tip. You will find that your harvest includes some leaves due to the way the flowers are held on the stems with some leaves between them. This is perfectly acceptable. The majority of your harvest will be flowers.

Passive drying   Cut long stems, and make small bunches to dry by hanging upside down in a warm, airy place. Alternatively, you can cut the flowers and lay them out on trays.

Active drying   Lay the flowers out loosely on dehydrator trays, and start the drying process

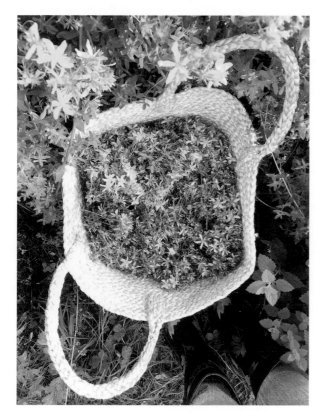

gamating batches from the same season into a larger container, as necessary. Once dried, the leaves should still be bright green and the flowers yellow. Your harvest will smell intensely of the particular sweet and bitter fragrance of fresh St John's Wort. After about 9 months in storage, you may notice that the colour starts to change and the plant material begins to take on a golden-reddish hue – the same colour as the dried seed heads of St John's Wort in winter. This is perfectly natural, and your harvest will still be excellent medicine at least until the next harvest is ready and even for 3–4 months beyond that.

Tincturing   I use dried herb and 60% alcohol.

at a temperature of 42ºC / 108ºF. Allow 12 hours before changing the trays around and continuing for additional 2-hour periods. The stalks are brittle when fresh, so the brittleness of the stalks is not a good guide as to when the crop is thoroughly dried. Until you become experienced, you will need to take extra care in judging when your crop is properly dry. Store each batch separately at first, and check it after two days in storage. If the flower stalks and leaves feel flexible and no longer brittle, replace them in the dehydrator and continue drying for at least a further 4 hours. Pack them away while still warm in a small container with minimal air gap, amal-

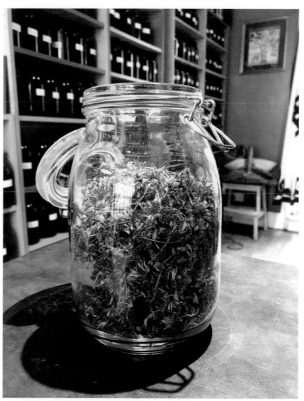

Borage (*Borago officinalis*) ❖ flowers and leaves

Hardy annual herb ✦ **full sun** ✦ **well-drained soil** ✦ **spacing: 60–90 cm / 24–36 in**

Growing Sow seeds in mid- to late spring. Successive sowings will give you a longer harvest period for flowers and young leaves.

Harvesting Harvest the flowers just as they open. You can also harvest young leaves. The fleshy stems and leaves can be difficult to dry, so it may be preferable to make a fresh tincture from the flowers and young leaves. Borage contains potentially toxic pyrrolizidine alkaloids that can affect the liver and the lungs. As a result, its medicinal use is either restricted or under review in many countries.

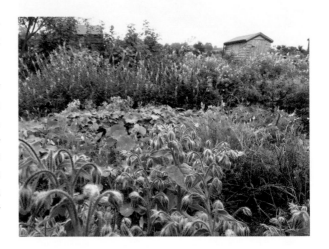

Tincturing I use dried herb and 45% alcohol.

Lady's Mantle (*Alchemilla mollis*) ❖ leaves and flowers

Hardy perennial herb ✦ **full sun to shade** ✦ **moist, well-drained soil** ✦ **spacing: 30–40 cm / 12–16 in**

Growing Sow seeds in late summer, or collect and repot self-sown seedlings. Large plants can be divided in early spring or autumn.

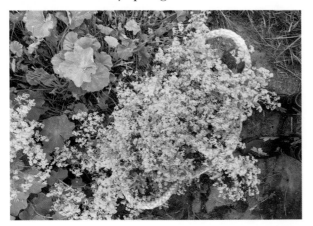

Harvesting Lady's Mantle is quite low-growing, so it can be harvested by bunching the leaves and stalks together before cutting. Avoid cutting too close to the base of the plant, in order to avoid soil contamination and also to avoid weakening the plant. By the time the plant is in full flower, the leaves are often past their best, so I sometimes prefer to take an early harvest for teas and a later harvest, including flowers, for use in sitz baths and other topical applications. If you are using Lady's Mantle for sitz baths, you will need to harvest quite a large quantity. Fortunately, it is very generous with its growth throughout the season and recovers well after cutting.

Passive drying   Remove stalks and spread the leaves loosely on trays to dry, or make small bunches to dry upside down using the leaf stalks.

Active drying   Remove stalks and spread the leaves loosely on dehydrator trays. Start the drying process at a temperature of 42°C / 108°F, allowing 12 hours before changing the trays around and continuing for additional 2-hour periods, if needed. Test for dryness by folding a leaf in half and seeing whether it snaps cleanly. Pack away into storage while still warm.

Tincturing   I use dried herb and 25% alcohol.

Raspberry (*Rubus idaeus*) ❖ leaves

Hardy perennial shrub ◆ full sun to partial shade ◆ well-drained, fertile soil ◆ spacing: 30–45 cm / 12–18 in

Growing   Establish from canes or cuttings. I usually wild harvest this crop. There is something really magical about seeing a patch of wild Raspberry in the moonlight. The underside of the leaves is a silvery colour, and this becomes particularly prominent under a full moon. I identified my best wild Raspberry gathering patch while I was returning home late at night along a very narrow rural lane. Being a committed forager, I stopped right there and then in the moonlight to fill a couple of large baskets.

Harvesting   Raspberry leaves are harvested during the summer. If you are harvesting from cultivated plants, wait until they have fruited, and then combine your harvest with a tidying up and cutting back of the canes. If you are wild harvesting, then you may want to enjoy some of the very sweet little fruit as you harvest. Cut stems above the last healthy leaf, and snip the leaves from the stems. You can do this in the field or back at your processing place. Always return the stems to the earth with gratitude.

Passive drying   Create small bunches of stems to dry the crop upside down, removing the

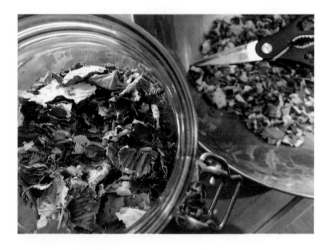

leaves once they are thoroughly dry. Alternatively, remove leaves from the stems and lay them out whole on trays to dry.

Active drying   Remove the leaves from the stems, and lay them out whole in a single layer on dehydrator trays. Start the drying process at 42°C / 108°F for 12 hours. Once the leaves are thoroughly dry and brittle, they can be put into storage.

Tincturing   I use dried leaves and 45% alcohol.

Calendula (*Calendula officinalis*)   ❖   flowers

Annual herb • full sun • wide range of soils • spacing: 24 cm / 10 in

Growing   Sow *in situ* in late spring. Plants self-seed readily.

Harvesting   Calendulas should be snipped off as near to the base of the flower as possible, so that you minimize the length of stalk in the harvest. If you do this, your cut flowers can be dried without further processing. It is time-consuming to go through your harvest trimming stalks once you get back to your processing area, and the more you handle your cut herbs, the greater the risk of bruising them. You will soon find your own rhythm in harvesting Calendulas, especially as you will be harvesting them every other day throughout the summer, weather permitting. I like to get each stem between two of the fingers of my left hand and run them up the stem towards the flower head until I am cupping the

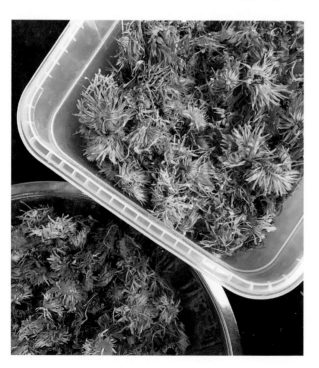

flower gently in my hand and then snip the stalk just below my fingers with my right hand. I repeat the process with 2–3 more flowers, forming a little stack in my left hand, before I bend down to place them gently into the basket. By stacking 2 or 3 before bending down, you make harvesting more efficient. Deadhead any flowers that have gone over in order to prolong your harvest. As soon as you allow your Calendulas to go to seed, they will produce fewer flowers.

Passive drying   Lay the flowers on trays, so that they do not touch each other. Leave to dry in a warm, airy place. If possible, finish the drying process in an airing cupboard. Ensure that the green calyces are thoroughly dried before storage.

Active drying   Place the flowers on dehydrator trays straight away, allowing space between flower heads. Start the drying process at a temperature of 42°C / 108°F, and allow 12 hours before changing the trays around. Continue for additional periods, for as long as needed. If the weather has been wet prior to harvest, the flowers will have a great deal of moisture in the calyces. Continue drying until the calyces feel thoroughly dry. In some years this may take over 36 hours of drying, but usually 24 hours would be more than adequate. If the ambient humidity is high, you may need to increase the temperature to 47°C / 116°F and continue drying for 4 hours at the higher temperature in order to complete the drying process. Once you are satisfied that they are properly dry, store them straight away in a small, temporary container. Check the calyces regularly until you become confident in assessing when they are thoroughly dry. As you build up quantities, amalgamate

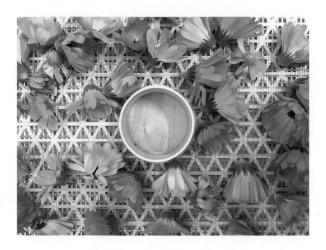

batches from the same season into a larger container. They should retain a bright orange colour and a bitter, resinous, sweet aroma. By the end of a year in storage, the orange colour of the flowers will be fading a little to a yellower colour, but the aroma should still be the same, and the medicine will be perfectly usable until the next season's crop is ready. If I have any flowers left over from the previous season, I use them in external treatments, sometimes mixed with some flowers from the new season. There is no need to throw them away if they still have the characteristic Calendula scent.

Tincturing   I use dried flowers and 25% alcohol.

Chamomile (*Matricaria recutita*) ❖ flowers

Hardy annual herb ◆ full sun ◆ light soil ◆ spacing: 10 cm / 4 in

Growing   Sow seeds *in situ* from late summer to autumn.

Harvesting Chamomile flowers are labour-intensive to pick by hand, but this is the way to get the best possible quality. Some people use a harvesting comb, which they pull through the leaves and stems, catching the flowers between the teeth and plucking them. The comb is pushed into the crop and then lifted up and back to create a plucking motion. As the flowers are plucked, they fall into a receptacle attached to the comb. I do not use combs myself, but if you have a very large quantity of Chamomile to harvest, you may find it helpful to experiment with different designs and harvesting techniques to get the best possible quality.

Passive drying   Spread the flowers out in a single layer on a tray, and leave to dry in a warm, airy place.

Active drying   Chamomile flowers should be spread out onto dehydrator trays and dried at a moderate temperature. Start at 38°C / 100°F for 8 hours and then re-assess as needed.

Tincturing   I use dried flowers and 45% alcohol.

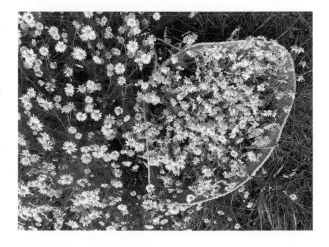

Rose (*Rosa* spp.)   ❖   petals

Hardy perennial shrub • full sun to partial shade • rich, moist, well-drained soil • spacing: 1.25–1.75 m / 4–6 ft

Growing Buy Rose plants from a reputable supplier, and plant according to their instructions. Any fragrant variety of Rose is suitable for medicine, provided that it has not been treated with chemicals. I instinctively choose red and pink versions, those being closer to the traditional Apothecary Rose and also just because I prefer them in the garden. I have never used yellow or orange Roses as medicines, so cannot comment on their comparative efficacy. If you are buying new Rose plants especially for your herb garden, ensure that they are scented.

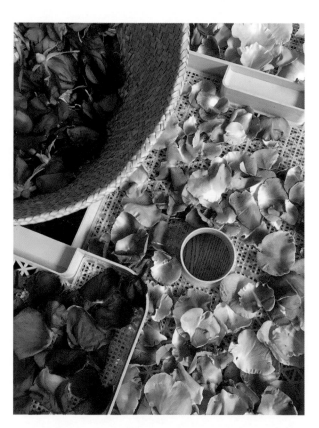

Many modern varieties are not. *Rosa rugosa* is excellent medicinally, is very hardy, and has a beautiful scent. Its flowers are used in traditional Chinese medicine.

Harvesting Gather Rose petals throughout the flowering period during the summer. Before harvesting, make sure that the flowers are completely dry, if at all possible. Take each flower, checking that there is no pollinating insect visiting it, gently gather up the petals from underneath the flower, and draw them together, as if to close the flower. Once you have the petals held between your thumb and fingers, support the calyx with your other hand, and gently pull to detach the petals in one go, leaving the calyx on the stem. Once you have placed the petals into your basket, snip off the calyx, so as to deadhead the Rose bush as you go. I find this method more convenient than going through my basket removing calyces once I get back to the processing area. Once I have harvested a sufficient volume of Rose petals, I leave the hips to develop on the bushes.

Passive drying Spread the petals thinly on mesh trays in the dark. Use a single layer on a surface that allows air flow from beneath. Aim not to move or touch the petals once they are on the tray. Finish the drying process in a warm place, such as an airing cupboard, if possible.

Active drying Rose petals need to be dried very gently in order to preserve their fragrance. Spread the petals in a thin layer on dehydrator trays, and start the drying process at 35°C / 96°F for 8 hours. Change the trays

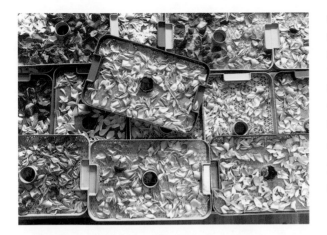

around and continue for 1-hour stints, for as long as necessary. Once dried, the petals should retain their colour and have a papery texture, but they will have reduced considerably in size. You should still be able to smell a definite Rose fragrance. This scent intensifies significantly in storage.

Tincturing   I use dried petals and 45% alcohol. I double-infuse my Rose tincture, using a second maceration of dried petals in the same tincture after it has been drained.

Goat's Rue (*Galega officinalis*)   ❖   aerial parts

Hardy perennial herb • **full sun to partial shade** • **rich, deep soil** • **spacing: 1–1.25 m / 3–4 ft**

Growing   Sow seeds in spring or transplant self-sown seedlings. This plant self-seeds very readily. Large plants can be divided in the autumn. Goat's Rue is a tall plant, reaching heights of 1–1.25 m / 3–4 ft. It benefits from some support in the border later on in the summer.

Harvesting   Harvest the flowering tops in high summer, when Goat's Rue is in full flower. Aim to cut flowering stems with younger leaves, but mature leaves in good condition are also fine. Place the base of the stems into your basket. The flowers and leaves will spill out, but you can transport your crop back to your processing area by carrying the basket in one hand and supporting the overflowing stems with the other.

Passive drying   Create small bunches of perhaps 8 stems, and hang them upside down in an airy place. Alternatively, you can remove the flowers and leaves from the stems and lay them

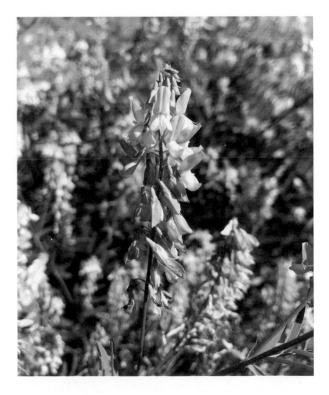

out on trays in a warm, airy place, away from direct light.

Active drying   Once you get back to your processing area, remove the leaves and the flowers from the stems, and lay them out on dehydrator trays. You may need to cut the larger leaves and remove fleshy leaf stalks, as these will not dry at the same rate as the rest of the plant material. Start the drying process at a temperature of 42°C / 108°F for 12 hours. Swap the trays around and reassess, continuing the drying process for 2-hour periods, for as long as necessary.

Tincturing   I use dried herb and 45% alcohol.

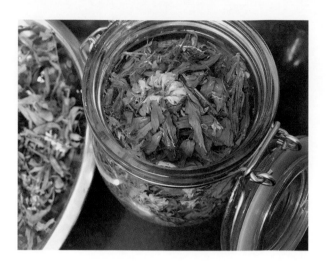

Yarrow (*Achillea millefolium*)   ❖   flowers

Perennial herb ◆ full sun ◆ well-drained soil ◆ spacing: 12.5–17 cm / 5–7 in

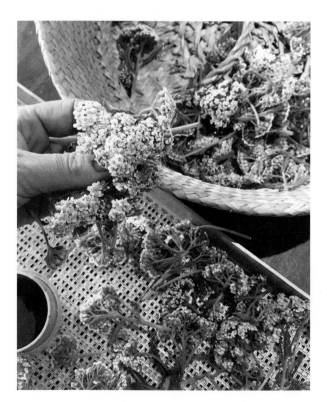

Growing   Many people will be able to wildcraft all that they need of this herb. If you do need to cultivate it, you can grow from seed or separate some rhizomes from an established clump and grow them in a pot until they are strong enough to be planted out. Once established, it spreads vigorously, so starting with a few plants will produce a reasonable patch in a couple of seasons.

Harvesting   I prefer to harvest mostly the flowers of this plant, although all parts are medicinal. Yarrow flowers over a long period during the summer, so you can return and take several cuts. In years where the Yarrow harvest has been sparse, I have also harvested young leaves in order to gather a sufficient amount for the needs of my patients. Cut the stems just below the flower heads or below the last healthy leaf, if you are including foliage.

Passive drying   Harvest stems below the last healthy leaf and suspend in small bunches to

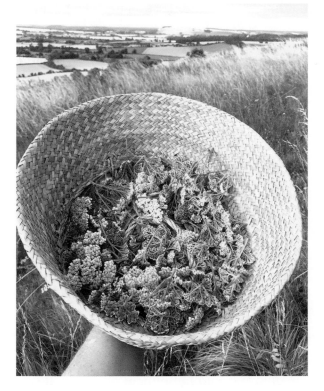

dry. Alternatively, place flower heads and leaves whole onto trays.

Active drying   Place the flowers onto dehydrator trays in a single layer. If you are including foliage, remove the leaves from the stalks by snipping them off with scissors. Resist the temptation to strip the leaves from the stalks by running your hand down the stalks and pulling them off in one go, even though this would be quicker. This method of leaf removal leads to crushing and bruising. Start the drying process at a temperature of 42°C / 108°F, allowing 12 hours before changing the trays around and continuing for additional 2-hour periods, for as long as necessary. Test for dryness by checking if a stalk snaps cleanly when you attempt to fold it. Leaves remain soft and flexible even when dry. They will retain their colour and smell very strongly of the scent of freshly picked Yarrow.

Tincturing   I use dried flowers and 45% alcohol.

Red Clover (*Trifolium pratense*)   ❖   flowers

Hardy perennial herb • full sun to partial shade • well-drained soil of moderate fertility • spacing: 20–30 cm / 8–12 in

Growing   Red Clover produces more flowers in soils with a relatively low nitrogen status. It is a nitrogen-fixing plant, so is an ideal crop to improve the fertility of your herb garden or to grow as a compost ingredient as well as for medicine. Direct sow in spring. Although I have grown Red Clover in the past, these days I wild harvest it due to lack of growing space.

Harvesting   Wild harvesting Red Clover is usually a case of picking little and often. I tend to walk through a particular meadow every 2–3

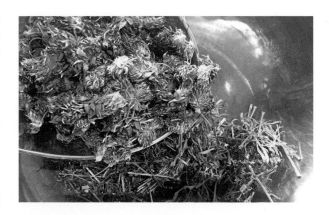

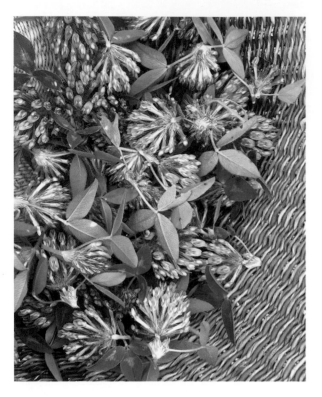

the flower head in order to minimize the inclusion of stalks. If you are consistent with your foraging activities over the summer, these small harvests will add up to a reasonable volume. If, however, you are able to grow your own crop, you may be able to harvest all that you need in one go. Cultivated Red Clover grows 20–78 cm / 8–31 in tall and is therefore easier on the back than harvesting wild-grown plants that lie close to the ground.

Passive drying Red Clover flowers dry very well passively. Spread the flowers on a tray, and leave in a warm, airy place, away from direct light.

Active drying As I gather small quantities at a time, I usually air-dry my Red Clover. I spread each little harvest on a tray in my clinic and leave it in a dark, airy place to dry. Once there are enough to fill a couple of dehydrator trays, I give them an hour or so at 42°C / 108°F in the dehydrator to finish them off before finally storing them.

Tincturing I use dried flowers and 45% alcohol.

days and gather any blossoms that are at their peak. Pick the flowers individually to avoid including grasses and other extraneous species in your basket. Nip each blossom off just below

Horsetail (*Equisetum arvense*) ❖ tops

Hardy perennial herb • full sun to partial shade • moist soil, with moderate fertility • spacing: 15–30 cm / 6–12 in

Growing Horsetail is rather invasive, so it is best to wild harvest it if you can. If you need to cultivate it, contain it in its own bed. Propagate from rhizomes in autumn.

Harvesting Horsetail has two types of stems. In early spring, it throws up a pale-green spike

terminated by a cylindrical spore-producing spike. In summer, the stems that we harvest for medicine grow: these are bright green, with whorls of jointed thread-like leaves. Gather the top 15 cm / 6 in or so of the shoots, using secateurs or scissors to cut through the silica-rich stems. They will feel dry to the touch but still

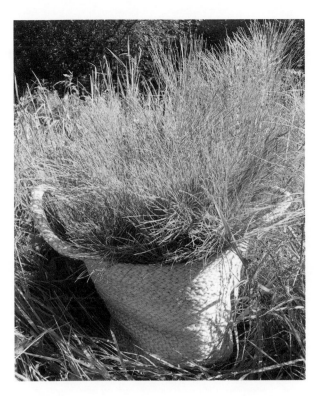

need further drying before storage, unless you are planning to use them while they are fresh.

Passive drying Form small bunches and hang them upside down in a warm, airy place, away from direct light. Place a tray or sheet beneath the bunches as the leaves are prone to breaking and dropping.

Active drying Cross-cut the stems into pieces approximately 7.5 cm / 3 in long. Lay them on dehydrator trays, and dry them for around 6 hours at 42°C / 108°F before assessing how much additional drying time will be needed: 8 hours in total is a reasonable estimate, but use your own judgement, as it does vary. Once they are thoroughly dry the leaves will be dark green and all of the plant material will be dry and brittle. Store your Horsetail while it is warm from the dryer.

Tincturing I use dried herb and 25% alcohol.

Eyebright (*Euphrasia* spp.) ❖ tops

Hardy annual semi-parasitic herb • full sun • meadows and well-drained and low-fertility soils

Growing There are around 450 species of Eyebright, and most can be used interchangeably as herbal medicine. The Eyebrights are semi parasitic, growing on grasses, Clovers, Vetches and Plantains and other plants commonly found in alpine and chalk downland meadows. Eyebright is under threat in the wild as it is very vulnerable to habitat loss. It needs to set seed each year in order to perpetuate itself, and it requires the presence of its preferred host plants in order to thrive. It is not easy to cultivate due to its

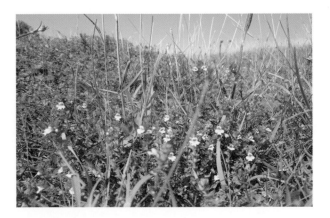

requirement for host plants although establishment within a wildflower meadow may be possible.

Harvesting   When wild harvesting Eyebright, only do so from places where it is abundant and do so sparingly. Cut the tops while it is in full flower, taking care not to uproot the plants so that they can regrow and produce more flowers later in the season.

Passive drying   Spread the stems onto trays in a single layer and leave to dry in a warm, airy place, away from direct light.

Active drying   Spread the plants out immediately and dry gently at 42°C / 108°F for at least 10 hours. Make sure they are thoroughly dry before storing.

Tincturing   I use dried herb and 45% alcohol.

California Poppy (*Eschscholzia californica*)   ❖   aerial parts

Annual herb (perennial in warm climates) ✦ full sun ✦ moderately fertile, well-drained soil ✦ spacing: 10–20 cm / 4–8 in

Growing   Direct sow and keep moist until plants established. Do not over-water as the plants are prone to mildew in damp conditions.

Harvesting   California Poppy is harvested when it is in full flower. You will be cutting whole plants, so each plant that you cut will include some open flowers, some flower buds, and some seed heads, as well as the feathery, fleshy leaves. All parts are medicinal. Cut the plant about 5 cm / 2 in from the base, taking care not to pull it out by the roots and avoiding faded or soil-splashed lower leaves. California Poppy is best used fresh. It does not seem to dry very well. In the past, I have dried batches of it, but despite it seeming to be thoroughly dry at the point of storage, it did not remain in good condition beyond 2–3 months. For this reason, I only use it to make fresh tincture these days.

Tincturing   I use fresh plant and 60% alcohol.

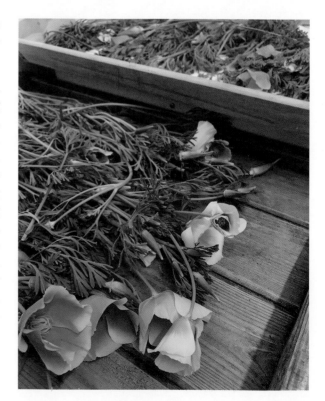

Nasturtium (*Tropaeolum majus*) ❖ flowers and leaves

Half-hardy annual herb ◆ full sun to partial shade ◆ rich, moist soil ◆ spacing: 30 cm / 12 in

Growing Nasturtium is very easy to grow from seed and produces prolific crops. Sow seeds under cover early in the spring, or direct sow after the last frost.

Harvesting Harvest when there is a high proportion of flowers on the plants. As I intend to dry my Nasturtium crops, I tend to cut individual leaves and flower heads, avoiding the fleshy stems, seed heads, and leaf stalks. If you are using your crop fresh, you can include all parts if you wish.

Passive drying Lay the flowers and leaves out on separate trays, in a single layer; do not overlap them. Leave them to dry in a warm, airy place, away from direct light.

Active drying Lay the flowers and leaves out on dehydrator trays, so that they do not overlap

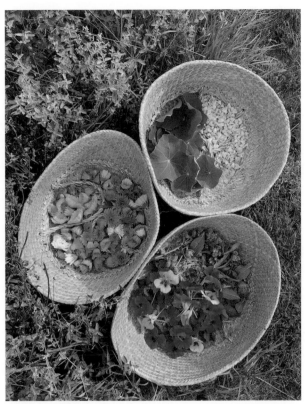

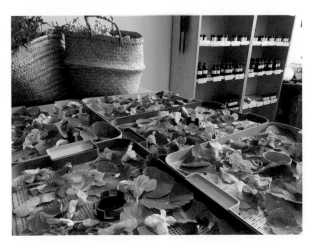

one another. Start the drying process at a temperature of 42°C / 108°F, and dry for 12 hours before rearranging the trays. The leaves may be completely or nearly dry at that point, but the flowers will need considerably longer: up to 24 or even 36 hours, depending on ambient humidity. Ensure that the flower stalks are thoroughly dried before storage. Store immediately, while still warm.

Tincturing I use dried herb and 45% alcohol.

Honeysuckle (*Lonicera periclymenum*) ❖ flowers

Hardy perennial climber ✦ **full sun to partial shade** ✦ **any fertile, well-drained soil** ✦ **grow on a wall or fence**

Growing Best grown from cuttings taken from non-flowering semi-hardwood shoots in summer. You can also propagate by layering.

Harvesting Gathering Honeysuckle flowers has to be one of the foraging highlights of the year. The scent of the flowers is absolutely divine. Honeysuckle is in flower over quite a long period, from the late spring to the autumn. The timing of the flowers will depend to some extent upon the microclimate in which the plant is growing, plants on a south-facing wall flowering earlier than those in a shadier location. Snip the flowers from the stems with secateurs or scissors. Choose vibrant open flowers and buds, avoiding old flowers

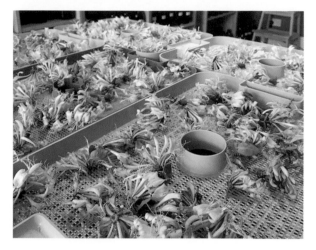

that are going over. Do not pile the flowers too deeply in your gathering basket as they will quickly deteriorate.

Passive drying Once back at your processing place, lay the flowers out thinly on trays straight away. Leave the trays in a warm, airy place, out of direct light.

Active drying Lay the flowers out onto dehydrator trays as soon as possible. Leave them for a couple of hours in a cool place, away from direct sunlight, in order to encourage any bugs present to leave the flowers and congregate on the inside of the windows, ready to be released. Start the flowers drying at a low temperature, say 38°C / 100°F, for 12 hours. If the ambient humidity is high, you may need to increase the temperature slightly for another few hours to achieve proper drying. Only store the flowers once the stems are brittle and the flowers feel totally dry.

Tincturing I use dried flowers and 45% alcohol.

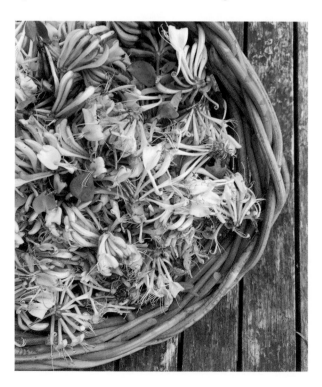

Lavender (*Lavandula angustifolia*) ❖ flowers

Hardy perennial ◆ full sun to partial shade ◆ slightly sandy loam ◆ dry soil ◆ spacing: 30–60 cm / 12–24 in

Growing Establish young plants in well-drained, moderately fertile soil. You can increase stock by taking softwood cuttings in spring or hardwood cuttings in autumn.

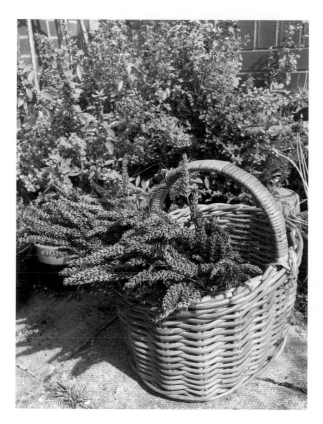

Harvesting For medicinal use, snip flowers from the stalks just before they open fully. For decorative and craft use, snip flower-bearing stalks of even lengths and create bundles.

Passive drying Lavender dries very well passively. Harvest flowers with their stalks, and hang bunches upside down, out of direct light. Posi-tion an open paper bag below each bunch, in order to catch any flower heads as they fall.

Active drying Spread flowers on dehydrator trays, and dry at a low temperature, 35°C / 96°F, for 4–8 hours. Continue drying for short periods, for as long as necessary. The time taken for the crop to become fully dried varies with the ambient humidity and the level of loading in the dehydrator.

Tincturing I use fresh flowers and 55% alcohol.

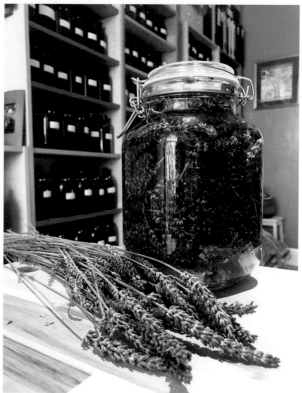

Rosemary (*Rosmarinus officinalis*) ❖ foliage

Hardy perennial shrub • full sun • sandy, dry soil • spacing: 60–90 cm / 24–36 in

Growing Take cuttings from non-flowering shoots in early summer. Once established, plant out in a sunny, sheltered spot.

Harvesting Combine harvesting with necessary pruning of established plants. Cut stems with secateurs and be conscious of maintaining a good shape.

Passive drying Hang bunches of stems upside down in a warm, airy, dust-free place, out of direct light. Alternatively, strip the needles from the stems, and lay them on a tray to dry.

Active drying Strip the needles from the stems, spread them evenly onto dehydrator trays, and dry at a low temperature of 35°C / 96°F for 8 hours before reassessing; continue to dry for short periods, for as long as necessary. The needles should be brittle before storage but still smell strongly of Rosemary.

Tincturing I use fresh herb and 50% alcohol. For making infused oil, I use fresh Rosemary.

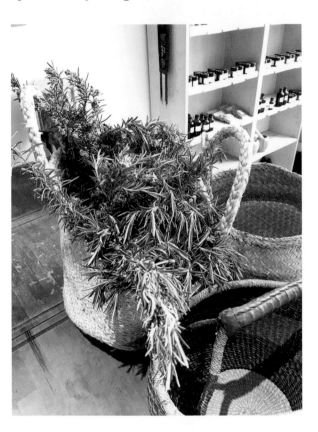

Boneset (*Eupatorium perfoliatum*) ❖ flowers and leaves

Hardy perennial herb • partial shade • moist, rich soil • spacing: 45–60 cm / 18–24 in

Growing Sow seeds in autumn. They require a period of cold before germination. Keep the seeds moist until they have germinated. This plant is very cold-hardy and will tolerate temperatures down to –25°C / –13°F.

Harvesting Cut the flower heads at full bloom, together with young leaves.

Passive drying Make small bunches, and hang these upside down in a warm, airy place, away from direct light.

Active drying Remove the leaves from the stems, and lay them out on dehydrator trays. Cut the flowers heads, if necessary, and lay them out in a thin layer. Start the drying process at

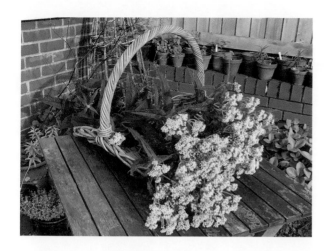

a temperature of 42°C / 108°F for 12 hours. Swap the trays around, and continue for 2-hour periods, as needed, until the leaves are brittle when folded.

Tincturing I use fresh herb that has been left to wilt for 12 hours on a tray and 50% alcohol.

Sage (*Salvia officinalis*) ❖ leaves

Hardy perennial herb ◆ full sun ◆ well-drained calcareous soil ◆ spacing: 50 cm / 20 in

Growing Sow seeds in late spring or early summer. Take cuttings in spring, or propagate by layering. Plant out in a sheltered location. Prune back the plants each winter in order to keep them from becoming leggy.

Harvesting Cut the upper, non-woody stems, using secateurs. Choose stems with healthy, unblemished, clean leaves, just as the plant is coming into flower.

Passive drying Make small bunches and hang them upside down in a warm, airy place, out of direct light.

Active drying Remove the leaves from the stems, and lay them out on dehydrator trays, together with the flower spikes. Dry at a temperature of 35°C / 96°F for a period of 10–12 hours. Continue for short periods if needed. The leaves and flower stalks should be brittle when thoroughly dry but they should retain a bright colour and strong scent.

Tincturing I use fresh herb that has been wilted for 12 hours and 50% alcohol.

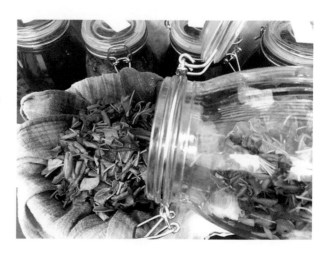

Vervain (*Verbena officinalis*) ❖ tops

Hardy perennial herb • **full sun** • **well-drained, moderately fertile soil** • **spacing: 30 cm / 12 in**

Growing Sow seed in pots in early spring, and plant out once established. Vervain self-seeds readily, so you can increase your colony by potting up and transplanting seedlings in the spring. Alternatively, you can divide large, established plants.

Harvesting Once the plant is in full flower, cut stems above the lowest healthy leaf. The lower leaves tend to become yellowish during the summer, as the plant puts all its energy into flowering. Avoid any upper stems that are discoloured or affected by mildew.

Passive drying Create small bunches of stems, and hang them upside down in a warm, airy place, away from direct light.

Active drying Cross-cut the stems into 7.5–10-cm / 3–4-in long sections complete with leaves and flowers. Spread the stems in dehydrator trays, and start the drying process at a tempera-

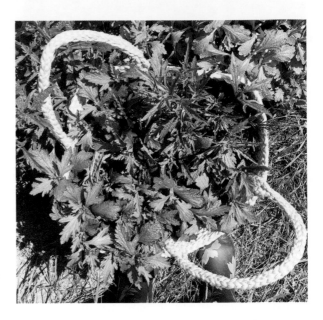

ture of 42°C / 108°F for 12 hours. The stems should be brittle when thoroughly dried.

Tincturing I use dried herb and 45% alcohol.

Mugwort (*Artemisia vulgaris*) ❖ aerial parts

Hardy perennial herb • **full sun** • **well-drained, moderately fertile soil** • **spacing: 30–45 cm / 12–18 in**

Growing Mugwort can be rather invasive and inhibits the growth of nearby plants, so it is better to wild harvest this rather than establishing it in your herb garden.

Harvesting Cut the flowering stems or stem tops during the summer.

Passive drying Create small bunches, and suspend them upside down in a warm, airy place, away from direct light.

Active drying Remove the leaves and flowers from the thickest stalks, and cut the upper softest stems into pieces approximately

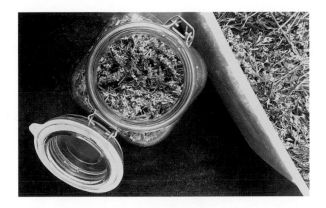

7.5–10 cm / 3–4 in long. Lay the leaves and stem pieces out onto dehydrator trays, and start the drying process at a temperature of 35°C / 96°F, provided that the ambient humidity is low. If the air is moist, increase the temperature to 42°C / 108°F, and dry for a period of 12 hours before reassessing. The stems should be brittle before the plant material is stored.

Tincturing   I use dried herb and 45% alcohol.

Thyme (*Thymus vulgaris*)   ❖   flowering tops

Hardy perennial herb • full sun • well-drained poor to moderately fertile soil • spacing: 25 cm / 10 in

Growing   Sow seed in spring, or propagate with soft-wood cuttings. Plant in a sheltered place, and cut back after flowering to prevent plants from becoming leggy.

Harvesting   I like to take a small harvest before the plants flower, and then take a second harvest once they are in flower.

Passive drying   Spread stems on trays, and leave them in a warm, airy place, away from direct light.

Active drying   Spread the stems on dehydrator trays. Start the drying process at 35°C / 96°F for 12 hours. Increase the temperature if the ambient humidity is high. Continue drying for short periods of time, if needed.

Tincturing   I use dried herb and 45% alcohol.

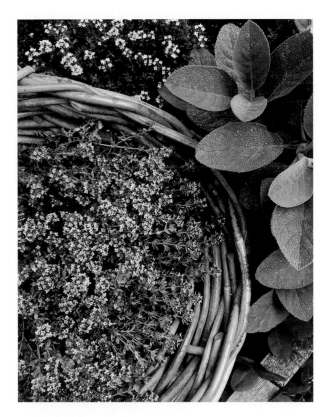

Comfrey (*Symphytum officinale*)   ❖   leaves and flowers

Hardy perennial herb • full sun to partial shade • moist, fertile soil • spacing: 1–1.25 m / 3–4 ft

Growing   Can be grown from seeds planted in spring, or divide large plants and take root cuttings. Cut back the dead leaves in the autumn or winter.

Harvesting   Cut perfect, healthy leaves on a dry day. Take care not to bruise them when transporting them back to your processing place.

Passive drying   Thread individual leaves and suspend them on a line in a warm, airy place, in the manner of drying Tobacco.

Active drying   Carefully remove the midribs from larger leaves, and cut the leaves into segments about 7.5–10 cm / 3–4 in wide. Small,

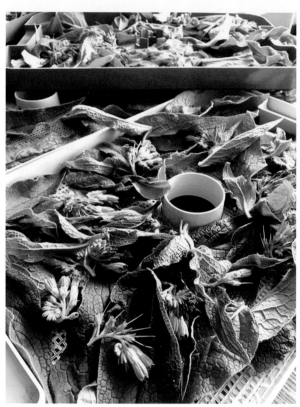

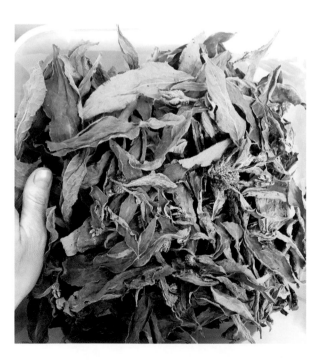

young leaves can be left whole, with the midribs in place. Lay the leaves and the leaf segments out onto dehydrator trays, and start the drying process at a temperature of 42°C / 108°F. After 12 hours rearrange the trays, and continue drying for 2-hour stints, as needed. The leaves should be brittle when thoroughly dried. Store immediately, while still warm.

Tincturing   I do not tincture this herb. I infuse it in oil or dry it for sitz baths.

Arnica (*Arnica montana*)   ❖   flowers

Hardy perennial herb ✦ **full sun** ✦ **well-drained soil** ✦ **spacing: 30 cm / 12 in**

Growing   Sow seed in spring, or divide large plants in the autumn. Arnica is an alpine herb, so it must be grown in a free-draining part of the garden. If your soil is heavy, create a raised alpine bed.

Harvesting   Pick individual flowers with their stalks just before they are at their peak. Mature flowers turn to fluffy seed heads, which are not convenient for medicine.

Passive drying   Lay the flowers out on trays, and leave them to dry in a warm, airy place, out of direct light.

Active drying   Lay the flowers out on dehydrator trays, and start them at a temperature of 38°C / 100°F for 12 hours. Increase the temperature if ambient humidity is high. Change the trays around, and continue drying for short periods of time, as needed. Store immediately in an airtight container.

Tincturing   I do not tincture this plant, I infuse it in oil for external treatments.

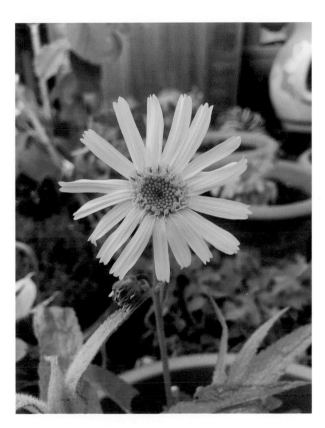

Red Poppy (*Papaver rhoeas*)   ❖   flowers

Hardy annual ✦ **full sun** ✦ **disturbed soils and as a weed of arable crops** ✦ **spacing: 7.5–10 cm / 3–4 in**

Growing   Poppies can be grown as part of a wildflower meadow, or they can be foraged from around the edge of organically managed arable crops. Scatter seeds onto disturbed ground in spring.

Harvesting   The ephemeral flowers only last one day. Snip the flowers into a shallow basket, and lay them out for drying within an hour of picking.

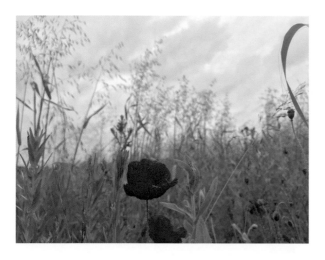

Passive drying Leave the flowers on trays in a warm, airy place, away from direct light. Be careful to avoid significant drafts, as they will blow the very light petals away.

Active drying Lay the flowers out on dehydrator trays, and start the drying at a temperature of 35°C / 96°F for a period of 6 hours. Change the trays around, and continue for periods of 1 hour, as needed. Ensure that the green calyces are thoroughly dry before storing the flowers. Use a small container, so that the air gap is minimized.

Tincturing I do not tincture this herb; I add dried flowers to prescription infusions.

Grape Vine (*Vitis vinifera*) ❖ leaves

Hardy perennial vine ◆ full sun ◆ deep, well-drained soil ◆ spacing: 1.25 m / 4 ft

Growing Establish young plants against a wall or other support, and water in the first year if there is a dry spell. Once the vines are established, they should not need watering.

Harvesting Pick young, vibrant leaves, taking care to handle them only by their leaf stalk, as they are prone to bruising. Lay them out on trays straight away.

Passive drying Lay the leaves out on trays, and leave in a warm, airy place until dry.

Active drying Start the drying process at a temperature of 42°C / 108°F. After 12 hours rearrange the trays, and continue drying for periods of 2 hours, as needed. The leaves should be brittle when thoroughly dried. Store immediately, while still warm.

Tincturing I do not tincture Grape Vine leaves, I use them in infusions.

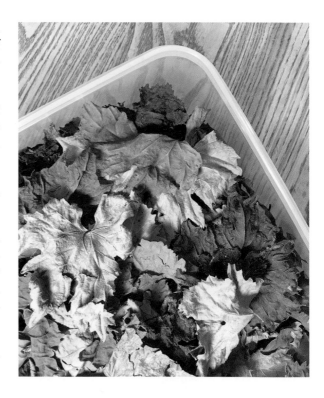

Nettle (*Urtica dioica*) ❖ seeds

Hardy perennial herb ⬥ **full sun to partial shade** ⬥ **moist, rich soil** ⬥ **spacing: 15–30 cm / 6–12 in**

Growing Most people will prefer to wild harvest from waste ground or field edges. The advantage of cultivating the crop is that it can be kept weed-free, making harvesting quick and efficient. I have cultivated Nettle in the past by planting root cuttings. Alternatively, transplant seedlings, or gather ripe seed and scatter in your chosen location in autumn.

Harvesting I first started harvesting Nettle seed years ago, after researching Roman ointments for a primitive archery event. Nettle flowers are held on little strings, and these gradually develop into green, disc-shaped seeds. Once they are plump and green, it is time to gather them. Nettle seed is quite time-consuming to harvest but well worth it, as it is such a wonderful medicine. Within the same patch of Nettles, the seeds ripen at different times. You will need to select the stems with the best seed development, and snip them off below the lowest bundle of seeds. Take the end of the stem in your left hand (if you are right-handed) and hold it over your basket, twisting it to allow each seed bundle to hang down freely below the stem. Using a pair of scissors in your

right hand, snip all the seed bundles off at the point where they are hanging freely below the stem. Rotate the stem again, so that more seed strings hang freely and can be snipped off into the basket. Keep rotating the stem until all the

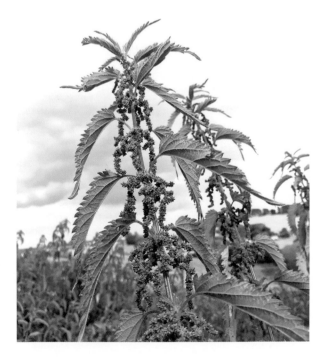

bundles are snipped off, and then start on the next one. This technique allows you to avoid snipping off mature leaves into your basket but is much quicker than snipping seed bundles off the plants directly. I prefer to do this work in the field, so that I can allow insects ample time to escape from the basket and I can return the stalks and leaves to the earth where they were growing. If you have a weather 'deadline' such as threatened rain, however, then you can do this work back at your processing area.

Passive drying   Once you have separated the seeds from the foliage, spread them out in a shallow layer on a tray. Leave them to dry in a warm, airy place, away from direct light.

Active drying   Spread the seed strings out on dehydrator trays. I usually leave an empty tray at the base of each stack in order to minimize the number of seeds that fall through the holes in the trays into the fan mechanism. Dry them for around 12 hours at 42°C / 108°F. In order to test whether they are dry, try to snap one of the seed-bearing stalks. It should snap cleanly. Gently rub the seeds in your fingers: they should not have any hint of moisture. Pack them away while they are still warm. Use a small container, so that there is not a large air gap that could act as a reservoir of moist air for rehydration of the seeds.

Tincturing   I use dried seeds and 45% alcohol.

Artichoke (*Cynara scolymus*)   ❖   leaves

Perennial herb ◆ full sun ◆ deep, well-drained soil ◆ spacing: 1.25–1.75 m / 4–6 ft

Growing   Sow seeds under cover in early spring, or divide large plants in autumn.

Harvesting   There is a particular moment when it is best to harvest Artichoke leaves. The ideal is when the leaves are large and mature, but not yet tattered and damaged by the early autumn storms. If you are growing your herbs in a community setting, you may have neigh-bouring gardeners who will happily spare you some Artichoke leaves once they have finished harvesting the flowers. Artichoke plants and the gardeners who grow them are generous with their leaves. Cut the leaves at the point where they join the main stem. Take them back to your processing area. Carefully cut along both sides of the fleshy mid-rib in order to remove it. It can be respectfully added to the compost later. Cut the leaves into smallish strips about 25 mm / 1 in wide.

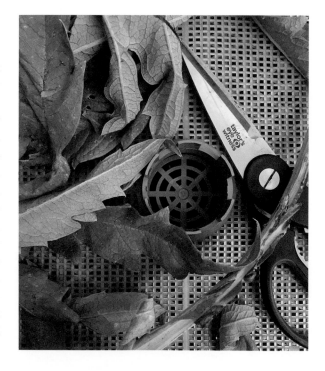

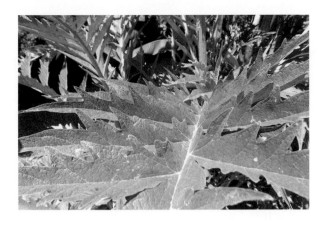

Passive drying   Lay the leaf strips out on trays, and leave them to dry in a warm, airy place, out of direct light.

Active drying   Lay the leaf strips out on dehydrator trays. Begin the drying process by setting the dryer to a temperature of 42°C / 108°F for 12 hours. After that time swap the trays around and continue for shorter periods, until the Artichoke leaf is thoroughly dry. Pack it away into storage while it is warm.

Tincturing   I use dried herb and 45% alcohol.

Hop (*Humulus lupulus*)   ❖   strobiles

Hardy perennial dioecious vine ⬧ full sun to partial shade ⬧ rich, fertile, moist soil ⬧ spacing: 1 m / 3 ft, against support

Growing   Sow seeds in summer or autumn or take cuttings in spring or early summer from a female plant. Plant in a location where you can provide support. Cut back mature plants in the autumn, and apply manure or compost.

Harvesting   If you are wild harvesting hops, you should already have identified your gathering areas and be watching for when the little clusters of strobiles start to form and ripen. I spent part of my childhood in Kent surrounded by hop gardens; where the hops are neatly trained up wires in a framework of poles. At harvest time the wires are released and the vines fall, allowing the hops to be gathered. One year I grew a hop plant over my shed at my allotment. I got a lovely crop of home-grown hops but lost my shed in the process, as the hop vine grew so vigorously! These days I prefer to wild harvest from particular locations where the hops grow along hedgerows at a height suitable for picking.

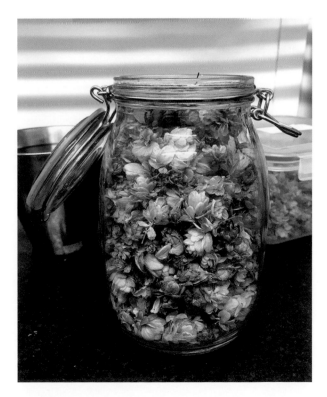

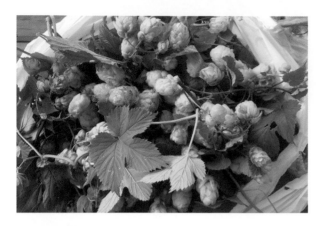

Harvesting Once the strobiles are turning pale green to amber, they are ready for picking. Snip the clusters off into your basket.

Passive drying Dry whole vines in a warm, dust-free place, or spread the strobiles onto trays, and leave them to dry in a warm, airy place.

Active drying Spread the strobiles out onto dehydrator trays, and dry them at a temperature of 42°C / 108°F for a period of 10 hours to start with. Further stints of 2 hours may be required, depending on the ambient humidity at the time of drying. Store them while they are still warm.

Tincturing I use dried strobiles and 60% alcohol.

Goldenrod (*Solidago canadensis* or *Solidago virgaurea*) ❖ aerial parts

Hardy perennial herb • full sun to full shade • well-drained, moderately fertile to poor soil • spacing: 3.5–5.5 m / 12–18 ft

Growing Sow seeds in spring or divide large plants in autumn.

Harvesting As soon as the flowers have opened, it is the time to harvest them, together with the youngest leaves, taking a length of around 60 cm / 24 in. Goldenrod flowers turn to fluffy seed heads later in the season, and for practical reasons these are best avoided in the dispensary. Keep an eye on the progress of the flowers, and do not leave it too late to take your harvest. I grow *Solidago canadensis* at my allotment, but I also have access to wild populations of *S. virgaurea* from which to wild harvest. Lay the flowering tops into your gathering basket in the same direction in order to avoid damaging

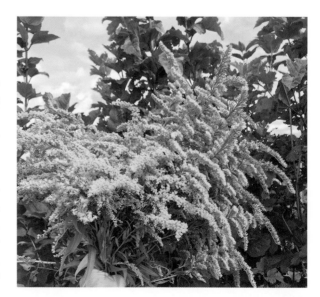

the flowers when you remove them for processing later.

Passive drying Hang small bunches upside down to dry in a warm, airy place, away from direct light, or spread the flowers and leaves on trays.

Active drying Once back at your processing place, carefully pull the leaves from the stems and snip each flower spike off. If you are working with *S. canadensis*, you may want to cross-cut the longest flower spikes to reduce their length in order to facilitate better drying. Spread the flowers and young leaves onto dehydrator trays, and start the process at a temperature of 42°C / 108°F for 12 hours before rearranging the trays and continuing the drying process for periods of 1–2 hours, as needed. Check that the flower stalks are brittle before storing.

Tincturing I use dried herb and 45% alcohol.

Couch Grass (*Agropyron repens*) ❖ rhizomes
Hardy perennial grass • full sun to partial shade • rich, well-drained soil

Growing Couch is very invasive, so I do not advise cultivating it intentionally in your herb garden. If you do wish to cultivate it, establish a small population from rhizome segments in a large tub of compost in spring. Keep it well watered, and at the end of the growing season you can tip it out onto a tarpaulin, to separate out the rhizomes. Beware of spreading the used compost onto your garden, as the tiniest fragment of Couch Grass will regrow into a vigorous colony. Either reuse the compost for your next crop of Couch, or add it to the compost heap and ensure that it reaches a high-enough temperature to deactivate any remaining plant material before spreading it onto your garden.

Harvesting If you already have a population of Couch as a weed, you can combine weeding with harvesting in the early spring, in summer, and in autumn. Gather up your Couch Grass, and place it in a tub, separate from the other weeds. Do not attempt to remove the rhizomes from the foliage at this stage. Rinse the Couch Grass a couple of times to remove soil, and pick out any extraneous material, such as twigs and dried leaves. Spread it out to air-dry on trays lined with absorbent kitchen paper. Turn the mass over a couple of times to allow each side to dry. Once it is surface-dry to the touch, go through it, removing the green foliage from the

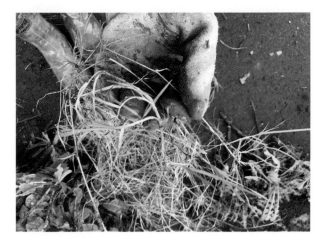

straw-coloured rhizomes. It is acceptable to have a low level of grass strands in your final harvest, but the majority of it should be rhizomes. The overall colour of the sorted material should be straw-coloured or brown.

Passive drying   Cut the rhizomes into sections around 10–13 cm / 4–5 in long and spread them out onto trays to dry.

Active drying   Cut the rhizomes into sections around 10–13 cm / 4–5 in long, and spread them out onto dehydrator trays. Start the drying process at a temperature of 42°C / 108°F, allowing 10 hours before changing the trays around and continuing for 1-hourly stints, if needed. Test for dryness by folding a rhizome in half and seeing whether it snaps cleanly. Pack away into storage while still warm.

Tincturing   I use dried rhizomes and 45% alcohol.

Sweetcorn or Maize (*Zea mays*) ❖ cornsilk

Half-hardy annual grass • full sun • well-drained fertile soil • spacing: 30–60 cm / 1–2 ft, in blocks

Growing   Sow seeds in pots indoors, and transplant into the growing position once the danger of frost is past. Maize is pollinated by the wind, so it is preferable to grow it in rectangular blocks rather than in simple rows. Once the plants are about 30 cm / 12 in high, earth them up a little, so that they form stronger roots.

Harvesting   Cornsilk is the green strands that enclose the developing seeds on the cob. The cobs ripen 3–4 weeks after flowering finishes. Ripe Sweetcorn has a tuft of brown cornsilk protruding from the top of each cob. The best time to harvest cornsilk is considered to be when the cobs are not yet ripe. This has always caused me a dilemma, since taking it at this stage means that you will sacrifice your home-grown crop of sweetcorn. At the scale I work with, I prefer to remove the cornsilk from ripe cobs and use that. I have always been very happy with its efficacy in practice, so will continue to harvest it at this time.

Passive drying   Spread out on trays, and leave to dry in a warm, airy place.

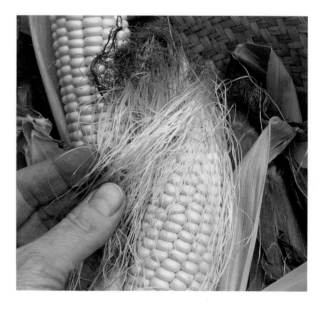

Active drying   Spread on dehydrator trays, and start with 6 hours at 42°C / 108°F. Continue until the strands are thoroughly dried. Store in a small storage container while still warm.

Tincturing   I use dried cornsilk and 45% alcohol.

Hyssop (*Hyssopus officinalis*)   ❖   flowers and tops

Hardy perennial ✦ full sun to partial shade ✦ sandy or loam, moderately dry soil ✦ spacing: 30 cm / 12 in

Growing Sow seeds in early spring, or take softwood cuttings from non-flowering stems in early summer. Once the new plants are established, plant them out in a sunny position in free-draining soil.

Harvesting Cut flowering stems, including leaves, while they are at their peak. Lay the stems carefully into the collecting basket to avoid bruising the flowers.

Passive drying If the stems are long enough, make small bunches and hang them upside down in a warm, airy place, out of direct light. Alternatively, cut the stems into sections 7.5–10 cm / 3–4 in long, and dry them on trays.

Active drying Cut the stems into sections that are 7.5–10 cm / 3–4 in in length, and lay them out onto dehydrator trays. Start the drying at a temperature of 38°C / 100°F for a period of 12 hours. Rearrange the trays, and continue drying for periods of 1–2 hours, for as long as needed.

Tincturing I use dried herb and 45% alcohol.

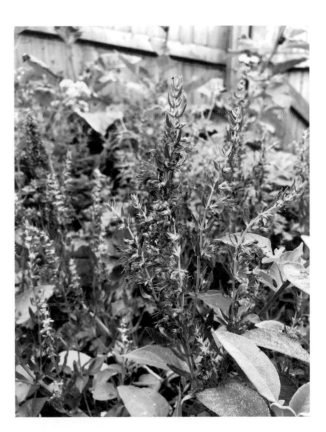

Fennel (*Foeniculum vulgare*)   ❖   seeds

Hardy biennial or perennial herb ✦ full sun ✦ well-drained soil ✦ spacing: 90 cm / 36 in

Growing Sow seeds *in situ* in late summer, or take cuttings in spring.

Harvesting Harvest seed heads in the second year. Cut the ripe seed heads, together with their stalks.

Passive drying Tie the seed heads in small bunches, and leave them hanging over a tray or large paper bag to catch the seeds as they fall.

Active drying Leave the seed heads whole, and spread them out on dehydrator trays. Leave an

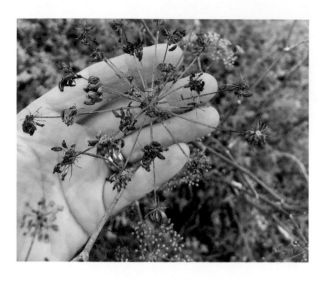

empty tray at the bottom of the stack to catch any stray seeds. Dry gently at 35°C / 96°F for 6–8 hours, and continue for short periods, as needed.

Tincturing   I use dried seeds and 45% alcohol.

Mallow (*Malva sylvestris*)   ❖   leaves and flowers

Hardy perennial herb • full sun to partial shade • well-drained soil • spacing: 1.2–1.5 m / 48–60 in

Growing   Collect ripe seeds and sow in your chosen location immediately.

Harvesting   Harvest when the plant is in full bloom. Cut young, healthy leaves, together with their leaf stalk. Cut individual flowers just below the calyx. Use a wide, flat basket to avoid crushing the flowers, and lay your crop out as soon as possible after cutting.

Passive drying   Lay the leaves and flowers out on trays, and dry in a warm, airy place, out of direct light.

Active drying   Lay the leaves and flowers out in a single layer onto dehydrator trays. Start the drying process at 42°C / 108°F for 12 hours, then continue for short periods, if needed. Check that the crop is fully dry by seeing if the leaf stalks and flower caly-ces are brittle. Store immediately while still warm.

Tincturing   I use dried herb and 25% alcohol.

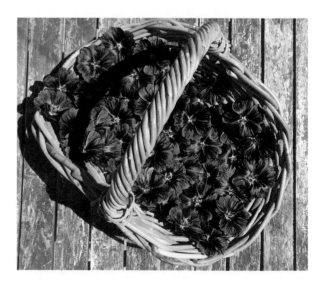

Kelp (*Laminaria digitata*) ❖ fronds

Brown algal seaweed • wild harvest from clean seawater

Harvesting Kelp can be gathered throughout spring and summer. It is included in the 'late summer' section due to the fact that in the United Kingdom this is when the sea temperatures are most pleasant for gathering, but you can harvest at any time, from April onwards. Wade or swim over seaweed beds and identify healthy, vibrant communities. Dive down and cut from the stipe or cut individual fronds. Place them into your gathering net or bag to keep them hydrated and safe while you continue gathering. Once you return to the shore, hang your net to drip until you are ready to return home. I tend to hang my newly harvested Kelp on the washing line for a day, in order to drip dry before I start the drying process.

Passive drying Leave your seaweed drying on a taut line in the shade. You may need to finish the drying process in an airing cupboard or in the presence of some active heat, such as a fan, if the ambient humidity is high.

Active drying Cut the fronds into sections approximately 7.5 cm / 3 in long. Spread them out onto dehydrator trays, and start the drying process at a temperature of 42°C / 108°F, for a period of 12 hours. Rearrange the trays, and continue drying for periods of 2 hours, until it is thoroughly dry. Store immediately in an airtight container.

Tincturing I use dried Kelp and 25% alcohol.

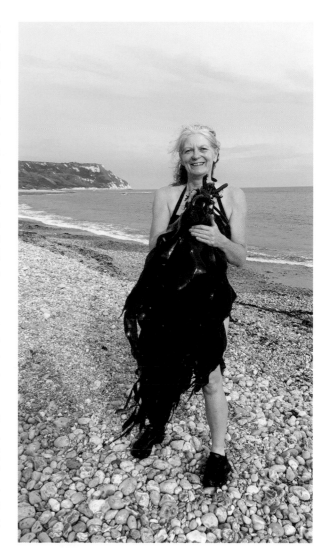

Autumn

Goji (*Lycium barbarum* / *Lycium chinense*) ❖ berries

Perennial shrub • full sun to partial shade • well-drained soil • spacing: 60–90 cm / 2–3 ft

Growing Goji berry is naturalized in the south of England, but it is easy to grow if you do not have access to a wild population. Cultivate from seeds inside a fresh berry, or take cuttings.

Harvesting Pick ripe berries carefully, taking care not to bruise them.

Passive drying Unless you live in a very dry, warm climate, I do not recommend passive drying of Goji berries. Use them added to food or make a fresh tincture.

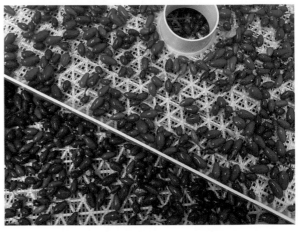

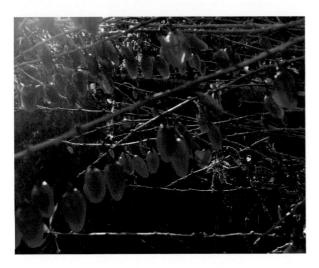

Active drying Lay the berries out in a single layer on dehydrator trays. Dry at a temperature of 43°C / 110°F for around 24–36 hours, depending on the ambient humidity and the efficiency of your dryer. The Goji berries will be dry and slightly sticky like raisins. Store in an airtight container immediately.

Tincturing I use dried berries and 25% alcohol.

Oregon Grape (*Mahonia aquifolium*)   ❖   roots

Hardy perennial shrub • full sun to dense shade • well-drained, moist soil • spacing: 1.5 m / 5 ft

Growing   Once the fruit is ripe, gather some seeds and sow them outdoors in pots. They require a period of exposure to cold in order to germinate, so by placing the pots out over winter, you will achieve this naturally. If you are in a very mild area, plant the seeds, and move the pots to a refrigerator for 3 weeks before moving outside. Germination can take up to 6 months. You can also propagate from semi-ripe wood cuttings in the autumn or divide established plants.

Harvesting   Oregon Grape root is harvested in autumn or in spring, by digging out a section of peripheral roots from an established shrub or tree. There is no need to uproot the plant. Provided that harvests are made from no more than one third of the total root area, the plant should recover well. If you are harvesting from a garden area with other plant species nearby, you will soon be able to identify which roots belong to the Mahonia. They are orange brown, and, on scraping away the outer bark, they are bright yellow. Younger roots are bright yellow, because they have not yet formed the brown outer bark. Thicker roots have higher levels of berberine, but young roots are still excellent medicine. Do not harvest roots from the same plant two years running. Wash the roots, and cut any thicker roots lengthways to make matchstick-shaped sections of equal thickness, leaving thinner roots whole. Air-dry them on trays lined with absorbent paper, away from direct light, for 12 hours.

Passive drying   Lay the roots out onto dry trays, and leave in a warm, airy place, away from direct light until thoroughly dried.

Active drying   Once the roots are dry to the touch, place them loosely on dehydrator trays, and start them off at 42°C / 108°F, allowing 12 hours before changing the trays around and continuing for additional 2-hour periods, if needed. Test for dryness by seeing if a root snaps cleanly. Pack away into storage while still warm.

Tincturing   I use dried roots and 45% alcohol.

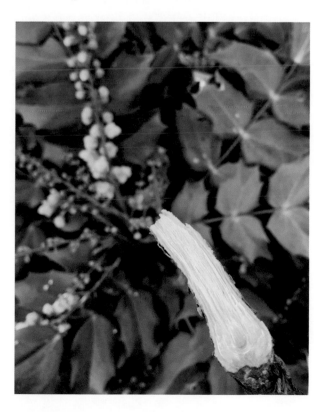

Burdock (*Arctium lappa*)   ❖   roots

Hardy biennial herb • full sun to partial shade • deep, rich, moist soil • spacing: 20 cm / 8 in

Growing Burdock is usually wild harvested, with permission from the landowner, but if you have the room to grow a crop every so often, you will find that you produce large, deep, easily harvested roots. Gather seeds and sow them *in situ* in the spring. Once established, thin to 12 cm / 5 in apart in rows 60 cm / 2 ft apart. Since you will be harvesting from first-year plants, you can grow them more densely than if you were growing them for seed.

Harvesting Burdock root should be harvested from first-year plants that have a rosette of large green leaves. Tall stems that bear flowers and seed heads do not develop until the second year. The roots of second-year plants are not suitable,

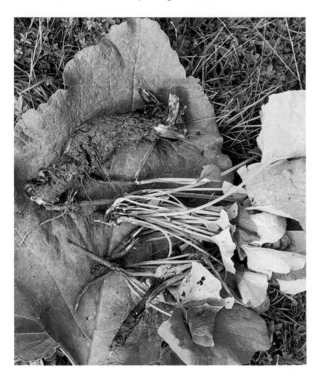

as they are woody and often much damaged by insect larvae. If you harvest in the autumn, the first-year plants will have the maximum level of inulin, and this can be helpful for certain therapeutic needs. If you prefer to maximize the bitterness of your harvest, dig them in the early spring. Burdock has a very deep tap root: you will need to be prepared to dig a large hole in order to harvest it. Work methodically to unearth as much as possible of the root in one piece. After you have removed the root, make sure that you replace the soil and the turf. One large root may be sufficient for the needs of a small practice, but since it is quite a common plant, you could consider harvesting two or three plants while you are at it. If they are dried carefully and stored well, they will keep well for at least two years, enabling you to save yourself the trouble the following year. Wash and scrub the roots, slicing them lengthways to form matchstick-shaped pieces of equal thickness.

Passive drying Air-dry them on trays lined with kitchen paper for a day, and then lay them out on their final drying trays. Leave them in a warm, airy place, out of direct light.

Active drying After 24 hours of air-drying on trays lined with kitchen paper, lay them out onto dehydrator trays. Dry at 43°C / 110°F for 12 hours to start with, swapping the trays around and continuing with additional 2–3-hour periods as needed. To test that they are dry, see if the root pieces snap cleanly. Store while still warm.

Tincturing I use dried roots and 25% alcohol.

Nettle (*Urtica dioica*) ❖ roots

Hardy perennial herb ✦ **full sun to partial shade** ✦ **moist, rich soil** ✦ **spacing: 15–30 cm / 6–12 in**

Growing Most people will prefer to wild harvest from waste ground or field edges. The advantage of cultivating the crop is that it can be kept weed-free, making harvesting quick and efficient. I have cultivated Nettle in the past by planting root cuttings. Alternatively, transplant seedlings or gather ripe seed and scatter in your chosen location in autumn.

Harvesting Officially, you can harvest Nettle roots at any time between autumn and early spring. This is handy, since it means that if you are weeding an area of your herb garden, you can reserve any Nettle roots that you remove. Digging the roots from an established Nettle patch is a tough job at any time of year. The roots run along the surface of the soil, forming impenetrable mats, but your challenge is made harder by the presence of the tall stinging foliage in high summer. You may prefer to concentrate your efforts in the autumn and early spring for this reason. Isolated plants that have established themselves among your herbs are generally easier to remove. Wash and scrub the roots, slicing them lengthways to form matchstick-shaped pieces of equal thickness. Air-dry them for a day away from direct sunlight.

Passive drying Lay the roots out onto dry trays, and leave in a warm, airy place, away from direct light. Turn the roots regularly.

Active drying Lay the roots out onto dehydrator trays. Dry at 43°C / 110°F for 12 hours to start with, swapping the trays around and increasing the drying time by periods of 2–3 hours, as needed. To test that they are dry, see if the root pieces snap cleanly. Store while still warm.

Tincturing I use dried roots and 45% alcohol.

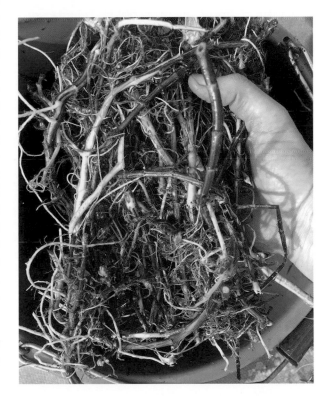

Dock (*Rumex crispus* and *Rumex obtusifolia*) ❖ roots

Hardy perennial herb ◆ full sun to partial shade ◆ most soils ◆ spacing:
12–45 cm / 5–18 in

Growing Most people will be able to source Dock roots through weeding gardens or allotments, or foraging on waste ground. If you do need to grow it, gather ripe seed, and scatter it in your chosen location in autumn, or take root cuttings in spring.

Harvesting Dock is usually harvested in late summer or autumn. It has a long tap root, and you need to dig quite a deep hole to get the roots out. Choose healthy-looking plants, and work steadily, aiming to minimize breakage of the roots. Be careful to replace the soil and the turf, so as not to leave a depression, which could be a hazard for horses and other grazing animals. The more yellow the roots, the more potent the medicine will be. Herbalist Henriette Kress observes that Dock roots growing in drier soils tend to be much more yellow than those growing on wet pastures. Wash and scrub the roots, then slice them lengthways to form matchstick-shaped pieces of equal thickness.

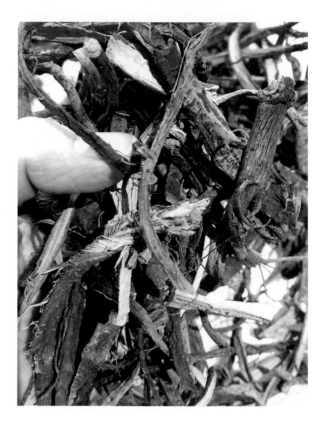

Passive drying Air-dry them on a tray lined

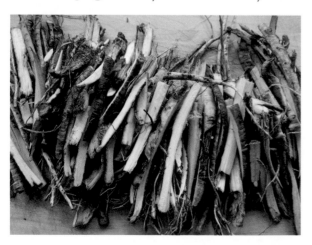

with absorbent paper after washing, then transfer to a dry tray. Leave in a warm, airy place to dry.

Active drying Air-dry them on a tray lined with absorbent paper for 24 hours after washing. Transfer to dehydrator trays, and dry at 43°C / 110°F for 12 hours to start with, swapping the trays around and increasing the drying time by periods of 2–3 hours, as needed. To test that they are dry, see if the root pieces snap cleanly. Store while still warm.

Tincturing I use dried roots and 45% alcohol.

Horse Chestnut (*Aesculus hippocastanum*) ❖ seeds

Hardy tree ◆ full sun to partial shade ◆ well-drained, moderately fertile soil ◆ spacing: 12 m / 40 ft

Growing Horse Chestnut seeds are otherwise known as 'conkers' after the children's game in which the seeds are used to bash competitor's seeds until one breaks. Trees can be grown from conkers in autumn, but it will be many years before your tree produces flowers and seeds.

Harvesting Locate trees that shed ripe conkers onto clean ground, and gather in autumn. Savvy children know that drying their conkers first makes them harder, and this is why it is better to break up the conkers before drying them. Take them out of their green spiky outer shells and use a large pestle and mortar or a mallet to break them up into pieces, preferably of a similar size. Only process a quantity that you can start to dry immediately after breaking up. Leave the others whole until you have drying capacity available.

Passive drying Spread the pieces out onto trays, and leave in a warm, airy place. Inspect regularly for signs of mould, and if this becomes an issue, remove affected pieces and move to a warmer place with better air movement, or place a fan by them. Alternatively, dry them whole and break them up later, using a mallet.

Active drying Spread the pieces on dehydrator trays, and start them off drying at 43°C / 110°F. Only place one tray in each dehydrator, otherwise drying is too slow. Even with only one tray per dehydrator, the drying process may take 36 hours. Set the dehydrator to run for 12-hour stints and reassess at the end of each one. Properly dried Horse Chestnut seeds will remain in good condition for several years.

Tincturing I use dried seeds and 45% alcohol.

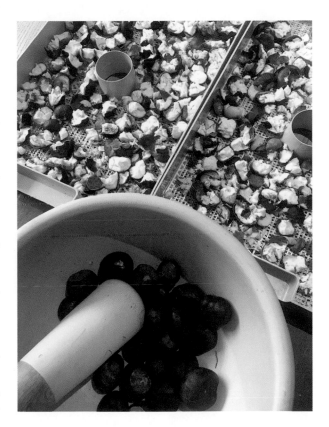

Horseradish (*Armoracia rusticana*)   ❖   roots

Hardy perennial herb ✦ full sun to partial shade ✦ any soil ✦ spacing: 20–30 cm /
8–12 in

Growing Establish new plants from root cuttings (known as thongs) in autumn. This plant requires a period of winter dormancy in order to be grown successfully. It can be grown as an annual in areas that do not experience a cold winter. Horseradish roots are very deep and persistent. You need to keep a close eye on them in the herb garden, so that you can keep them from spreading too much. For this reason, if you are cultivating your own Horseradish you will know exactly where it is growing in your herb garden. If you are wild harvesting your Horseradish, it is recommended that you have likely sources marked on your mental foraging map, so you know where to look. In late autumn or early spring there can be little sign of where the plants are growing, but if you look carefully among the other vegetation, you will see tiny greenish-purplish spiky shoots.

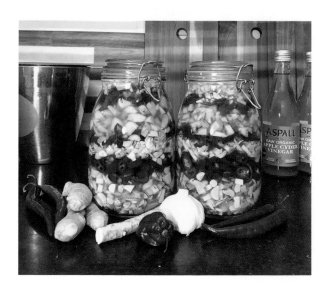

Harvesting Dig carefully, and aim to remove all of the root from each plant, including the small sucker roots. Remove the tops from the roots, and brush the soil off them before taking them back to your processing area. The autumn is an ideal time to produce a winter tonic, which is known as 'Fire Cider'. For this you can use fresh Horseradish roots after they have been washed and air-dried. If you have harvested more than you need for tincture making or Fire Cider making, you can dry the remaining roots. Drying Horseradish root does mean that you will lose some of the aromatic compounds, so it is best to make preparations using fresh root. However, carefully dried root can still be quite potent, and it can be useful to have it available in the dispensary, for example to add to capsule blends.

Passive drying Cut the roots into matchstick-shaped pieces and leave them to dry on a tray in a warm, airy place.

Active drying Cut the roots into matchstick-shaped pieces and dry them for 3 hours at 43°C / 110°F; then reduce the heat to 38°C / 100°F for further drying for 4–5-hour periods, for as long as necessary. You may need to increase this temperature if ambient humidity is high. To test that they are dry, see if the root pieces snap cleanly. Store while still warm.

Tincturing I use fresh root that has been air-dried for 24 hours and 60% alcohol; out of season, I use dried root and 45% alcohol.

Ashwagandha (*Withania somnifera*)   ❖   roots

Tender perennial (grown as an annual outdoors in the United Kingdom) • full sun • deep, moist, fertile soil • spacing: 22–30 cm / 9–12 in

Growing   Ashwagandha is a tender, frost-sensitive plant, but in the United Kingdom and in other temperate regions it can be grown as an annual or as a protected crop, much as you would cultivate tomatoes. If you are growing it as an annual, you will need to promote the strongest possible root growth in the one growing season that is available to you. Start the seedlings off indoors in early February under a grow light, then plant them out in a sunny position in a deep, fertile, moisture-retentive soil. Using cloches or other temporary protection will help to extend the growing season a little by allowing them to be planted out slightly earlier once the soil has warmed up in spring. Irrigate the plants as necessary to avoid any check to growth. In the autumn allow the plants to set seed, and gather some ripe seeds to ensure a continued supply in your herb garden.

Harvesting   Wait until the first frost is forecast before harvesting the roots, since you want to get the maximum possible growing season. Pull the plants out and cut the foliage from the roots. The foliage is a strong emetic and cannot be used as an internal medicine, although there are some traditional uses as a topical treatment. Wash the roots and cut the largest ones into even-sized lengths. Cut thicker roots lengthways to make even thicknesses of the pieces that you are drying. Save even the tiniest roots: they are valuable medicine.

Passive drying   Allow the roots to air-dry for 24 hours on a tray covered with absorbent kitchen paper, and then transfer them to a dry tray, and

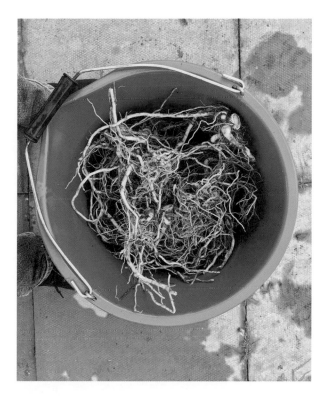

leave to dry in a warm, airy place, away from direct light.

Active drying   Allow the roots to air-dry for 24 hours on a tray lined with absorbent kitchen paper, and then transfer them to dehydrator trays, and start them off at a temperature of 43°C / 110°F. After 12 hours swap the trays around and continue at 42°C / 108°F for additional 2-hour periods, until the largest pieces snap cleanly and feel thoroughly dry. Store them immediately while they are still warm.

Tincturing   I use dried root and 45% alcohol.

Elecampane (*Inula helenium*) ❖ roots

Hardy perennial herb ◆ **full sun to partial shade** ◆ **moist, rich soil** ◆ **spacing: 1 m / 40 in**

Growing Elecampane self-seeds vigorously, but I find it best to establish new plants from root cuttings in autumn at the time of harvest.

Harvesting Elecampane develops a very large root system. Depending on the size of your practice, you may only need to harvest one or two plants in order to have sufficient root for an entire year. It is easiest to remove the aerial parts before starting to dig. This is not the sort of plant that you can simply pull out of the ground. Use a fork and dig around the outside of the chosen plant, gently excavating the roots as they become exposed. Do your best to avoid damaging the roots. Once the surface root system has been loosened, you may need to use a narrow spade to excavate the deeper roots. Gradually lever the plant out of the ground. It can be helpful to enlist the help of a friend who can work at the same time on the opposite

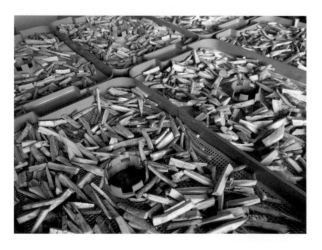

side of the plant. If the amount that has been unearthed is too great for your needs, you can divide the crown and replant some of the sections, as long as they have a healthy bud on the top. Brush off the soil as much as possible *in situ*, and then rinse the roots a couple of times before taking them back to your processing area in a tub. Cut away and discard any damaged roots and roots that are impossible to clean, scrubbing the remaining ones until they are clean. Leave them to air-dry whole for 12–24 hours on a tray lined with absorbent kitchen paper, then cut them into matchstick-shaped pieces.

Passive drying Place the root pieces onto trays, and leave them to dry in a warm, airy place, away from direct light.

Active drying Place the root pieces onto dehydrator trays. Elecampane has high levels of aromatic constituents, and therefore the drying and processing technique needs to take this into account to minimize the loss of these. Start the roots off for 3 hours at 43°C / 110°F, then reduce the heat to 38°C / 100°F for a further 12 hours. You may need to increase this temperature if ambient humidity is high. To test that they are dry see if the root pieces snap cleanly. Store while still warm. They should still smell significantly of the characteristic aroma of Elecampane.

Tincturing I use dried roots and 45% alcohol.

Jerusalem Artichoke (*Helianthus tuberosum*)   ❖   tubers

Hardy perennial herb ◆ **full sun** ◆ **rich, fertile, well-drained soil** ◆ **spacing: 1–1.25 m / 3–4 ft**

Growing Jerusalem Artichoke is very easy to grow and can be a useful crop to break in a newly cultivated area. Establish by planting tubers. They are not commonly used in herbal medicine these days, but I was taught that this herb is a specific for salivary gland stones. When I first started growing my own herbs, I enthusiastically planted a large amount of Jerusalem Artichoke, but unless you are planning to eat them as a vegetable, you will probably only need one or two plants to provide you with all the medicine that you will need for each year.

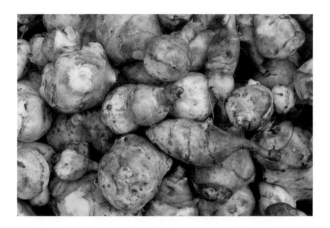

Harvesting Jerusalem Artichoke tubers are easy to unearth in cultivated soil and can simply be pulled out of the ground by the main stem. Any tubers left in the soil can be easily lifted with a fork and added to the collecting tub. Wash and scrub the tubers, and then slice them evenly. Jerusalem Artichokes have a reputation for causing intestinal gas, but this issue is much reduced when the tubers remain uncooked. The dehydrated slices can be eaten raw, tinctured, or ground and made into capsules.

Passive drying Lay the slices out on a tray in a single layer. Leave in a warm, airy place to dry, turning the slices every 2–3 days.

Active drying Lay the slices out onto dehydrator trays to air-dry for 24 hours before starting the active drying process. Dry for 12 hours at 42°C / 108°F and then continue for additional 2-hour periods, for as long as needed.

Tincturing I use dried tubers and 45% alcohol.

Marshmallow (*Althaea officinalis*)   ❖   roots

Perennial herb ◆ **full sun** ◆ **moist, rich soil** ◆ **spacing: 90 cm / 36 in**

Growing Divide roots and replant in spring or autumn. This is a good candidate for growing in a moist part of the herb garden.

Harvesting I am always torn when it comes to harvesting Marshmallow root. I have such great need for the foliage each year that I usu-

ally leave the roots in the ground. Ideally, I would dedicate a much larger area to growing Marshmallow plants, but at the moment I do not have the luxury of sufficient growing space. The way that I get around this is to harvest one or two plants every 2–3 years. I can use these home-grown roots to produce a good batch of

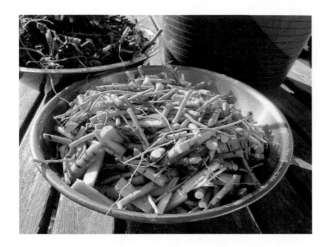

tincture, and I buy in additional Marshmallow root to use as a powder in capsules, since I require a very large volume for this. Use a fork to unearth the chosen plant or plants, working around each plant to free up the root system without damaging it. Use a narrow spade to unearth the deeper roots. If there is any foliage remaining on the plant, cut it off and place it safely to one side to avoid contaminating it with soil. Marshmallow leaves are precious. Brush off as much soil as possible, and then rinse the roots a couple of times before taking them back to your processing area for thorough washing. Do not leave them soaking in the water for too long, as you will lose mucilage. Scrub them and cut them into matchstick-shaped pieces of even thickness.

Passive drying   Air-dry them for about 24 hours on a tray lined with absorbent paper, and then lay them out onto trays. Leave to dry in a warm, airy place, out of direct light.

Active drying   Air-dry them for about 24 hours, and then dry them at 43°C / 110°F for 12 hours. After this time, swap the trays around, and continue drying for further 2-hour periods, for as long as necessary. Make sure that the pieces snap cleanly and are thoroughly dry before storage. Put the roots into storage while they are still warm.

Tincturing   I use dried roots and 25% alcohol.

Ginkgo (*Ginkgo biloba*)   ❖   leaves

Hardy deciduous tree ◆ full sun to partial shade ◆ well-drained soil ◆ spacing: 6 m / 20 ft

Growing   Ginkgo can be grown from seed or cuttings, or young plants can be purchased for planting. The mature tree reaches a height of up to 40 m / 130 ft, so if you do not have room for one in your garden, you can forage leaves from those that do, or from trees in public green spaces.

Harvesting   The leaves should be gathered when they are golden in autumn. If your tree is in a clean spot, you may be able to gather the

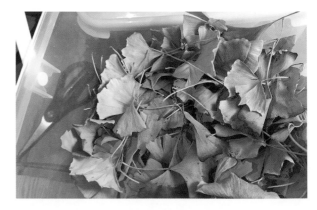

leaves from the ground, but if you have doubts, pick clean leaves from the lower branches.

Passive drying Lay the leaves out on trays in an airy place, away from direct light. The leaves are resilient to gentle handling, so you can turn them regularly throughout the drying process.

Active drying Lay the leaves out on dehydrator trays, and start the drying process at a temperature of 42°C / 108°F for a period of 12 hours. Increase drying time in short bursts, if needed. Make sure that both the leaves and the leaf stalks are thoroughly brittle before storage.

Tincturing   I use dried leaves and 45% alcohol.

Valerian (*Valeriana officinalis*)   ❖   roots

Hardy perennial ✦ full sun to partial shade ✦ moist soil ✦ spacing: 45 cm / 18 in

Growing Sow seed in spring, or divide large plants in autumn. Valerian self-seeds readily, so you can also pot up and relocate seedlings as you find them. Choose a moist area of the herb garden.

Harvesting Dig up second- or third-year plants. Trim the aerial parts from the mass of fragrant fibrous roots, and put them into a bucket or tub for washing. Do 2–3 rinses on site, returning the water to the garden if possible. Bring them back to your processing area in order to do a final, very thorough clean. Spread the roots out onto trays lined with absorbent kitchen paper to air-dry for 24 hours.

Passive drying Spread the roots out onto trays, cutting the longest ones, if necessary, into pieces approximately 7.5–10 cm / 3–4 in long. Leave in a warm, airy place, away from direct light, in order to dry.

Active drying Spread the roots out onto dehydrator trays, and begin the drying process at a temperature of 35°C / 96°F for 12 hours, increasing the temperature to 42°C / 108°F if the ambient humidity is high. The dried root should snap cleanly and smell strongly of the

characteristic Valerian aroma. Store immediately, while still warm.

Tincturing   I use dried roots and 45% alcohol.

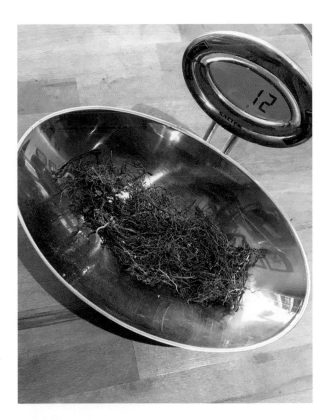

Elder (*Sambucus nigra*)   ❖   berries

Hardy perennial shrub • full sun to shade • moderately fertile, moist, well-drained soil • spacing: 1.8–4 m / 6–13 ft

Growing   It is usually possible to gather all that you need of this abundant wild medicinal, but it can be grown in the garden if gathering is difficult in your location. Grow from seed, or buy in a young plant.

Harvesting   Pick clusters of berries and when back at your processing place, remove them from the stems using a fork. I think that Elderberries are best used fresh to make syrup, as they take some time to dry.

Passive drying   This is not recommended unless you live in a very dry and warm climate.

Active drying   It may take some time for the berries to be properly dry. Start with a temperature of 43°C / 110°F and change the trays around after 12 hours. Continue drying for further 12-hour periods, for as long as needed: until the fruit is like hard raisins.

Tincturing   I do not make tincture of Elderberries.

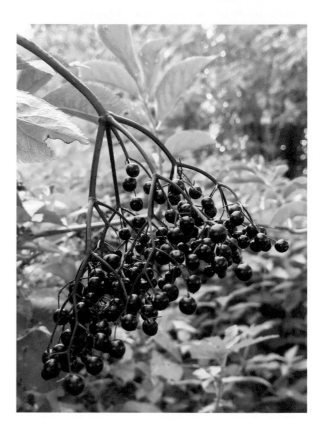

Hawthorn (*Crataegus monogyna*)   ❖   berries

Hardy perennial shrub or small tree • full sun to partial shade • any well-drained soil • spacing: 30 cm / 12 in for hedging, and up to 10 m / 30 ft for trees

Growing   Hawthorn grows abundantly in waste ground, in hedges, and on woodland edges. It can be grown as a hedge or shelter belt for the herb garden.

Harvesting   In order to avoid damaging the branches, support them with one hand while you pick the berries off with the other. Hawthorn berries are quite resilient if you are picking them before they have been exposed to frost.

Passive drying   Spread the fruit out on trays,

and leave to dry in a warm, airy place, away from direct light.

Active drying   Lay the fruit out on dehydrator trays, and start the drying process at a temperature of 43°C / 110°F for at least 12 hours; then change the trays around and continue for periods of 3–4 hours, as needed. When they are thoroughly dry, they should be dark red and very hard. Store immediately, while still warm.

Tincturing   I use dried berries and 45% alcohol.

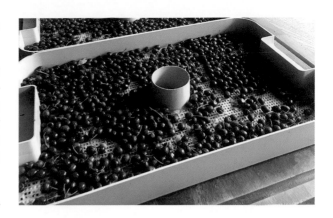

Phytolacca (*Phytolacca americana* or *Phytolacca polyandra*) ❖ roots

Hardy perennial herb ◆ **full sun to partial shade** ◆ **sheltered site with moist, rich soil** ◆ **spacing: 1.25–1.75 m / 4–6 ft**

Growing   This is a tall plant: it can reach 1.5 m / 5 ft in height. Choose a sheltered spot where it has room to spread. It dies down each winter, but avoid the temptation to tidy up the dead stems. The stems are hollow, and if you cut them in the autumn, they will hold water over winter, causing the crown to rot. It can be grown from seed in autumn, but it is easiest to take root divisions at the time of harvest.

Harvesting   Dig carefully around the chosen plant in order to free the root system. Remove the roots whole, if possible. Brush off the soil, and trim off the aerial parts. Wash the roots a couple of times *in situ*, so that you can return the earthy water to your garden. Once back at your processing place, wash them thoroughly, removing any damaged pieces and scrubbing them clean. Cut the larger roots lengthways, into even thicknesses. Leave small roots whole. Spread the

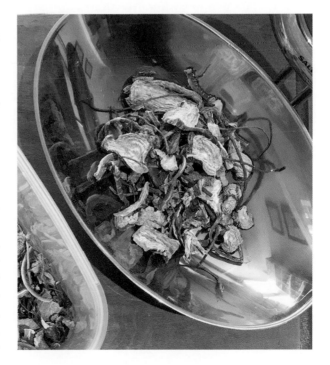

roots out onto trays lined with absorbent paper to air-dry for 24 hours before starting the drying process. This is a potentially toxic plant, so wash your hands thoroughly after handling freshly cut roots, or wear gloves.

Passive drying Spread the roots out evenly onto trays, and leave in a warm, airy place, away from direct light.

Active drying Spread the roots onto dehydrator trays. Dry at 43°C / 110°F for 12 hours before rearranging the trays and continuing for further periods of 3–4 hours, as needed. The root pieces should snap cleanly and feel dry before storage.

Tincturing I use dried roots and 45% alcohol.

Echinacea (*Echinacea purpurea, Echinacea angustifolia, Echinacea pallida*) ❖ roots

Hardy perennial herb ◆ full sun ◆ fertile, free-draining soil ◆ spacing: 30–45 cm / 12–18 in

Growing Divide plants and replant sections of root in autumn. This can be done at the time of harvest. The young spring growth of Echinacea is a great delicacy to slugs and snails, so be very vigilant or take protective measures, especially when plants are not fully established.

Harvesting Dig the roots of third- or fourth-year plants in autumn. Remove as much soil as possible on site, and do one or two rinses, so that the water can be returned to the herb garden. Once back at your processing place, wash the roots thoroughly, and slice the thicker roots lengthways so that drying times will be even throughout the crop. Leave the roots on trays lined with absorbent paper for 24 hours to air-dry before starting the drying process. I often take a harvest of flowers in the summer to dry and use in infusions.

Passive drying Transfer the roots to a dry tray and leave in a warm, airy place, away from direct

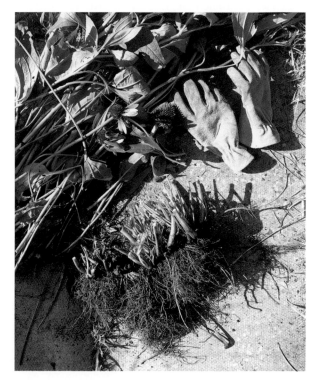

light. Turn the roots regularly to ensure even drying.

Active drying Spread the roots onto dehydrator trays, and start the drying process at a temperature of 43°C / 110°F for a period of 12 hours. After this time, rearrange the trays, and continue drying for further periods of 2 hours, as needed. Ensure that the roots snap cleanly before storage.

Tincturing I use dried roots and 45% alcohol.

Culver's Root (*Veronicastrum virginicum*) ❖ roots

Hardy perennial herb ◆ full sun ◆ fertile, moist soil ◆ spacing: 1–1.5 m / 3–5 ft

Growing Culver's Root is best propagated by dividing established plants or replanting root cuttings in the autumn, at the same time as your harvest. The plant needs plenty of moisture and does well on heavier soils.

Harvesting Choose well-established plants 3–4 years old. Dig around them, to unearth the whole plant. The central, dense crown is unsuitable for medicine making as it is difficult to clean, but the straight side roots can be trimmed away. Replant the remaining central crown. Clean the harvested roots on site, before taking them back to your processing place for a final wash. Once they are clean, split the roots lengthways to form pieces of an even thickness. Lay them out on a tray lined with absorbent paper to air-dry for 24 hours.

Passive drying Move the roots to a dry tray, in a warm, airy place, away from direct light. Turn the roots regularly to ensure even drying.

Active drying Spread the roots out onto dehydrator trays. Start the drying process at a temperature of 43°C / 110°F for a period of 12 hours. Rearrange the trays, and continue drying for additional 2-hour time periods, for as long as needed. Store when thoroughly dry, indicated by the roots snapping cleanly.

Tincturing I use dried roots and 45% alcohol.

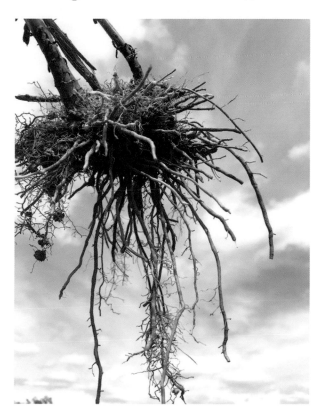

Golden Seal (*Hydrastis canadensis*) ❖ roots

Hardy perennial herb ◆ partial shade ◆ rich, free-draining moist soil with a thick hardwood leaf mulch ◆ spacing: 15–30 cm / 6–12 in

Growing Golden Seal is not native to the United Kingdom. Its natural range is south-eastern Canada and the eastern United States, growing in temperate hardwood forests with a slightly acidic soil and plenty of precipitation, which drains away readily after rain. Sloping sites are helpful in that they encourage better drainage, but they are not essential. Golden Seal requires dappled shade at a level of around 70% and a significant cold period of 3–4 months in order for it to thrive. If you live in a temperate climate and have a suitable shaded location, it is well worth trying to grow it, since it is so valuable and endangered. If you do not have natural shade, you can create it using shade cloths or companion planting. This plant can be grown from seed, but it is probably easiest to buy in a mother plant and increase your colony from root cuttings. Slugs absolutely love

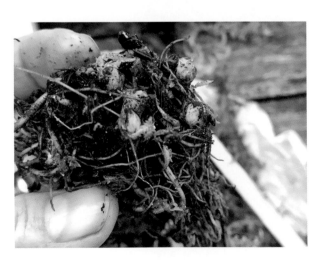

Golden Seal – something that I still cannot get my head around since it is so intensely bitter to our human palate. It can be difficult to establish shady, undisturbed growing conditions with a thick mulch of hardwood leaf mould without creating a slug paradise. Constant vigilance is essential. I have found that container-grown plants survive best in my current location, but naturalized populations would be ideal for the best yield of roots.

Harvesting Plants 3–4 years old can be dug up to harvest. Pot up several root cuttings from each plant immediately, and nurture them until they are ready to be replanted *in situ*. Gently wash the harvested roots, saving even the tiniest ones. This medicine is like gold.

Passive drying Lay the roots out on trays, and dry in a warm, airy place. Inspect frequently for signs of mould, and if drying is not efficient enough, move the trays near a source of dry heat, so that they dry properly without deteriorating.

Active drying Allow the roots to air-dry for a period of 24 hours on a tray lined with absorbent paper. Lay the roots out on dehydrator trays, and begin the drying process at a temperature of 42°C / 108°F for a period of 12 hours. Continue drying for short time periods, for as long as needed. Store the roots whole while still warm, in an airtight container.

Tincturing I use dried root and 60% alcohol.

Soapwort (*Saponaria officinalis*) ❖ roots

Hardy perennial herb ⋆ **full sun** ⋆ **moderately fertile to poor, well-drained soil** ⋆ **spacing: 60–90 cm / 24–36 in**

Growing Soapwort is best propagated using root cuttings. It spreads vigorously, especially in fertile soil, and can easily become invasive. Do not plant it near ponds, as its root secretions can adversely affect water quality.

Harvesting If you are anything like me, you grow more Soapwort than you need because it looks so heavenly when it is in full flower. Each autumn the harvest of roots can be combined with an operation to keep it from taking over more than its allotted space in the herb garden. The roots are easily unearthed, but be aware that the slightest root fragment will quickly form a new plant, so aim to be thorough in your removal process. Rinse the roots and transport them back to your processing area for washing. Ensure that you do not leave the roots in the water any longer than is absolutely necessary, as you will be leaching out the valuable saponins. Cut away and discard any damaged or discoloured sections of root. Leave to air-dry on a tray lined with absorbent paper for 24 hours before you start the drying process.

Passive drying Spread the roots out onto trays, and leave in a warm, airy place, out of direct light.

Active drying Spread the roots on dehydrator

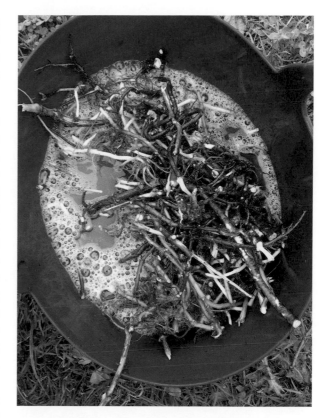

trays, and start the drying process at a temperature of 43°C / 110°F for a period of 12 hours before moving the trays around and continuing as necessary.

Tincturing I use dried roots and 25% alcohol.

Comfrey (*Symphytum officinale*)   ❖   roots

Hardy perennial herb • **full sun to partial shade** • **moist, fertile soil** • **spacing: 1–1.25 m / 3–4 ft**

Growing   Can be grown from seeds planted in spring, or divide large plants and take root cuttings. Cut back the dead leaves in the autumn or winter.

Harvesting   Excavate around the plant with a border fork, and loosen individual large roots with a trowel, if needed. The idea is to keep the roots as intact as possible, so that if you are lifting a plant you remove all of it. Root cuttings can be replanted after the plant has been lifted. Brush off surplus soil *in situ*, and hose the plants or rinse in a tub a few times, returning the dirty water to your growing site. Once the roots are reasonably clean, you can take them back to your processing area in order to give them a final scrub. Lay the whole roots out on a tray lined with absorbent paper for 24 hours in order to surface-dry, before cutting them lengthways to form sections of an even thickness. These should dry at the same rate.

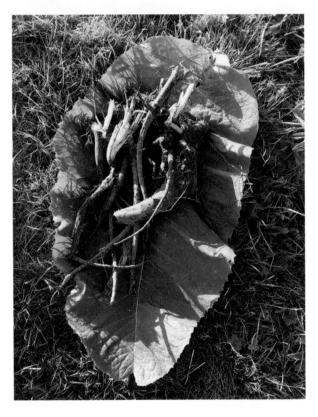

Passive drying   Lay the root segments out on trays, and leave them in a warm, airy place, away from direct light. Turn the roots regularly. If possible, finish the drying process in an airing cupboard, or with the addition of a warm fan, for the last 24 hours.

Active drying   Lay the root segments on dehydrator trays. Start the drying at 43°C / 110°F for at least 12 hours. It may take up to 36 hours for roots to be fully dry, depending on their moisture content and the size of the load in the dehydrator.

Tincturing   I do not tincture Comfrey root but if I were to I would use dried root and 25% alcohol.

Ginger (*Zingiber officinale*) ❖ roots

Tender herbaceous perennial (which grows annual pseudostems) • **partial sun** • **free-draining, fertile soil** • **spacing: 30–60 cm / 12–24 in, or individual containers**

Growing In the United Kingdom, this plant can be grown indoors as a house plant, or in a heated greenhouse. Establish your plants from root cuttings taken from organic Ginger rhizomes. Cut the rhizomes into sections containing 2–3 buds, and plant them 5–10 cm / 2–4 in deep, with the buds uppermost. If you are cultivating your Ginger in a container, use a good-quality, free-draining potting medium. Ginger requires high temperatures (21–25 °C / 71–77°F) in order to break dormancy and start to grow. Once shoots develop, keep the soil watered, but not too wet, as this can cause the rhizomes to rot. Place the pot in a warm, partially shaded spot. Mulch the surface of the soil during colder weather to protect it. In colder weather and lower light levels, the foliage turns yellow and dies back. At this point gradually reduce watering and let the soil dry out, until the following growth season, when the rhizomes will re-sprout. Once the plants have had 3–4 growing seasons, they will be ready to harvest.

Harvesting Take a harvest when repotting your Ginger plants. You can cut sections of larger roots and replant the rest straight away to continue your colony. Clean the harvested roots and slice them into thin rounds. There is no need to peel them.

Passive drying Lay the slices out onto trays, and leave them to dry in a warm, airy place, away from direct light.

Active drying Lay the slices out onto dehydrator trays. Start the drying process at a temperature of 42°C / 108°F for a period of 12 hours initially. It may take 15–24 hours of drying for the roots to be perfectly dry. They should be brittle and have a strong, fiery aroma.

Tincturing I use fresh root and 90% alcohol.

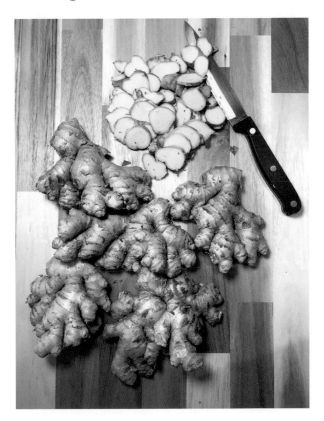

Karela (*Momordica charantia*)   ❖   fruit

Tender perennial vine • full sun • fertile, moist, free-draining soil • spacing:
1–1.25 m / 3–4 ft

Growing Karela or Bitter Gourd can be grown in the United Kingdom as an annual under cover, in the way we cultivate many tomatoes. Start your plants from seed in early spring under warmth in order to maximize the growing season. Plant the seeds out under cover, and provide them with support. The vines will reach 1.75–2.5 m / 6–8 ft if well watered. In ideal growth conditions the vines flower 40–50 days after planting. To increase the fruit yield, pinch out side-shoots, similar to the method used when growing vine tomatoes. If you are unable to grow your own Karela, you can purchase fruit from continental grocery stores.

Harvesting The gourds are harvested while unripe and green. The seeds inside the green cucumber-like fruit are not ripe. If you wish to

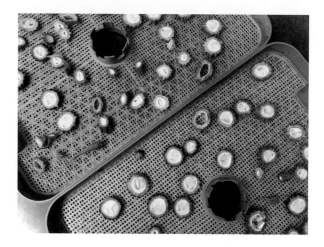

save your own seed, allow some of the fruit to reach maturity, at which stage they burst open and take on the appearance of the roof of a pagoda.

Passive drying It is not recommended that you dry Karela fruit passively, as they are extremely prone to going mouldy.

Active drying Slice the gourds into thin even-thickness rounds and lay them out onto dehydrator trays in a single layer, with space between them. Start the drying process at a temperature of 42°C / 108°F for a period of 12 hours. Continue for further short time periods, if needed. The dried fruit slices should be brittle.

Tincturing I do not tincture Karela. I use the dried fruit in capsules.

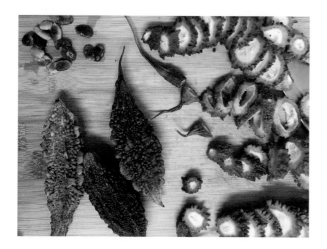

Solomon's Seal (*Polygonatum officinale*)   ❖   roots

Hardy perennial herb • partial shade • fertile, moist, well-drained soil • spacing: 30 cm / 12 in

Growing   Sow fresh seeds in autumn, or divide established plants in spring or autumn. This can be combined with harvesting. The plants may need irrigation during dry spells, as they do not like to dry out. Keep them well mulched with compost or hardwood leaves.

Harvesting   Dig the roots in autumn, and replant root cuttings with healthy buds to maintain your colony. Wash the roots; split thick ones lengthways so that they are all of an even thickness. Lay them out to air-dry on a tray lined with absorbent paper for 24 hours.

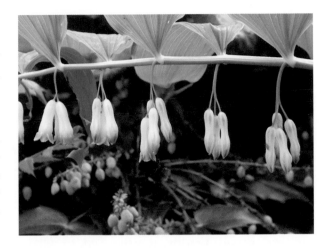

Passive drying   Lay the roots out on trays in a warm, airy place, out of direct light. If possible, finish the drying process in an airing cupboard for 24 hours.

Active drying   Lay the roots out onto dehydrator trays. Dry at a temperature of 42°C / 108°F for a period of 12 hours before rearranging the trays and continuing as needed. The roots should snap cleanly when they are thoroughly dry. Store immediately.

Tincturing   I use dried roots and 25% alcohol.

Liquorice (*Glycyrrhiza glabra*) ❖ roots

Hardy perennial herb ⬩ **full sun to partial shade** ⬩ **rich, fertile, moist soil** ⬩ **spacing: 60–90 cm / 24–36 in**

Growing Liquorice was once a major crop around Pontefract in Yorkshire. Although it did not flower readily, it produced excellent roots. Liquorice roots can reach 1.25 m / 4 ft in length. Establish plants in deep, well-prepared soil, using root cuttings, in the autumn and early winter. Be aware that Liquorice can be very slow to emerge in spring. Every spring, without fail, I conclude that my plant has been lost, and every year, without fail, it emerges long after everything else has done so and it is more or less summer.

Harvesting Plants that are 3–4 years old are ready for a harvest. Dig them up before the ground is frozen, in late autumn or early winter. Unearth them carefully, excavating the roots individually, in order to avoid breaking them. Carry out the first washing *in situ*, so you can return the washing water to the herb garden. Once back at your processing place, wash the roots thoroughly, and cut them lengthways into segments of equal thickness. Leave small roots intact. Lay them out on a tray lined with absorbent paper and let them air-dry for 24 hours.

Passive drying Spread the roots out onto a dry tray, and place it in a warm, airy place, out of direct sunlight.

Active drying Spread the roots out onto dehydrator trays, and start the drying process at a temperature of 43°C / 110°F for 12 hours. Rearrange the trays, and continue drying at 42°C / 108°F for further periods of 2 hours, as needed. When properly dried, the roots should have the characteristic sweet Liquorice scent and snap readily. Store immediately, while still warm.

Tincturing I use dried root and 25% alcohol.

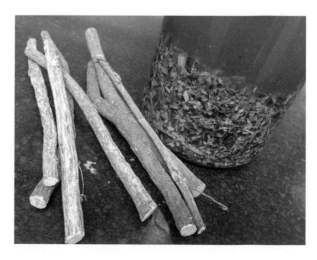

Turkey Tail (*Trametes versicolor*)   ❖   mushrooms
Saprophytic fungus growing on dead logs in woodland

Harvesting   Turkey Tail can be harvested throughout the year, but it is a good candidate for winter harvesting, as this is when you will have spare drying capacity. Pull off the fans gently in order to keep them in one piece, or cut them away using a sharp knife. Once back at your processing place, carefully brush off any debris and, if necessary, wipe the mushrooms with a damp piece of kitchen paper. Do not wash them. Place them whole onto a tray or slice larger specimens.

Passive drying   Spread them onto a tray, and allow them to air-dry in a warm, well-ventilated place.

Active drying   Spread them onto dehydrator trays, and start the drying process at a temperature of 42°C / 108°F for a period of 12 hours. Rearrange the trays and continue, if needed,

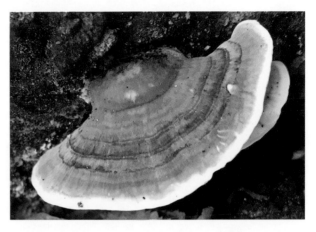

for shorter periods of 1–2 hours. When dried, the mushrooms are light but are still somewhat pliable. Store in an airtight container.

Tincturing   Turkey Tail is prepared by a double-extraction technique as described in Chapter 12.

Mistletoe (*Viscum album*)   ❖   leaves and stems (not berries)
Parasitic plant growing mostly on Apple trees but also found on Lime, Hawthorn, and Poplar

Harvesting   Mistletoe is a potent magical plant, and many landowners believe that it should not be cut. You will need to rely on obtaining permission from landowners who do not mind. Alternatively, you can search for fallen branches after heavy storms in winter or ask wood merchants in your neighbourhood. One

year a patient of mine brought in two enormous sacks of Mistletoe from one of her Apple trees, which had fallen in a storm.

Harvesting   If cutting from a living colony on a tree, cut the main stem with secateurs and place it into your basket before it touches the ground.

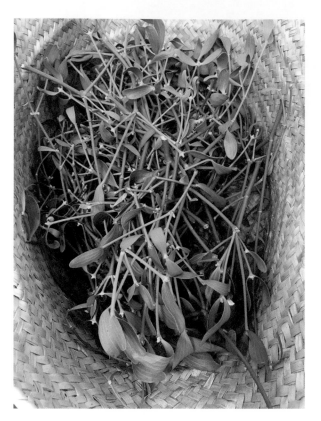

Once back at your processing place, go through your harvest, removing any berries (which are toxic) and any damaged or faded leaves. Cut the stalks and leaves into manageable sections ready for drying.

Passive drying   Spread the Mistletoe pieces out onto trays, and leave to dry in a warm, airy place, away from direct light. Alternatively, you can leave the bunches whole and hang them to dry.

Active drying   Spread the plant material onto dehydrator trays, and start the drying process at a temperature of 42°C / 108°F for 12 hours. Rearrange the trays, and continue drying as needed. Store while warm.

Tincturing   I use dried herb and 45% alcohol.

The notes in this Calendar are intended to serve as a useful starting point and guide for those just beginning on the path of self-sufficient herbalism. The herbs that I work with and the methods that I use to dry and process them are much influenced by climatic factors and by my way of working with them as medicines for patients. In other areas and with different herbal end uses, other ways of working with and preparing herbs will seem more appropriate and will work better. Now that you understand the principles involved in the creation of high-quality dried herbs and herbal medicines, you can adjust the techniques that I have shared to suit your own working set-up, climate and preferred end uses. If you are working with herbs that are not included here there is no need to be daunted, you now have the ability to extrapolate from what you have learnt so far and apply it to your own situation. At no point am I suggesting that my way is the only way. This is your journey, and I hope that you will make it your own.

Index of herbs

Page numbers marked in **bold** indicate main entries in The Herbal Harvesting Year section.